Musculoskeletal Surgery for Cancer

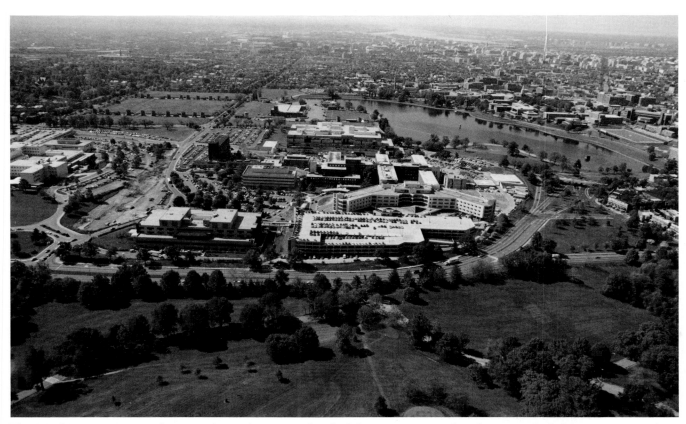

The Washington Hospital Center (WHC), National Rehabilitation Hospital and National Children's Hospital are located due north of the U.S. Capitol Building in Washington, D.C. These combined institutions are uniquely qualified to treat and rehabilitate patients with musculoskeletal cancer.

Musculoskeletal Surgery for Cancer

Principles and Techniques

Paul H. Sugarbaker, M.D.
Medical Director
The Cancer Institute
Washington Hospital Center
Washington, D.C.

Martin M. Malawer, M.D.
Director, Orthopedic Oncology
The Cancer Institute
Washington Hospital Center

Associate Professor of Surgery
Department of Orthopedics
Children's National Medical Center, and
The George Washington University
School of Medicine and Health Sciences
Washington, D.C.

Consultant in Surgery
National Institutes of Health
Bethesda, Maryland

With 21 contributors.

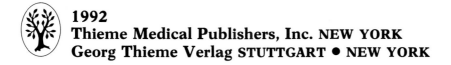

1992
Thieme Medical Publishers, Inc. NEW YORK
Georg Thieme Verlag STUTTGART ● NEW YORK

Thieme Medical Publishers, Inc.
381 Park Avenue South
New York, New York 10016

**MUSCULOSKELETAL SURGERY FOR CANCER:
PRINCIPLES AND TECHNIQUES**
Paul H. Sugarbaker, M.D.
Martin M. Malawer, M.D.

Library of Congress Cataloging-in-Publication Data

Sugarbaker, Paul H.
    Musculoskeletal surgery for cancer: Principles and techniques /
Paul H. Sugarbaker, Martin M. Malawer with 21 contributors.
        p. cm.
    Includes bibliographical references and index.
    ISBN 0-86577-368-8 (Thieme Medical Publishers).—ISBN
3-13-764801-7 (Georg Thieme Verlag)
    1. Extremities (Anatomy)—Cancer—Surgery. 2. Musculoskeletal
system—Cancer—Surgery. I. Malawer, Martin M. II. Title.
    [DNLM: 1. Extremities—surgery. 2. Sarcoma—surgery. 3. Soft
Tissue Neoplasms. WE 800 S947m]
RD674.S84 1991
616.99′4059—dc20
DNLM/DLC
for Library of Congress   91-4850
                                                              CIP

Some portions of this book previously appeared in *Atlas of Extremity Sarcoma Surgery*, edited by Paul H. Sugarbaker and Trudy Nicholson, published in 1984 by the J.B. Lippincott Company.

Important note: Medicine is an ever-changing science. Research and clinical experience are continually broadening our knowledge, in particular our knowledge of proper treatment and drug therapy. Insofar as this book mentions any dosage or application, readers may rest assured that the authors, editors, and publishers have made every effort to ensure that such references are strictly in accordance with the state of knowledge at the time of production of the book. Nevertheless, every user is requested to carefully examine the manufacturers' leaflets accompanying each drug to check on his own responsibility whether the dosage schedules recommended therein or the contraindications stated by the manufacturers differ from the statements made in the present book. Such examination is particularly important with drugs that are either rarely used or have been newly released on the market.

Some of the product names, patents, and registered designs referred to in this book are in fact registered trademarks or proprietary names even though specific reference to this fact is not always made in the text. Therefore, the appearance of a name without designation as proprietary is not to be construed as a representation by the publisher that it is in the public domain.

Printed in the United States of America.

5 4 3 2 1

TMP ISBN 0-86577-368-8
GTV ISBN 3-13-764801-7

Contents

Dedication

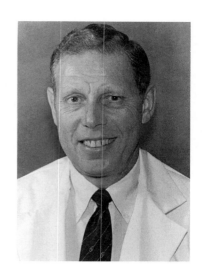

RICHARD EMANUEL WILSON, M.D.

After gradation from Medical School at SUNY Medical Center in his hometown of Syracuse, New York, Dick Wilson spent his professional career and most of his waking hours at the Peter Bent Brigham Hospital. Work was his passion and his recreation. He was Director of the Surgical Research Laboratory, Harvard Medical School, from 1969 to 1975 and Director of the Transplant Service at the Peter Bent Brigham Hospital from 1972 to 1975. His initial research interest in transplantation immunology gradually changed to the related field of tumor immunology. His clinical interest ran parallel with his research endeavors and in 1975 he became Chief of Surgical Oncology at the Peter Bent Brigham Hospital, later the Brigham & Women's Hospital. Trained in molecular genetics by the Noble laureate James Watson, Dick represented the vangaurd of individuals seeking to apply the ideas of molecular biology to the field of surgical oncology. A major factor in Dick's career change from transplantation to surgical oncology was the change in the treatment of soft tissue sarcomas occurring during the early 1970s. A surgeon who believed totally in the virtues of adequate surgical resection, Dick recognized the potential and virtues for multidisciplinary approaches to the treatment of many cancers of which soft tissue sarcomas were a paradigm. His many papers on the treatment of sarcomas emphasized innovative surgical resections carefully coordinated with radiation therapy and chemotherapy and based on exhaustively examined pathology. Dick's legacy is a large literature, a collection of challenging ideas, and a group of skilled enthusiastic trainees.

Robert T. Osteen, M.D.

Dedication

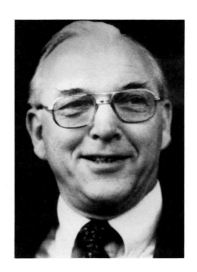

WILLIAM FISHER ENNEKING, M.D.

William Fisher Enneking, M.D., received his medical degree from the University of Wisconsin. He was a resident in orthopedics at the University of Chicago. After a brief time at the University of Mississippi, he arrived in Gainesville, Florida, where he spent the majority of his professional career. He has held the Eugene L. Jewett Professorship in Orthopedic Surgery from 1977 until the present. Before William Enneking, bone cancer studies were confused and lacked direction. From around 1960 until the present, he has been the point person for the development of orthopedic oncology. His personal innovations have advanced the field in concept and in practice. His teaching has resulted in a score of clinical and laboratory oncologists who dominate the field in both practice and research activity. His dedication, patience, and intellect have provided the scientific basis for the new discipline of orthopedic oncology.

Paul H. Sugarbaker, M.D.

Contributors

Alan R. Baker, M.D.
Senior Investigator
Surgery Branch
National Cancer Institute
National Institutes of Health
Bethesda, Maryland

Kim J. Burchiel, M.D.
Professor and Head
Division of Neurosurgery
Oregon Health Sciences University
Portland, Oregon

Paul B. Chretien, M.D.
Professor
Department of Surgery
University of Maryland
Baltimore, Maryland

Tapas K. Das Gupta, M.D., Ph.D.
Professor of Surgery
Head, Division of Surgical Oncology
University of Illinois at Chicago
Chicago, Illinois

Harald J. Hoekstra, M.D.
Division of Surgical Oncology
University Hospital Groningen
The Netherlands

Constantine P. Karakousis, M.D., Ph.D.
Associate Chief
Department of Surgical Oncology
Roswell Park Memorial Institute
Buffalo, New York

Heimen Schraffordt Koops, M.D.
Division of Surgical Oncology
University Hospital Groningen
The Netherlands

Marsha H. Lampert, R.P.T.
Director
Physical Therapy Service
Grosvenor Rehabilitation Service
Bethesda, Maryland

Martin M. Malawer, M.D.
Director, Orthopedic Oncology
The Cancer Institute
Washington Hospital Center

Associate Professor of Surgery
Department of Orthopedics
Children's National Medical Center, and
     The George Washington University
School of Medicine and Health Sciences
Washington, D.C.

Consultant in Surgery
National Institutes of Health
Bethesda, Maryland

Dinesh M. Mehta, M.D.
Department of Radiotherapy
University Hospital Groningen
The Netherlands

Robert T. Osteen, M.D.
Associate Professor of Surgery
Harvard Medical School

Associate Surgeon
Brigham and Women's Hospital
Boston, Massachusetts

Dennis A. Priebat, M.D.
Chairman
Section of Medical Oncology
Washington Hospital Center
Washington, D.C.

Steven A. Rosenberg, M.D., Ph.D.
Chief of Surgery
National Cancer Institute
National Institutes of Health
Bethesda, Maryland

Jack A. Roth, M.D.
Professor and Chairman
Department of Thoracic Surgery
MD Anderson Cancer Center
Houston, Texas

Richard S. Schulof, M.D., Ph.D.
Professor of Medicine
Division of Hematology and Oncology
George Washington University
School of Medicine and Health Sciences
Washington, D.C.

Barry M. Shmookler, M.D.
Director of Surgical Pathology
Washington Hospital Center
Washington, D.C.

Juliana Simmons, M.D.
Chairman
Department of Radiation Oncology
Washington Hospital Center
Washington, D.C.

Paul H. Sugarbaker, M.D.
Medical Director
The Cancer Institute
Washington Hospital Center
Washington, D.C.

Ram S. Trehan, M.D.
Attending in Medical Oncology
Washington Hospital Center
Washington, D.C.

René P.H. Veth, M.D.
Department of Orthopaedic Surgery
University Hospital Groningen
The Netherlands

Pax H. B. Willemse, M.D.
Division of Medical Oncology
University Hospital Groningen
The Netherlands

James C. Yang, M.D.
Senior Investigator
Surgery Branch
National Cancer Institute
National Institutes of Health
Bethesda, Maryland

Foreword

The therapy of patients with soft tissue sarcomas of the extremities has changed drastically in recent years and in many ways has mirrored changes in the entire field of oncology. In the early 1970s the standard treatment for patients with high-grade soft tissue sarcomas of the extremities involved amputation at or above the joint proximal to the tumor. After surgery a period of watchful waiting ensued during which over half of the patients suffered recurrence with pulmonary metastases and died from their disease. Surgeons unfamiliar with the aggressive local invasiveness of soft tissue sarcomas often treated patients with local excision as the sole therapy, and local recurrence occurred in about 50% of these cases as well.

The following recent developments have improved treatment results dramatically in patients with high-grade soft tissue sarcomas.

1. Limb-sparing surgery is emphasized, with reliance on multimodality treatments to improve local control rates.
2. Surgical procedures based on a knowledge of the natural history of the disease are planned carefully and performed expertly by experienced specialists.
3. Chemotherapy may be administered in the perioperative period to eliminate micrometastatic disease and enforce local control.
4. The quality of life of patients is maximized by attempting to spare the extremity when possible but also by applying vigorous rehabilitation techniques to maximize the function of residual tissue.
5. Metastatic disease is vigorously treated by the resection of metastatic pulmonary nodules. The resection of pulmonary metastases in patients with high-grade sarcomas results in the long-term survival of approximately 25% of these patients.

These principles are being actively applied to the treatment of other cancers as well.

In 1975 the Surgery Branch of the National Cancer Institute began a series of controlled clinical trials designed to improve the survival and the quality of life of patients with high-grade soft tissue sarcomas. Since May, 1975 over 1000 patients with the diagnosis of soft tissue sarcoma have been referred to the Surgery Branch for evaluation. Experience gained from treating the large number of patients has helped produce the refinements in surgical techniques reflected in this atlas.

It is our conviction that advances in understanding and treating soft tissue sarcomas will eventuate from carefully designed prospective randomized trials. Our experiences to date have reinforced this conviction. An important aspect of the conduct of these clinical trials is the expert performance of the surgical resection. Because soft tissue sarcomas are uncommon, most general surgeons are not familiar with the details of their surgical management. The appropriate performance of the correct surgical procedure plays a major role in the quality of life as well as the survival of patients with soft tissue sarcomas. It is hoped that the surgical procedures described in this book will be of value to surgeons in their approach to patients with extremity sarcomas.

Steven A. Rosenberg, M.D., Ph.D.

Preface

There are few surgical procedures that the well-trained orthopedic or general surgeon cannot routinely perform. The surgical techniques taught in this book are an exception. Experience, self-confidence, and much technical skill are required to bring about the optimal long-term result when a patient needs a major musculoskeletal procedure. Indeed, the ability to perform the dissections and reconstructions shown in this volume may be one feature that distinguishes a surgical oncologist or orthopedic oncologist from his or her generalist colleagues. These procedures are not taught in surgical training programs. They can only be mastered through intensive postgraduate training. These major ablative and reconstructive procedures are not frequently required and, therefore, are not commonly encountered by the general surgeon or general orthopedist. However, when they must be performed, the greatest care must be exercised. For only if the surgeon's technical maneuvers approach perfection will the oncologic and long-term functional result be uniformly good and the patient's potential for an acceptable quality of life be maximized.

The technical aspects of treatment are emphasized in this text. It is designed to provide the orthopedic and surgical oncologist with an up-to-date approach to bone and soft tissue sarcomas of the extremities. Moreover, a wide variety of extremity tumors of many different histologic types require the use of the procedures illustrated. Many of the surgical procedures have never been displayed as a step-by-step presentation in a surgical atlas. Nor has such a complete collection of musculoskeletal procedures for extremity cancer been compiled in a single volume. With the concentration of clinical problems presented by the large number of sarcoma patients at the Surgery Branch, National Institutes of Health, and at the Washington Hospital Center, Cancer Institute, it was natural that a surgical atlas of this nature would come into existence.

The present volume published by Thieme had its inception in two previous projects. The text evolved from a series of eight journal articles published as peer-reviewed technical presentations in the surgical literature. These individual journal articles were not produced quickly, but they represent our efforts to develop a smooth sequence for the procedure worked out in multiple patients over nearly a decade. These journal articles were revised and integrated with eight additional chapters as the *Atlas of Extremity Sarcoma Surgery*. This volume presented a high standard of excellence in design and presentation of the surgical anatomy. The atlas was published in 1984 by J. B. Lippincott, and 2,500 volumes were distributed. The book went out of print in 1988, as the sales volume diminished. This volume ran up against severe competition, since many other texts on sarcoma were published in the latter half of the 1980s. In 1983 Lawrence, Neifeld, and Terz produced the *Manual of Soft-Tissue Tumor Surgery* (Medical College of Virginia, Richmond, Va.), published by Springer.

In 1983 Enzinger and Weiss produced *Soft Tissue Tumors*, Armed Forces Institute of Pathology, Washington, D.C., published by C. V. Mosby Company. In 1984 the National Institutes of Health sponsored a Health Consensus Development Conference on Extremity Sarcoma. This resulted in a *Cancer Treatment Symposium*, published by the Public Health Service in 1985. In 1984 Marcove (Memorial Sloan-Kettering Hospital, New York City) produced *The Surgery of Tumors of Bone and Cartilage*, published by Grune and Stratton. In 1984 Das Gupta (University of Illinois, Chicago) produced *Tumors of the Soft Tissues*, published by Appleton-Century-Croft. Karakousis in 1985 (Roswell Park Memorial Institute, Buffalo, N.Y.) produced the *Atlas of Operations for Soft Tissue Tumors*. In 1986 van Oosterom and van Unnik (European Organization for Research for Treatment on Cancer Monograph No. 16) produced *Management of Soft Tissue and Bone Sarcomas*. Arlen and Marcove in

1987 (North Shore Hospital, Cornell University, Manhahaset, N.Y.) produced *Surgical Management of Soft Tissue Sarcomas*, published by W. B. Saunders. In 1987 Eilber, Morton, Sondak, and Economou (University of California, Los Angeles) produced *The Soft Tissue Sarcomas*, published by Grune and Stratton. In 1987 Enneking (University of Florida, Gainesville, Fla.) produced *Limb Salvage in Musculoskeletal Oncology*, published by Churchill Livingston. Raaf (Cleveland Clinic Foundation, Cleveland, Ohio) has in press *Management of Soft Tissue Sarcomas*, to be published by Year Book Medical Publishers.

Despite its out-of-print status, the quality of the *Atlas of Extremity Sarcoma Surgery* remained secure. In this volume, numerous intraoperative photographs and artist's sketches were refined into anatomic drawings of great precision and complete accuracy. In this regard the painstaking efforts of Trudy Nicholson need to be acknowledged. Trudy Nicholson and PHS designed the drawings and text to take the reader through the procedure step by step. We realized that these procedures are not frequently performed by any one surgeon. It was not uncommon for me, along with the very complete text provided by the *Atlas of Extremity Sarcoma Surgery*, to coach by telephone a surgeon in another country through one of these procedures. Often the surgeon had never performed the procedure by himself. Often it was the first time that this procedure had ever been performed in his native land.

Our aim was to develop a conceptual approach but never to compromise technical detail. Careful selection of landmarks in the anatomic drawings together with a complete description in the accompanying text provide a convenient display for operative guidance without memorizing steps in detail.

As new treatment strategies evolved for extremity sarcoma over the past five years, it became clear that a major revision of the *Atlas of Extremity Sarcoma Surgery* was needed. In order to ensure an international distribution and several translations of our book into other languages, Thieme Medical Publishers was selected as the new publisher. The new volume was to be greatly expanded and completely updated. Our new title was considerably more general, *Musculoskeletal Surgery for Cancer: Principles and Techniques.*

It was natural that Martin M. Malawer, M.D., would be selected as coauthor of the second edition. He had contributed generously to the first edition. He has been one of the pioneers in orthopedic surgery with bone and joint replacement for cancer. He has developed a modular segmental replacement system for the hip, knee, and shoulder joints that is widely

utilized (Howmedica, Inc., Rutherford, N.J.). These procedures and internal prosthetic devices now available have markedly improved the quality of life of patients with musculoskeletal cancer.

Also, the immense contribution of Constantine Karakousis to this second edition merits special comment. Constantine Karakousis brings innovation and experience to our surgical team. His leadership throughout the world in the treatment of extremity and truncal sarcoma is generated from the high level of expertise that is demonstrated at the soft tissue sarcoma service at Roswell Park Memorial Institute in Buffalo, New York.

The second volume has been designed for use by surgeons interested in treating musculoskeletal cancer, by all surgical oncologists, by orthopedic surgeons treating cancer, and by physical therapists. It also provides new background information for medical oncologists and radiation therapists who deal with these difficult malignancies. Throughout this volume, we have provided pictures of patients who demonstrate the complete procedure to provide a standard by which readers can evaluate their own efforts. They also demonstrate to the physical therapist and physiatrist the anatomic end result of the surgery. The anatomic end result (often an amputation stump) is of utmost importance to rehabilitation, for it provides the base on which a prosthesis must rest. The usable prostheses presently available are described and pictured in the text.

A companion text also published by Thieme should be mentioned. *Atlas of Amputation Surgery*, authored by Walther H. O. Bohne, presents a most usable presentation of the multiplicity of amputative procedures. It should be consulted for help in amputations through and distal to the wrist and through and distal to the ankle. Drs. Sugarbaker and Malawer congratulate Dr. Bohne on his excellent contribution.

Nowadays the treatment of musculoskeletal cancer more than ever demonstrates effectively the requirements for a multimodality approach to the malignant process. The clinician must integrate his or her knowledge of the anatomic location of the tumor, the biologic character of the malignancy, and the likelihood of a response to chemotherapy and radiation therapy. Optimization of the treatment process demands a multimodality approach. The plan that must be clearly defined prior to the initiation of therapy is the one most likely to give local control and yet not necessarily sacrifice function or quality of life. The treatment decision must be reached after radiation therapist, chemotherapist, rehabilitation physician, physical therapist, and surgeon have become familiar with the patient's clinical situation and been given an opportunity to make a judgment. This multidisciplinary group must have a close working relationship and must be willing to compromise to realize a true multimodality approach to the treatment of musculoskeletal cancer. More than providing a second or third opinion, this group effort represents a desire to create an optimal treatment plan based on the natural history of the disease and the varied experience of the members of the group.

This multimodality group must adhere to four steps required for progress in cancer therapy. First, communication is essential. The multimodality group must get along, they must meet on a regular basis, and they must interact in a scholarly fashion. Second, through their collective intellectual energies, written protocols for patient management must evolve. If changes in management are made on a frequent basis, then no plan can ever be evaluated. The discipline of writing down the optimal approach is an absolute necessity for progress to occur. Third, data managers must be employed in order to allow frequent and timely analysis of results. Physicians by themselves do not characteristically collect carefully enough data in a timely fashion and as accurately as is necessary for evaluation of a treatment plan. Another group of data management persons must work with the physicians in this regard. Fourth, there must be patient accrual. Even the most carefully designed protocol study cannot receive its due credits unless generous numbers of patients are treated so that the improvements in either survival or quality of life can be demonstrated with statistical validity. The treatment of musculoskeletal cancer provides oncologic problems that will challenge the multimodality group to work together for optimized results of therapy.

Musculoskeletal Surgery for Cancer has two introductory chapters. Chapter 1 covers the principles and practice of treating soft tissue sarcoma, and chapter 2 does the same for osteogenic sarcoma. These chapters are authored by surgeons from the Surgery Branch, National Institutes of Health, Bethesda, MD. Doctors Yang, Rosenberg and Baker deal with sarcoma patients on a daily basis as they conduct the prospective sarcoma trials in progress at the Surgery Branch. They command a unique position from which to comment on the natural history of extremity sarcoma and to give an overview of diagnostic and treatment options.

Chapter 3 is a new chapter and concerns the pathology of sarcomas. Doctors Shmookler and Malawer have worked together for nearly a decade at the Washington Hospital Center. This chapter represents a collection of their integrated experience, as well as a comprehensive review of the pathology literature.

Chapter 4 concerns rehabilitation of patients with extremity sarcoma and is a collaborative effort of Marsha Lampert, P.T., and myself. This chapter has been revised and updated to include all of the new procedures. Rehabilitation is usually discussed at the end of a book of this type. We include it near the beginning to emphasize that the rehabilitation process must begin before the patient gets to the operating theater. Rehabilitation efforts are essential not only for patients with prosthetic devices after amputation but also to preserve mobility and function for patients undergoing radiation therapy or bone replacement. Without proper physical therapy, the extremity (especially a lower extremity) that has had surgery followed by high-dose wide-field radiation may become contracted and motionless and ultimately less functional than an artificial limb.

"Phantom Limb Pain" is a new chapter authored by Dr. Burchiel. Often, the only lasting quality-of-life debit in a patient with a major amputation is persistent phantom limb pain over many years. New theory and procedures by which to deal with this severe problem are described by Dr. Burchiel.

Throughout the United States, extremity soft tissue sarcomas are most commonly treated by wide excision followed with high-dose radiation therapy. Good local control is expected if there is proper patient selection, careful surgery, and expert radiation therapy. The multidisciplinary group must consider a wide spectrum of procedures, including both amputation and limb salvage procedures. A patient's life may be lost, whereas it might have been saved if treatment decisions were made that resulted in local recurrence. It seems hard to escape the fact that local recurrence is frequently an accompaniment of systemic disease dissemination. Amputation is the time-honored treatment affording local control in nearly 100% of patients. All other local treatment plans must be compared with these results. The combination treatment with which the greatest amount of experience has been gained, that conserves the largest amount of tissue, is wide local excision of the primary tumor mass followed by postoperative radiation therapy.

Chapter 7 presents a new and exciting concept in the treatment of extremity cancer. Induction chemotherapy is used prior to to surgery to shrink the tumor mass. Frequently, an extremity that would require amputation because of positive surgical margins can be treated with a limb salvage procedure after 2 or 3 cycles of induction chemotherapy preoperatively. The intra-arterial route is often utilized to maximize local responses. It should be emphasized that induction chemotherapy provides not only markedly improved local responses but early systemic treatment of micrometastatic disease equivalent to the intravenous route of chemotherapy. We think that the application of induction chemotherapy will have profound consequences for all modern treatment plans for musculoskeletal surgery in the extremity.

Chapters 8 through 14 concern the treatment of tumors of the upper thigh, hip, buttock, and pelvis. Both limb salvage and ablative procedures are described. The sometimes complicated decisions required to select the optimal surgical procedure are reviewed in chapter 13, "Summary of Alternative Approaches to Hemipelvectomy."

Chapter 15 is by Constantine Karakousis and concerns sacrectomy. This is one of the few chapters that does not concern an extremity tumor. However, the principles of management are completely similar to the other pelvic procedures described in this book. It was thought essential to include it to complete the discussion concerning the surgical treatment of pelvic malignancy.

Chapters 16, 18, 25, and 29 present our thoughts on some routine amputative procedures, but these procedures are presented from an oncologic perspective. Patients with extremity cancer requiring these amputative procedures present a special problem in management. These chapters emphasize these special problems.

Chapters 6, 17, 19, and 27 present our approach to limb-sparing surgery for malignant bone tumors and highlight Dr. Malawer's contribution to this edition. The development of internal prosthetics and bone and joint replacement has revolutionized the orthopedic surgeon's approach to arthritic joints. It also revolutionized our approach to tumors of the proximal humerus, distal femur, and proximal tibia. Also, occasionally, a very low grade malignancy of the proximal femur may be treated with a prosthetic bone replacement. With the combined use of induction chemotherapy and prosthetic limb replacement, amputations are much less frequent for extremity osteosarcoma. The extensive experience of Dr. Malawer collected in this text should prove invaluable to orthopedic oncologists and surgical oncologists around the world who are beginning to use these procedures.

Chapters 20–22 present a technique for muscle group excision of the three compartments of the thigh. Occasionally there may be other muscle group excisions performed within the upper or lower extremity, but these have not been encountered with any frequency in our experience. The muscle group excisions should be viewed as amputative procedures that are complete in and of themselves as definitive procedures for the treatment of extremity cancer. Especially if combined with induction chemotherapy so that surgical margins of excisions are negative, radiation therapy does not need to be used following these surgical procedures.

Chapters 23 through 28 concern the treatment of tumors of the upper arm, shoulder, and scapula. Treatment of these tumors may be as radical as the "radical forequarter amputation with chest wall resection" or as wide as local excision supplemented by radiation therapy. Chapter 28 presents a "Summary of Alternative Approaches to Forequarter Amputation."

Chapter 30 is on the treatment of bone metastases and it is another new contribution. It comes from the interdisciplinary experience of over a decade in ths field of endeavor. It serves to complete the subject of musculoskeletal surgery and so it is our final chapter.

One may conclude from the contents of *Musculoskeletal Surgery for Cancer* that these authors may consider it a grave mistake not to include amputation as a treatment option for these malignancies. If the multimodality team cannot bring themselves to recommend an amputation to a patient, then they should not be treating sarcoma patients. Sometimes amputation must be performed to make survival possible. The need for an amputation should be explained to a patient and family in terms of body economy: the diseased extremity is being traded for a chance at long-term survival. The major amputation procedures described in this book are sometimes the only reasonable treatment for an extremity cancer.

When a major restorative or amputative procedure is thought necessary, the surgeon must proceed after fully informing the patient. Of course, the surgeon must be confident that he or she has the experience, the expertise, and the team to perform the procedure as well as any other physician. If the morbidity and mortality of these procedures are kept low through meticulous attention to technical detail, the results in terms of survival and quality of existence can be rewarding.

Paul H. Sugarbaker, M.D.

Acknowledgments

Permission to use illustrations from the following sources is gratefully acknowledged.

Anatomic drawings in Chapter 8: Chretien PA, Sugarbaker PH: Surgical technique of hemipelvectomy in the lateral position. *Surgery* 1981;90:900–909.

Anatomic drawings in Chapter 9: Sugarbaker PH, Chretien PA: Surgical technique for anterior flap hemipelvectomy. *Ann Surg* 1983;197:106–115.

Anatomic drawings in Chapter 14: Sugarbaker PH, Chretien PA: A surgical technique for hip disarticulation. *Surgery* 1981;90:546–553.

Anatomic drawings in Chapter 12: Sugarbaker PH, Chretien PA: A surgical technique for buttockectomy. *Surgery* 1982;91:104–107.

Anatomic drawings and tables in Chapter 20: Mentzer SJ, Sugarbaker PH, Chretien PA: Surgical technique for excision of the adductor muscle group. *Surgery* 1982;91:662–668.

Anatomic drawings in Chapter 21: Sugarbaker PH, Lampert MH: Quadriceps muscle group excision. *Surgery* 1983;93:462–466.

Anatomic drawings in Chapter 24: Roth JA, Baker AR, Sugarbaker PH: Radical forequarter amputation with chest wall resection. *Ann Thorac Surg* 1984;37:423–427.

Anatomic drawings in Chapter 26: Modified from Das Gupta TK: Scapulectomy: Indications and technique. *Surgery* 1970;67:601–606.

Anatomic drawings in Chapter 27: Malawer MM, Sugarbaker PH, Lampert M, Baker AR, Gerber NL: Limb salvage surgery for tumors of the proximal humerus and shoulder girdle: The Tikhoff-Linberg procedure and its modifications. *Surgery* 97:518–528, 1985.

We would also like to thank the illustrators of the book: Trudy H. Nicholson (Chaps. 5, 6, 8, 9, 10, 12–14, 20, 21, 23, 24, 26–28), Patsy A. Bryan (Chaps. 10, 11, 15, 16, 18, 19, 22, 25, 29), and Joyce Hurwitz, AMI (Chaps. 17, 19).

Paul H. Sugarbaker, M.D.
Martin M. Malawer, M.D.

Musculoskeletal Surgery for Cancer

Surgical Treatment of Soft Tissue Sarcomas of the Extremities

JAMES C. YANG, M.D.
STEVEN A. ROSENBERG, M.D., Ph.D.

OVERVIEW

Two major surgical strategies are available for patients with high-grade soft tissue sarcomas of the extremities as the initial component of a multimodality treatment approach. Radical local excision alone (including amputation) can be utilized in selected patients and can result in local control rates of approximately 80%. It appears that similar local control rates can be achieved when smaller local excisions are performed followed by adjuvant radiation. Trials from the Surgery Branch of the National Cancer Institute provide evidence that adjuvant chemotherapy can improve the disease-free survival, overall survival, and local control in patients with high-grade soft tissue sarcomas of the extremities. Although new evidence exists that adjuvant radiation therapy can reduce local recurrence in patients receiving local excision and chemotherapy, this benefit may have a minimal to negligible impact on overall survival.

INTRODUCTION

The term *soft tissue sarcomas* refers to a group of malignant tumors that arise in the extraskeletal soft connective tissues of the body. These tumors are grouped together because of similarities in pathologic appearance, clinical presentation, and behavior. Approximately 5,000 new cases of soft tissue sarcomas are reported in the United States each year, resulting in an annual age-adjusted incidence rate of 2 per 100,000. Soft tissue sarcomas constitute 0.7% of all cancers, though these tumors constitute 6.5% of all cancers in children under the age of 15.[1]

Approximately 60% of all soft tissue sarcomas arise in the extremities, with over two thirds of these being in the lower extremity. Table 1–1 summarizes the sites of occurrence of soft tissue sarcomas in four major series.[2–5]

More than 30 different histologic types of soft tissue sarcomas have been identified. Table 1–2 presents the characteristic distribution of the most common histologies.[1] The criteria for assigning a precise histologic cell of origin is an area of controversy among pathologists. The histologic cell of origin, however, does not have a major impact on the prognosis of patients with soft tissue sarcomas of the extremities. By far the most important prognostic indicator is the histologic grade of the primary tumor.[3,6] Grade I tumors are well-differentiated lesions with a very low tendency to spread from the local site. Higher-grade lesions (grades II and III) tend to metastasize primarily to the lungs early in their clinical course. The site and size of the primary lesion are other prognostic indicators that appear to impact on prognosis, either through local control issues, metastatic behavior, or response to adjuvant therapy. Table 1–3 presents a common schema for the staging of soft tissue sarcomas of the extremities.[3] This staging system depends predominantly on the grade of the lesion, although other factors, such as the size of the primary lesion and the presence of lymph node metastases, also play a role in assigning clinical stage.

The therapeutic approach to the treatment of patients with soft tissue sarcomas depends on the natural history of this disease. Because many treatment options are based on the most common natural history of these sarcomas, a very brief summary follows.

NATURAL HISTORY

The two features that characterize the natural history of high-grade soft tissue sarcomas are their tendency to aggressively invade surrounding local tissues and a tendency to form micrometastases in the lung early in the clinical course. Grade I, or well-differentiated, soft tissue sarcomas have a tendency to aggressively invade local tissues but a very low tendency to spread to distant sites. Therefore the following discussion applies only to high-grade (grades II and III) soft tissue sarcomas.

The local spread of soft tissue sarcomas tends to occur along anatomic planes such as nerve fibers, muscle bundles, and fascial planes. Approximately 10% of patients present for the first time with clinical metastases in the lung evident on chest x-ray or chest tomograms. Following local surgical excision alone, local recurrence rates are high. Excision of a soft tissue sarcoma through its pseudocapsule is associated with about a 90% recurrence rate. A wide local excision alone—that is, an excision of the tumor with a small surrounding rim of normal tissue—is associated with approximately a 40% local recurrence rate. Radical local excision (compartmental or muscle group excision or amputation) is associated with

Table 1-1.   Sites of Soft Tissue Sarcomas

	SHIEBER AND GRAHAM 1962[2]	RUSSELL ET AL 1977[3]	LINDBERG ET AL 1975[4]	ROSENBERG ET AL 1978[5]	TOTAL
Number of patients	125	1215	166	113	1,619
Site		(% of total cases)			
Head & Neck	12.8	15	9.0	4.4	12
Trunk	31.2	32	25.9	34.5	30
(mediastinum)		(1)		(0.9)	
(retroperitoneum)		(13)	(9)	(15.0)	
Upper Extremity	16.0	13	25.9	10.6	16
Lower Extremity	40.0	40	39.2	50.5	42
(at/above knee)		(32)		(38.0)	
(below knee)		(8)		(12.4)	

Table 1-2. Relative Incidence of Histologic Types of Soft Tissue Sarcomas*

HISTOLOGIC TYPE	INCIDENCE (%)
Unclassified	17.4
Liposarcoma	22.6
Rhabdomyosarcoma	10.4
Synovial sarcoma	11.3
Neurofibrosarcoma	6.1
Fibrosarcoma	1.7
Angiosarcoma	1.7
Leiomyosarcoma	11.3
Mesenchymoma	0.1
Malignant Fibrous Histiocytoma	17.4
Other	0

*From Rosenberg et al.[1]

local recurrence rates between 10% and 15%.[1] In almost all reported series, approximately 80% of recurrences (both local and disseminated) occur by two years after definitive treatment.[4,7,8]

Spread to draining lymph nodes is an uncommon finding in the natural history of patients with soft tissue sarcomas. In a review of well over 3,000 patients, only 5.8% developed lymph node metastases sometime during their course.[9] The presence of lymph node metastases is a very poor prognostic sign, and a few patients with positive lymph nodes are long-term survivors.

The lungs are almost always the first site of metastases of soft tissue sarcomas. Without vigorous resection of pulmonary metastases, the median survival following the onset of pulmonary metastases is about 12 months. Resection of pulmonary metastases can cure about 25% of patients.[10,11] The overall five-year survival in most reported series of patients with soft tissue sarcomas treated by surgery alone is about 40%, and the results of several reported series are presented in Table 1–4.[2,3,5,12–16]

DIAGNOSIS

Most patients with a soft tissue sarcoma of the extremity present with an asymptomatic mass in the soft tissues. As this tumor mass grows, it compresses normal tissue at its periphery and forms a "pseudocapsule." This pseudocapsule is always invaded by microscopic tumor, and thus "shelling out" soft tissue sarcomas is rarely curative.

The proper histologic diagnosis of a soft tissue mass is important, because errors in obtaining a diagnosis can greatly affect the ability to apply curative surgical therapy. Aspiration or needle biopsy

have not been of value in the diagnosis of soft tissue sarcomas. A large representative sample of tissue is usually necessary for the accurate diagnosis of soft tissue sarcomas, and special studies such as electron microscopy may often be needed as well. For these reasons, the traditional technique for diagnosing a soft tissue sarcoma is an incisional biopsy. Excisional biopsies should be avoided for any lesions greater than about 4 cm because of the likelihood that excisional biopsies of these large masses will spread the tumor to other sites and compromise subsequent definitive surgical procedures. A careful incisional biopsy of the lesion should be performed to obtain a wedge of tissue. Care should be taken to avoid hematomas or other iatrogenic spread of the tumor. Incisional biopsies of soft tissue masses in the extremity should always be performed through longitudinal, not transverse, incisions, and the use of drains is to be avoided. The biopsy site will need to be removed in any definitive surgical excision, and large transverse incisions or remote drain exit sites can render this difficult or impossible.

Because all approaches to the therapy of soft tissue sarcomas depend on the surgical excision of the soft tissue sarcoma with some normal surrounding tissue, it is important to localize anatomically the soft tissue sarcoma within the extremity as well as possible. By far, the most helpful diagnostic procedures in assessing the anatomic areas of involvement of extremity soft tissue sarcomas are computerized tomography (CT) and magnetic resonance imaging (MRI) (Fig. 1–1). These scans can often precisely localize the lesion to a muscle group and carefully delineate the proximity of the lesion to vital nerves, vessels, and bone. MRI can offer significant advantages even over CT scanning in differentiating the tumor from normal tissue.[17] Conventional soft tissue x-rays of the extremities are rarely of value in the diagnosis of these lesions.

Soft tissue sarcomas rarely invade bone and rarely cause periosteal changes even when directly adjacent to bone. To assess the proximity of soft tissue sarcomas to bone, a bone scan can be helpful. A positive bone scan does not mean that the tumor is directly adjacent to the bone; it usually means that there is a soft tissue reaction to the tumor near the bone (Fig. 1–2).

Arteriography is of limited value, although in selected cases proximity to major vessels can be ascertained by appropriate angiographic studies (Fig. 1–3).

Once the precise diagnosis and location of the soft tissue sarcoma in the extremity is determined, the treatment strategy can be delineated. The two major surgical strategies for treating patients with soft

Table 1–3. Schema for Staging Soft Tissue Sarcomas by T, N, M, G*

T	Primary tumor
	T1 Tumor less than 5 cm
	T2 Tumor 5 cm or greater
	T3 Tumor that grossly invades bone, major vessel, or major nerve
N	Regional lymph nodes
	N0 No histologically verified metastases to regional lymph nodes
	N1 Histologically verified regional lymph node metastasis
M	Distant metastasis
	M0 No distant metastasis
	M1 Distant metastasis
G	Histologic grade of malignancy
	G1 Low
	G2 Moderate
	G3 High

Stage I
___Stage IA___

G1, T1, N0, M0	Grade 1 tumor less than 5 cm in diameter with no regional lymph nodes or distant metastases

___Stage IB___

G1, T2, N0, M0	Grade 1 tumor 5 cm or greater in diameter with no regional lymph nodes or distant metastases

Stage II
___Stage IIA___

G2, T1, N0, M0	Grade 2 tumor less than 5 cm in diameter with no regional lymph nodes or distant metastases

___Stage IIB___

G2, T2, N0, M0	Grade 2 tumor 5 cm or greater in diameter with no regional lymph nodes or distant metastases

Stage III
___Stage IIIA___

G3, T1, N0, M0	Grade 3 tumor less than 5 cm in diameter with no regional lymph nodes or distant metastases

___Stage IIIB___

G3, T1, N0, M0	Grade 3 tumor 5 cm or greater in diameter with no regional lymph nodes or distant metastases

___Stage IIIC___

Any G, T1-2, N1, M0	Tumor of any grade or size (no invasion) with regional lymph nodes, but no distant metastases

Stage IV
___Stage IVA___

Any G, T3, N0-1, M0	Tumor of any grade that grossly invades bone, major vessel, or major nerve with or without regional lymph node metastases but without distant metastases

___Stage IVB___

Any G, T, N, M1	Tumor with distant metastases

*From Russell et al.[3]

Table 1–4. Soft Tissue Sarcomas: Five-Year Survival

GROUP	NUMBER OF PATIENTS	SURVIVAL (%) 5-Year	SURVIVAL (%) 10-Year
Task Force, AJC[3]	1,215	41	30
Surgery Branch, NCI (before 1975)[5]	66	48	44
Gerner et al[12]	155	50	26
Shieber and Graham[2]	125	27	22
Martin et al[13]	183	40	—
Pack and Ariel[14]	717	39	—
Hare and Cerny[15]	200	39	—
Shiu et al[16]	297	55	41

tissue sarcomas will be considered in the next section.

SURGICAL TREATMENT

Two major types of treatment strategies have evolved in the local therapy of patients with soft tissue sarcomas of the extremities:

1. The use of radical surgical excision alone to obtain local control
2. The use of surgery combined with adjuvant treat-

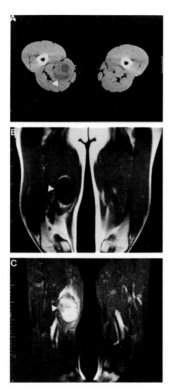

Figure 1–1. (A) Transverse computerized axial tomographic scan through the thigh of a patient with grade III soft tissue sarcoma (arrow). The lesion is demarcated by fat planes and displacement of normal tissues. (B) A T1-weighted MRI of the same patient reconstructed in the coronal plane. Again a well-demarcated lesion is seen as well as adjacent normal structures such as large vessels. (C) A T2-weighted MRI vividly differentiating this tumor from normal muscle by magnetic resonance characteristics.

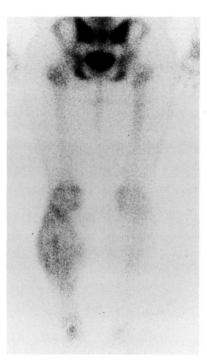

Figure 1–2. Bone scan of a patient with a soft tissue sarcoma of the proximal leg. The tumor diffusely incorporates the radionuclide. Note that there is some increased uptake in the knee, hip, and ankle joints on the side of the tumor. This increased uptake in joints proximal and distal to the tumor is commonly seen and is not indicative of a tumor at these sites.

ment modalities designed to improve local control rates

When surgery alone is used to obtain local control, radical local excisions are necessary. These excisions must encompass the tumor and all of the anatomic structures in the anatomic compartment occupied by the tumor. Muscle group excisions, compartmental excisions, or amputations are often used when surgery alone is being considered for the local treatment of patients with soft tissue sarcomas. When local excisions, in conjunction with adjuvant modalities, are utilized, an attempt is made to remove all gross tumor with a small (1- to 2-cm) rim of normal tissue around the sarcoma in all directions. No attempt is made to remove the entire muscle group or the anatomic compartment involved with the tumor. In the postoperative period, adjuvant radiation therapy and chemotherapy can be used to aid in the control of any residual cells remaining at the local site.[8,16]

When radical resection surgery is used as the sole treatment for soft tissue sarcomas of the extremities,

local control rates of about 80% can be achieved. In about half of the patients, amputation will be necessary. Two large reported series of radical surgical excision as a primary treatment strategy for the

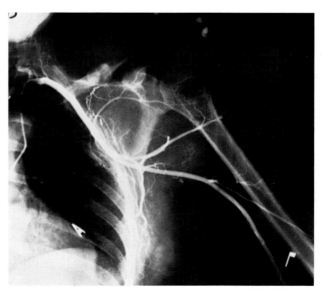

Figure 1–3. Axillary arteriogram of a woman with a large soft tissue sarcoma presenting behind and superior to the clavical with extensive local invasion. Note the deviation of the axillary artery caused by the tumor.

treatment of patients with soft tissue sarcomas are presented in Table 1–5.[8,16] As can be seen, both of these groups utilized amputation in about half of the patients with extremity soft tissue sarcomas. The remaining patients received radical local resections designed to remove the entire anatomic area containing the tumor. Local control rates in these series were about 80%. The extensive anatomic areas involved when radical local resections are utilized in the treatment of patients with soft tissue sarcomas generally precludes the use of postoperative radiation therapy. Substantial morbidity is seen when large radiation fields are treated following compartmental or muscle group excisions. Many tissue flaps, such as hemipelvectomy or hip disarticulation flaps, do not tolerate radiation therapy well. When amputations are used to treat patients with these lesions, radiation therapy often cannot be used as an adjuvant treatment.

A second approach to the treatment of patients with soft tissue sarcomas of the extremities involves a wide local excision with a rim of surrounding normal tissue followed by adjunctive radiation with or without chemotherapy. In many reported series the use of this type of local excision results in local control rates as good as those reported with radical local resection or amputation.[4,18,19] However, when wide local excision is utilized, adjunctive therapy is necessary.

Regardless of the type of surgical procedure used for treating soft tissue sarcomas, several principles of surgical excision of these lesions should be adhered to. The most important are the following:

1. Previous biopsy sites and any areas that may have contained hematomas or areas of iatrogenic spread from previous biopsies should be excised along with the local tumor.
2. Removal of the sarcoma should be achieved without visualizing the tumor during the surgical excision. Spilling of the tumor during a major surgical excision greatly increases the incidence of local recurrence.

3. Resection of the draining lymph nodes is not recommended unless these lymph nodes are clinically suspicious for the presence of a tumor.
4. Metallic clips should be placed as a guide to the limits of the surgical dissection. This is essential in all local sarcoma resections to enable the radiation therapist to adequately plan subsequent therapy.

The Surgery Branch of the National Cancer Institute conducted a prospective randomized trial in which patients with extremity soft tissue sarcomas were randomized to receive amputation at or above the joint proximal to the tumor, or else they were randomized to receive local excision with removal of gross tumor and a margin of surrounding normal tissue followed by adjuvant radiation therapy to the potential areas of spread and the tumor bed.[20] Both groups received adjuvant chemotherapy with doxorubicin, cyclophosphamide, and high-dose methotrexate. The results of this clinical trial with a median follow-up in excess of eight years are presented in Figures 1–4, 1–5, and 1–6. There were no significant differences in disease-free or overall survival or incidence of local recurrence in patients randomized to receive either radical amputation or wide local excision plus radiation therapy.

This result, as well as others in the literature from nonrandomized trials, strongly suggests that local

Table 1–5. Radical surgical excision as the sole treatment for extremity soft tissue sarcoma

	SIMON AND ENNEKING[8]	SHIU ET AL[16]
Total Number of Patients	54	297
Radical Local Resection	25 (46%)	158 (53%)
Amputation	29 (54%)	139 (47%)
Local Control		
Radical Local Resection	88%	72%
Amputation	79.3%	93%
Overall	83.3%	82%

*From Rosenberg et al.[1]

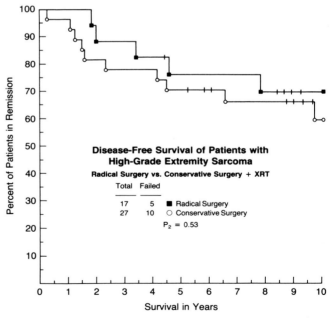

Figure 1–4. Actuarial analysis of continuous disease-free survival of patients with extremity soft tissue sarcomas randomized to receive either radical surgery or conservative surgery in the Surgery Branch, National Cancer Institute trial. No difference was seen between these two patient groups.

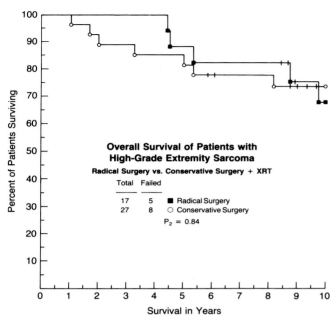

Figure 1–5.   Actuarial analysis of overall survival of the same patients shown in Figure 1–4. No difference was seen between these two patient groups.

surgical excision followed by adjunctive therapy can produce levels of local control equivalent to that of major radical surgical excisions without the morbidity of these latter procedures. As emphasized earlier, however, adjunctive therapy is essential, and the role of radiation therapy and chemotherapy will now be considered.

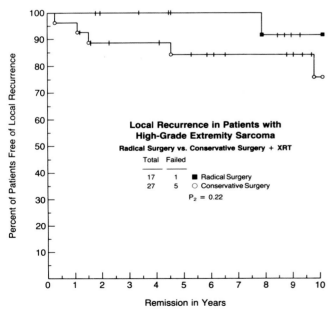

Figure 1–6.   Local recurrences in patients shown in Figures 1–4 and 1–5. A small statistically insignificant difference in local recurrences did not affect overall survival.

ADJUVANT CHEMOTHERAPY

Adjuvant chemotherapy has long been considered for patients with soft tissue sarcomas of the extremities because of the high propensity of these lesions to spread hematogenously from the local site early in the clinical course. The Surgery Branch of the National Cancer Institute conducted a prospective randomized trial of the value of adjuvant chemotherapy in the postoperative period compared with no chemotherapy.[20–22] Patients were prospectively randomized to receive either chemotherapy with doxorubicin, cyclophosphamide, and high-dose methotrexate, or else they were randomized to receive local therapy alone with no adjuvant chemotherapy. Chemotherapy was begun when the surgical wound was healed. The first dose was given three days prior to the initiation of any radiation therapy. Doxorubicin and cyclophosphamide were given on day 1 of a 28-day treatment cycle. The initial dose of doxorubicin was 50 mg/m^2, and this dose was escalated to a maximum of 70 mg/m^2, depending on bone marrow toxicity. Cyclophosphamide was also started, at a dosage of 500 mg/m^2 given simultaneously with the doxorubicin and was escalated to a maximum of 700 mg/m^2, depending on toxic side effects. Cumulative doxorubicin doses up to 530 mg/m^2 were administered. When the maximum cumulative doxorubicin dose was achieved, usually about eight months after the definitive surgery, the patient was switched to a course of high-dose methotrexate with leucovorin rescue for 5 cycles. Toxicity associated with the use of this chemotherapy regimen included alopecia and nausea and vomiting, although doxorubicin-induced cardiomyopathy was the most troublesome side effect. Approximately 10% of the patients treated with full doxorubicin and cyclophosphamide doses on this regimen developed congestive heart failure, and approximately 50% of the patients developed a subclinical decrease in the left ventricular ejection fraction as evaluated by ECG-gated radionuclide angiography. Despite cardiotoxicity, this chemotherapy regimen was effective in improving disease-free survival and overall survival in patients with high-grade soft tissue sarcomas.[20–22] Figures 1–7 and 1–8 show the disease-free and overall survival of patients (as of 1989) randomized to receive either chemotherapy or no chemotherapy. Long-term follow-up supports improvement in disease-free and overall survival in patients receiving chemotherapy.

A subsequent randomized trial has demonstrated that this improved long-term disease-free and overall survival in patients with high-grade extremity sarcoma is unchanged by a reduction in the total doxorubicin and cyclophosphamide doses to 350 mg/m^2

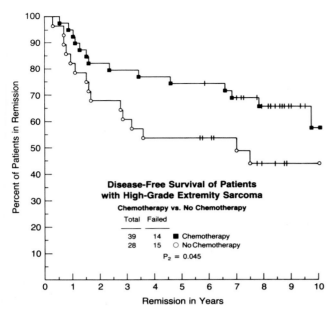

Figure 1–7. Actuarial analysis of continuous disease-free survival of patients with extremity soft tissue sarcomas in a prospective randomized trial conducted by the Surgery Branch, NCI. Patients were randomized to either receive or not receive chemotherapy following surgery. An improvement in continuous disease-free survival was seen in patients randomized to receive chemotherapy.

and 3,500 mg/m^2, respectively, along with elimination of methotrexate[22] (Fig. 1–9). Radionuclide cardiac studies on patients in this subsequent study revealed that the incidence of cardiac impairment as well as the incidence of clinically evident cardiomyopathy was much reduced by the decrease of doxorubicin. Therefore, this modified lower-dose regimen is now the standard adjuvant chemotherapy used for high-grade extremity soft tissue sarcomas in the Surgery Branch at the National Cancer Institute.

A variety of other adjuvant chemotherapy regimens have been studied by other investigators. These studies utilize a variety of chemotherapy agents and dose schedules, and the regimens are begun at varying times following surgery. Some studies include both low-grade and high-grade tumors and both extremity and truncal lesions. This may account for some of the variability in the results. Although some trials have not confirmed a survival benefit with the use of adjuvant chemotherapy,[23] one study, confined to high-grade extremity sarcomas and using a doxorubicin regimen, has confirmed an increased survival of patients receiving adjuvant chemotherapy.[24]

The use of preoperative chemotherapy (also termed *neoadjuvant* chemotherapy) has become increasingly popular. Several groups have described favorable long-term survival rates as well as low local

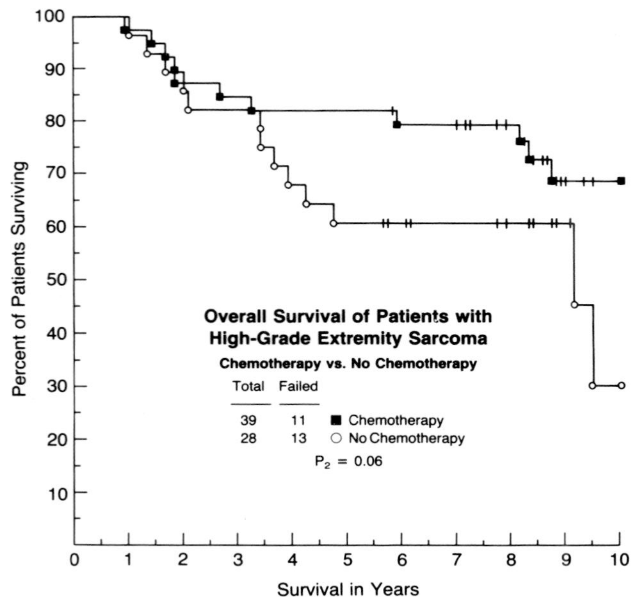

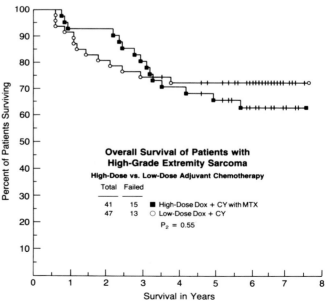

Figure 1–8. Actuarial analysis of overall survival for the same patients presented in Figure 1–6. An improvement in overall survival was seen in patients randomized to receive chemotherapy.

Figure 1–9. Overall survival of patients randomized to a high-dose, three-agent postoperative chemotherapy regimen (used in study shown in Figs 1–7 and 1–8) *v* a low-dose, two-agent regimen. There was no significant difference in the long-term survival of these patients, and the low-dose regimen resulted in significantly less cardiotoxicity.

recurrence rates for high-grade extremity sarcomas using this approach.[25] It is also postulated that this strategy may reduce the need for radical surgery. Thus far, there have been no randomized prospective trials comparing neoadjuvant with postoperative adjuvant chemotherapy. Excellent long-term results have been obtained with both approaches, and randomized trials are necessary to conclude that preoperative chemotherapy has benefits in either long-term survival or the need for radical surgery.

RADIATION THERAPY

Soft tissue sarcomas are responsive to radiation therapy.[1,4,18,19,26] The role of adjuvant radiation therapy following local surgical procedures in patients with soft tissue sarcomas of the extremities has been studied by several groups. These studies have strongly suggested that adjuvant radiation therapy improves local control rates.[1,4,18,20] Certainly it is a modality that is widely used and has clinically significant activity against sarcomas. The appropriate application of radiation therapy is essential if good results are to be achieved.

It is often necessary to use large fields surrounding the local lesion in order to minimize the risk of missing possible areas of local spread.[26] Fields should generally provide approximately 10-cm margins above and below the area of resection. Ideally, the radiation therapist attempts to treat entire muscle groups that have been involved with the tumor and that would have been removed by the surgeon had radical surgical excision been utilized. Computerized axial tomographic scans and the prior placement of clips by the surgeon are the most valuable tools for sophisticated treatment planning.

After the gross tumor is excised, a dose of about 5,500 rads is usually recommended in fractions of 180 to 200 rads per day. Shrinking-field techniques are then utilized to treat the tumor bed to approximately 6,500 rads. Close collaboration and discussion between the surgeon and the radiation therapist are required to identify areas at potential risks due to contamination by the surgical procedure. In most cases, ideal dose distribution requires some combination of photons and electrons in the treatment plan. A thorough rehabilitation plan that begins in the postoperative period and extends through and after radiation therapy is essential if maximal functional results are to be achieved following the combination of surgery and radiation therapy.[27]

In general, one attempts to limit the radiation therapy to about half of the cross-sectional volume of the extremity. Although this is not always possible, it is essential that a small strip of skin in normal tissue be spared radiation therapy, to provide lymphatic drainage from the extremity. Circumferential radiation therapy often results in severe distal edema.

Recently, increasing interest is being exhibited in the use of radiation therapy prior to the surgical excision.[1] There is currently no evidence that the use of preoperative radiation therapy is superior to postoperative radiation therapy, although this question may well deserve a critical evaluation.

Despite the proven ability of radiation to affect sarcomas, its use is associated with significant acute and chronic toxicity. Extremities treated to 6,000 R can show a significant incidence of long-term edema, limitation of motion, fracture, pain, induration, and fibrosis. The cost of these sequelae must be balanced against the effectiveness of radiation (versus other adjuncts) in preventing local recurrence or the consequences of those local recurrences. Possible effects of chemotherapy on local recurrences and the contention by some investigators that local recurrences have minimal impact on the overall prognosis of patients with sarcoma[28] prompted a critical assessment of the benefits of postoperative radiation in patients receiving chemotherapy for high-grade extremity lesions. Patients with high-grade extremity sarcomas amenable to wide local excision (WLE) were randomized to receive WLE and postoperative chemotherapy *v* WLE with postoperative radiation and chemotherapy. The chemotherapy consisted of doxorubicin and cyclophosphamide begun after initial wound healing and given in five monthly doses to a cumulative total of 350 mg/m^2 and 3,500 mg/m^2, respectively. Patients randomized to radiation began therapy concurrently and were treated to a maximum dose of 6,300 R with a shrinking-field technique. With a median follow-up of 4.4 years, there have been 6 local recurrences in 39 patients treated with surgery and chemotherapy, and 0 of 40 patients treated with surgery, radiation, and chemotherapy have locally recurred ($p_2 = 0.02$). Interestingly, because most patients recurring locally have done so with simultaneous or prior metastatic recurrences, the disease-free survival of the two treatment groups is not significantly different at three years (74% in irradiated patients and 67% in nonirradiated patients), nor is overall survival. In addition, all isolated local recurrences have been resectable without requiring amputation, and none have thus far appeared again. These results suggest that the local recurrence rate in patients treated with surgery and chemotherapy is similar to reported rates of local recurrence in patients treated with surgery and radiation. Although the addition of radiation to surgery and chemotherapy may further reduce these recurrences, the prognosis of these patients is primarily determined by the development of metastatic disease.

Another recent randomized trial has investigated the benefit of postoperative adjuvant brachytherapy (delivered by afterloading catheters placed at the time of surgery and loaded five to six days postoperatively) in patients with high- and low-grade sarcomas of the extremities and superficial trunk.[29] After a median follow-up of 16 months, 2 of 52 patients receiving radiation via brachytherapy had suffered local recurrences v 9 of 65 not receiving radiation. No difference in overall survival was demonstrable. Because factors such as the administration of adjuvant chemotherapy was not controlled and because the consequences of these local recurrences are not yet clear, the precise role of radiation in a multimodality therapy approach to primary sarcomas still requires further investigation. Therapeutic decisions on the use of radiation in these patients must balance the reduction in local recurrences in a minority of patients with the toxicity of radiation given to all patients. Ultimately, if no differences in survival are identified, quality-of-life issues may determine the role of radiotherapy in the treatment of these patients.

SUMMARY

The treatment of sarcoma has undergone a dramatic improvement over the last several decades. The primary reason for this has been the implementation of multimodality treatment plans for addressing sarcoma when it presents in its initial stage. Refinement of surgical techniques combined with critical coordination with both radiotherapy and chemotherapy adjuncts have improved the overall survival of these patients while dramatically improving their function by avoiding the need for ablative surgery.

REFERENCES

1. Rosenberg SA, Suit HD, Baker LH, et al: Sarcomas of the soft tissue and bone, in DeVita VT, Hellman S, Rosenberg SA (eds): *Principles and Practice of Oncology.* Philadelphia, JB Lippincott Co, 1982, pp 1037–1093.
2. Shieber W, Graham P: An experience with sarcomas of the soft tissues in adults. *Surgery* 1962;52:25.
3. Russell WO, Cohen J, Enzinger FM, et al: A clinical and pathological staging system for soft tissue sarcomas. *Cancer* 1977;40:1562–1570.
4. Lindberg RD, Martin RG, Romsdahl MM: Surgery and postoperative radiotherapy in the treatment of soft tissue sarcomas in adults. *Am J Roentgenol Rad Therap Nucl Med* 1975;123:123–129.
5. Rosenberg SA, Kent H, Costa J, et al: Prospective randomized evaluation of the role of limb-sparing surgery, radiation therapy, and adjuvant chemoimmunotherapy in the treatment of adult soft-tissue sarcomas. *Surgery* 1978;84:62–66.
6. Costa J, Wesley R, Glatstein E, et al: The grading of soft tissue sarcomas: Results of a clinico-histopathologic correlation in a series of 163 cases. *Cancer,* to be published.
7. Cantin J, McNeer GP, Chu FC, et al: The problem of local recurrence after treatment of soft tissue sarcoma. *Ann Surg* 1968;168:47–52.
8. Simon MA, Enneking WF: The management of soft-tissue sarcomas of the extremities. *J Bone Joint Surg* 1976;58-A:317.
9. Weingrad DN, Rosenberg SA: Early lymphatic spread of osteogenic and soft tissue sarcomas. *Surgery* 1978;84:231–240.
10. Putnam JB, Roth JA, Wesley MN, et al: Analysis of prognostic factors in patients undergoing resection of pulmonary metastases from soft tissue sarcomas. *J Thorac Cardio Vasc Surg,* to be published.
11. Ultmann JE, Phillips TL: Treatment of metastatic cancer, in DeVita VT, Hellman S, Rosenberg SA (eds): *Principles and Practice of Oncology.* Philadelphia, JB Lippincott Co, 1982, pp 1534–1581.
12. Gerner RE, Moore GE, Pickren JW: Soft tissue sarcomas. *Ann Surg* 1975;181:803–808.
13. Martin RG, Butler JJ, Albores-Saavedra J: Soft tissue tumors: Surgical treatment and results, in *Tumors of Bone and Soft Tissue.* Chicago, Year Book Medical Publishers, 1965.
14. Pack GI, Ariel IM: Treatment of cancer and allied diseases, in *Tumors of the Soft Somatic Tissues and Bone.* New York, Harper and Row, 1964, vol VIII.
15. Hare HF, Cerny MF: Soft tissue sarcoma: A review of 200 cases. *Cancer* 1963;16:1332.
16. Shiu MH, Castro EB, Hajdu SI, et al: Surgical treatment of 27 soft tissue sarcomas of the lower extremity. *Ann Surg* 1975;182:597.
17. Chang AE, Yvedt L, Matory MD, et al: Magnetic resonance imaging versus computed tomography in the evaluation of soft tissue tumors of the extremities. *Ann Surg* 1987;205:340–348.
18. Suit HD, Russell WO, Martin RG: Sarcoma of soft tissue: Clinical and histopathologic parameters and response to treatment. *Cancer* 1975;35:1478–1483.
19. Yang JC, Rosenberg SA: Surgery for adult patients with soft tissue sarcomas. *Sem Oncol* 1989;16:289–296.
20. Maurer HM, Moon T, Donaldson M, et al: The intergroup rhabdomyosarcoma study. *Cancer* 1977;40:2015.
21. Rosenberg SA, Tepper J, Glatstein E, et al: Prospective randomized evaluation of adjuvant chemotherapy in adults with soft tissue sarcomas of the extremities. *Cancer* 1983;52:424–434.
22. Chang AE, Kinsella T, Glatstein E, et al: Adjuvant chemotherapy for patients with high-grade soft-tissue sarcomas of the extremity. *J Clin Oncol* 1988;6:1491–1500.
23. Antman K, Suit H, Amato D, et al: Preliminary results of a randomized trial of adjuvant doxorubicin for sarcomas: Lack of apparent difference between treatment groups. *J Clin Oncol* 1984;2:601–608.
24. Picci P, Bacci G, Gherlinzoni F, et al: Results of a

randomized trial for the treatment of localized soft tissue tumors (STS) of the extremities in adult patients, in Ryan JR, Baker LO (eds): *Recent Concepts in Sarcoma Treatment*. Dordrecht, Netherlands, Kluwer Academic, 1988, pp 144–148.

25. Eiber FR, Morton DL, Eckardt J, et al: Limb salvage for skeletal and soft tissue sarcomas. *Cancer* 1984;53: 2579–2584.

26. Tepper J, Rosenberg SA, Glatstein E: Radiation therapy technique in soft tissue sarcomas of the extremity: Policies of treatment at the National Cancer Institute. *Intl J Rad Oncol* 1982;8:263–273.

27. Sugarbaker PH, Bartofsky I, Rosenberg SA, et al: Quality of life assessment of patients in extremity sarcoma clinical trials. *Surgery* 1982;1:17–23.

28. Rööser B, Gustafson P, Rydholm A: Is there no influence of local control on the rate of metsatases in high-grade soft tissue sarcoma? *Cancer* 1990;65:1727–1729.

29. Brennan MF, Hilaris B, Shiu MH, et al: Local recurrence in adult soft-tissue sarcoma. *Arch Surg* 1987;122:128–132.

2

Osteogenic Sarcoma

ALAN R. BAKER, M.D.
PAUL H. SUGARBAKER, M.D.
MARTIN M. MALAWER, M.D.

OVERVIEW

Definitive surgical treatment of osteogenic sarcoma of an extremity is usually accomplished by amputation. However, a limb salvage procedure with or without prosthetic replacement of bone should always be considered. The level of amputation is determined by careful physical examination and preoperative bone scan. Improvement in survival of osteogenic sarcoma patients is due to (1) a trend toward earlier diagnosis and an aggressive approach to pulmonary metastatic disease by thoracotomy and wedge excision of tumor nodules, and (2) growing experience with a chemotherapeutic approach to primary and recurrent disease. Adjuvant chemotherapy protocols now studied within randomized controlled clinical trials continue to explore the optimum use of combined treatments.

DIAGNOSIS

Primary neoplasms of bone are uncommon. Current estimates suggest that there are approximately 2,000 new cases of bone cancer in the United States each year.[1] This figure represents only 0.2% of the total number of serious malignancies occurring each year. By far the majority of these bone tumors were osteogenic sarcomas.

The demographic features associated with osteogenic sarcoma are summarized in Table 2–1. Typically, the tumor presents as a painful mass in and about the involved bone of a young person. The mass usually has been present for a period of days to weeks. It is not at all uncommon to elicit a history of trauma, the insult having served to uncover the underlying problem. After a traumatic musculoskeletal injury, signs or symptoms that persist warrant inquiry and explanation. If left unattended, the destructive process continues, with progressive loss of function of the afflicted part and, on occasion, the occurrence of a pathologic fracture.

Plain x-rays of the symptomatic area should be the initial study done. If properly interpreted, these films take the problem out of the simple sprain and strain category and raise the specter of more serious diagnostical alternatives. The x-ray appearance of a classical osteogenic sarcoma is seen in Figure 2–1. This femoral lesion is metaphyseal in location and shows evidence of mixed blastic and lytic changes. The margins of the bony pathologic process are ill-defined, and cortical disruption is visible. An associated soft tissue mass is readily recognizable, with extensive malignant calcification giving rise to the "sunburst" appearance of the tumor. Periosteal reaction is notable with the formation of a Codman's triangle. The roentgenographic abnormalities can naturally be much more subtle and less highly specific than those in the illustration, and give rise to a fairly long list of differential diagnostic possibilities.

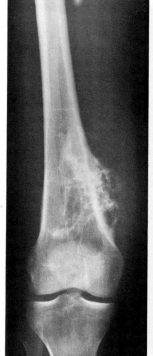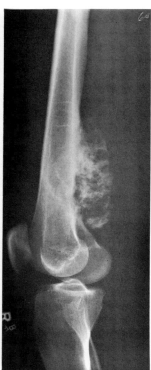

Figure 2–1. These anteroposterior and lateral x-ray projections of the knee illustrate many of the features of a "classical" osteogenic sarcoma. The Codman's triangle includes (1) metaphyseal location, (2) mixed blastic and lytic changes with ill-defined borders within the bone, and (3) cortical disruption and a large soft tissue mass with associated malignant calcification.

The alternatives that should be considered are summarized in Table 2–2. Both benign and malignant pathologic processes as well as infection are possibilities that must be entertained. Because the treatment for these different entities differs dramatically, the specific pathologic diagnosis must be sought by biopsy with appropriate histologic and microbiologic assessment of the sampled tissue. Prior to biopsy the patient should undergo the workup outlined in Table 2–3.

The biopsy should provide definitive information about the nature of the pathologic process and thereby permit selection of appropriate therapy. Although seemingly a "little operation," the details of its conduct are far from trivial, and difficulties ensuing from it can seriously complicate a patient's subsequent care. The incision should be carefully planned in such a way that it does not compromise subsequent therapeutic surgical options. For extremity lesions this almost always means a longitudinal, rather than a transverse, incision. The surgical strategy should be to keep the operation as small as

Table 2–1. Demographic Features in Osteogenic Sarcoma

VARIABLES	FEATURES
Age	60% Occur in Second and Third Decades
Sex	60% Male, 40% Female
Site	50% Arise about the Knee
	42% Femur
	18% Tibia
	10% Humerus
	8% Pelvis
Predisposing Factors	Bone Irradiation
	Paget's Disease
	Retinoblastoma
	Ollier's Disease

Table 2-2.   Differential Diagnostic Possibilities Raised by Abnormal Plain X-ray*

TUMOR		
Malignant†	*Benign*	*Infection*
Osteogenic Sarcoma	Osteoidosteoma	Pyogenic
	Osteoblastoma	Mycobacterial
		Fungal
Chondrosarcoma	Osteochondroma	
	Enchondroma	
	Chondroblastoma	
Ewing's Sarcoma		
Parosteal Osteogenic Sarcoma	Myositis Ossificans	
Periosteal Osteogenic Sarcoma		
Lymphoma		
Giant Cell Tumor	Giant Cell Tumor	
Chordoma		
Malignant Fibrous Histiocytoma of Bone	Hyperparathyroidism	
	Desmoplastic Fibroma	
Hemangiosarcoma of Bone	Hemangioma	
Mesenchymal Chondrosarcoma		
	Aneurysmal Bone Cyst	
	Unicameral Bone Cyst	
	Eosinophilic Granuloma	
	Paget's Disease	

*From Marcove[2] and Mirra.[3]
†Listed roughly in order of frequency of occurrence.

possible, compatible with ensuring adequacy of material sampled to provide definitive diagnosis. Fine-needle aspiration and cytology almost never provide diagnostic material and hence should be avoided. Although frequently useful in primary soft tissue sarcoma diagnosis, "true-cut" or similar needle biopsy cannot sample the bony component of the lesion and hence usually provides inadequate tissue. A percutaneous Craig needle biopsy core or an open procedure in which a Michelle trephine is used to obtain a 4- to 10-mm core of tissue is usually a satisfactory technique. Errors frequently involve sampling an insufficient quantity of material to make the diagnosis, failing to sample the lesion at all, or sampling an unrepresentative portion of it. Performing the biopsy under fluoroscopic guidance, if intraoperative fluoroscopy is available, placing a stainless steel clip in the biopsy defect, and confirming its superimposition with the preoperative x-ray abnormality by obtaining intraoperative anterior-posterior and lateral views are frequently quite helpful and preclude the occasional need for a second biopsy.

Table 2-3.   Workup of Patient with Bony Pathologic Process

PREBIOPSY	POSTBIOPSY (if osteogenic sarcoma)
History and Physical Examination	CT Scan and/or MRI of Involved Area*
Specifically query	Arteriogram*
recent trauma	Full-Lung Tomography or Chest CT Scan
any recent infection	
constitutional symptoms—anorexia, weight loss, fever, chills, sweats	
Plain X-rays	
AP and lateral views of entire involved bone	
prior x-rays of involved area	
Hematologic profile	
sedimentation rate	
CBC and differential	
alkaline phosphatase	
Radionuclide bone scan	
Arthrograms and arthroscopy are rarely useful	

*If limb-sparing operation is contemplated.

Pathologic assessment of the biopsy material by frozen-section techniques is also often quite helpful. Although the pathologist is frequently unable or unwilling to give a definitive specific diagnosis in this setting, he or she can often comment on the "adequacy" of the material sampled. If a tumor appears to be present, the pathologist may suggest that with a "high degree of probability" a malignant diagnosis will be forthcoming on permanent sections.

Prophylactic preoperative antibiotic coverage is used whenever, by prebiopsy assessment, the lesion is thought likely to be neoplastic. The biopsy material, in addition to wound swabs, should always be sent for appropriate culture. This will permit delineation of an infectious etiology.

Infection as a complication of the biopsy procedure is a very serious problem, often compromising the optimal timing and conduct of subsequent treatment. Both gentle surgical technique and careful hemostasis should further minimize the risk of wound infection secondary to tissue trauma or hematoma collection, and should prevent extensive tumor contamination of tissue planes by hematoma tracking. On occasion, when wax or absorbable gelatin sponge do not provide hemostasis, methyl methacrylate can be used to plug the biopsy defect to control bleeding. The biopsy wound should be closed per primum. Open-wound drainage should be avoided. On rare occasions, small-catheter suction drainage is useful. Because the bone is further weakened by the biopsy procedure, additional care should be taken postbiopsy to avoid pathologic fracture. Crutch gait, casts, splints, and slings can all be useful as postbiopsy adjuncts to minimize undue stress and its adverse sequelae.

Radiologic Studies

If the biopsy reveals osteogenic sarcoma, additional studies need to be performed before proceeding with a therapeutic surgical procedure. The postbiopsy workup is outlined in Table 2–3. About 15% of patients with osteogenic sarcoma will have clinically detectable pulmonary metastases at the time of presentation. About 90% of these patients will have metastases that will be apparent on routine plain x-rays of the chest, and 10% of these patients will have metastases that will be seen only on full-lung tomograph or computed tomography of the chest. Even if the results are negative, these two studies will prove clinically useful as baseline determinations for subsequent follow-up. Pulmonary nodules, although an adverse prognostic feature, still represent a surgically curable situation, provided that they are clinically appreciated at the earliest possible time and the

patient can be rendered free of pulmonary metastases by wedge excision at thoracotomy.

NATURAL HISTORY

Osteosarcoma of bone has characteristic patterns of behavior and growth that distinguish it from other malignant lesions.[4,5] These patterns form the basis of a staging system and current treatment strategies.

Primary Tumor

The three mechanisms of local progression of bone tumors are compression of normal tissue, resorption of bone by reactive osteoclasts, and direct destruction of normal tissue. Benign tumors grow and expand by the first two mechanisms, but invasion directly into adjacent tissue is characteristic of malignant bone tumors. Local anatomy influences tumor growth by providing the natural barriers to extension. Growth of all cancers takes the path of least resistance. Most benign bone tumors are unicompartmental; they remain confined and may expand within the bone in which they arose. Malignant bone tumors are bicompartmental; they destroy the overlying cortex and invade the adjacent soft tissue. The precise determination of anatomic extension has become increasingly important with the advent of limb preservation surgery.

Metastases

Bone tumors, unlike carcinomas, disseminate almost exclusively through the blood; bones lack a lymphatic system. There have been only rare reports of early lymphatic spread to regional nodes.[6,7] Lymphatic involvement, which has been noticed in 10% of cases at autopsy, is a poor prognostic sign.[8] McKenna et al reported that 6 (3%) of 194 patients with osteosarcoma who underwent amputation demonstrated lymph node involvement. None of these patients survived five years. Hematogenous spread is manifested in its early stages by pulmonary involvement and secondarily by bony involvement.[9,10] Bone metastases are occasionally the first sign of dissemination. With the use of adjuvant chemotherapy, the skeletal system has become a more common site of initial relapse.[11]

Skip Metastases

Skip metastases are tumor nodules located within the same bone as the main tumor but not continuous with it. They are most often seen with high-grade sarcomas. Transarticular skip metastases are located in the joint adjacent to the main tumor.[12] A skip lesion develops by the embolization of tumor cells within the marrow sinusoids; in effect, they are local micrometastases that have not passed through the circulation. Transarticular skips are believed to occur through periarticular venous anastomoses. The clinical incidence of skip metastases is less than 1%.[13] These lesions predict poor survival.[12,13]

STAGING BONE TUMORS

In 1980, the Musculoskeletal Tumor Society (MSTS) adopted a Surgical Staging System (SSS) for bone sarcomas (Table 2–4). The system is based on the fact that all types of mesenchymal sarcomas of bone behave similarly. The SSS described by Enneking and colleagues[14] is based on the GTM classification: grade (G), location (T), and lymph node involvement and metastases (M).

- Surgical grade (G): G represents the histologic grade of a lesion and other clinical data that are used to make a surgical determination of low grade (G1) or high grade (G2).
- Surgical site (T): T represents the site of the lesion, which may be intracompartmental (T1) or extracompartmental (T2). A compartment is an anatomic structure or space bounded by natural barriers to tumor extension. The significance of T1 lesions is easier to define clinically, surgically, and radiographically than that of T2 lesions, and there is a higher chance of adequate removal of T1 tumors by nonamputative procedures. In general,

low-grade bone sarcomas are intracompartmental (T1), and high-grade sarcomas are extracompartmental (T2).
- Lymph node involvement and metastases (M): Lymphatic spread is a sign of wide dissemination. Regional lymphatic involvement is equated with distant metastases.

SURGICAL APPROACH

The first major decision required after biopsy shows osteogenic sarcoma concerns the possibility of a limb salvage procedure. Around the world the definitive surgical treatment for the primary osteogenic sarcoma is most often accomplished by amputation. However, surgeons in several centers are providing local control for the primary tumor by performing an extensive en bloc excision of the tumor and surrounding soft tissues with reconstruction by endoprosthetic implants. The technical details of the procedures themselves are reviewed in chapters 13, 17, 19, and 27. If a limb-sparing procedure is contemplated, a preoperative computer tomography (CT) scan, magnetic resonance imaging (MRI), and arteriogram of the involved region provide information essential to the determination of local resectability. Table 2–5 itemizes the contraindications for limb-sparing surgery.

The second major surgical judgment concerns the level of amputation. Although it is critical to provide an adequate margin proximal to the tumor to ensure

---

Table 2–4. Surgical Staging of Bone Sarcoma*

STAGE	GRADE†	SITE
IA	Low (G1)	Intracompartmental (T1)
IB	Low (G1)	Extracompartmental (T2)
IIA	High (G2)	Intracompartmental (T1)
IIB	High (G2)	Extracompartmental (T2)
III	Any G Regional or Distant Metastasis (M1)	Any (T)

*From Enneking WF et al.[14]
†G = grade: G1 is any low-grade tumor; G2 is any high-grade tumor. T = site: T1 intracompartmental location of tumor; T2 extracompartmental location of tumor. M = regional or distal metastases: M0 = no metastases; M1 = any metastases.

Table 2–5. Contraindications for Limb-Sparing Surgery

1. *Major neurovascular involvement:* Although vascular grafts may be used, the adjacent nerves are usually at risk, making successful resection less likely. In addition, the magnitude of resection in combination with vascular reconstruction is often prohibitive.
2. *Pathologic fractures:* A fracture through a bone affected by a tumor spreads tumor cells by the hematoma beyond accurately determined limits. The risk of local recurrence increases under such circumstances.
3. *Inappropriate biopsy sites:* An inappropriate or poorly planned biopsy jeopardizes local tumor control by contaminating normal tissue planes and compartments.
4. *Infection:* The risk of infection following implantation of a metallic device or allograft in an infected area is prohibitive. Sepsis jeopardizes the effectiveness of adjuvant chemotherapy.
5. *Immature skeletal age:* The predicted leg-length discrepancy should not be greater than 6 to 8 cm. Upper-extremity reconstruction does not depend on skeletal maturity.
6. *Extensive muscle involvement:* There must be enough muscle remaining to reconstruct a functional extremity.

that local control will be achieved, it is equally important that the operation done be consistent with maximal rehabilitative potential for the patient.

Two factors play a critical role in determining the level of amputation. The first factor is the extent of the soft tissue component of the tumor. This is best assessed on simple physical examination. On occasion, computed tomography of the involved region provides additional useful information. Figure 2–2 is a CT scan made through an osteogenic sarcoma of the distal femur. It shows the extensive soft tissue component of the tumor encroaching on the distal femoral neurovascular bundle. The second factor in determining the level of amputation is the extent of bony tumor involvement and, more importantly, intramedullary tumor spread. This is best determined preoperatively by a technetium 99m phosphorate radionuclide bone scan. It is quite helpful if,

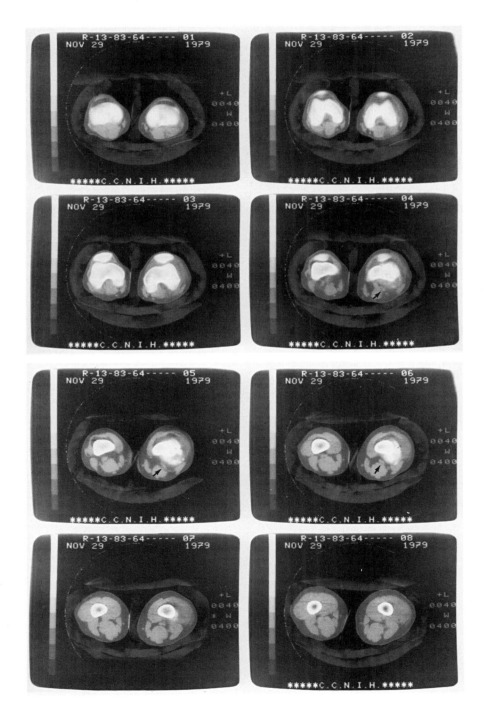

Figure 2–2. CT scan of a primary osteogenic sarcoma of the left distal femur. The black arrow in panels 4 to 6 points to the neurovascular bundle that is displaced and abutted by the large soft tissue component of the tumor erupting out of the lateral femoral condyle.

during the radionuclide bone scan, the surgeon, using the small amount of tracer in a test tube as a localization guide, marks off on the patient's skin the site corresponding to the most proximal area of enhanced radionuclide uptake by the underlying involved bone. As a general rule, the level of amputation should be about 6 cm proximal to the most proximal extent of both the soft tissue component and the intramedullary component of the tumor. Intramedullary spread is usually more extensive than either soft tissue spread or cortical involvement. The radionuclide bone scan of a distal femoral osteogenic sarcoma is illustrated in Figure 2–3. Note that although the lesion by plain x-ray (Fig. 2–1) appears confined to the distal femur, intramedullary extension, indicated by increased tracer uptake, extends to the mid-femur. The appropriate level of amputation in this instance would be a very high above-knee amputation (AKA) done at the level of the lesser femoral trochanter. Although this creates a very short AKA stump, with the help of an able prosthetist it proves to be functionally superior to what is seen when a hip disarticulation is performed. Table 2–6 summarizes the guidelines for level of amputation used by the Surgery Branch of the National Cancer Institute (NCI). From 1973 to 1983, under these

guidelines, only one AKA stump recurrence was recorded in more than 50 such transbone amputations for primary osteogenic sarcoma of the femur.

Several specific additional points should be made about the management of these amputations. Our practice has been to do these procedures under preoperative prophylactic antibiotic coverage. A tourniquet is not used. The proximal margin of all transbone amputations is assessed by frozen section during the procedure by making a "touch preparation" of the marrow at the level of bone transection. The stump wounds are managed with closed-system catheter suction drains for two to three days postoperatively. All extremity amputations are handled with a rigid plaster postoperative dressing in an effort to minimize wound edema and stump swelling, promote patient comfort, and encourage early functional rehabilitation. Because these amputations for the most part have been done for young patients free of vascular insufficiency, no complications secondary to the use of rigid dressings have occurred. Once uneventful wound healing has been accomplished, the patient's functional recovery is encouraged through frequent interaction with the rehabilitation therapist and the use of a temporary prosthesis. By six to eight weeks postamputation,

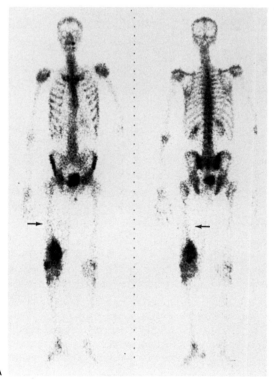

A

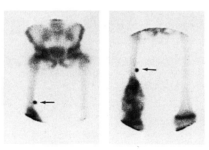

B

Figure 2–3. (A) Technetium 99m phosphorate bone scan of an osteogenic sarcoma of the right distal femur shows increased radionuclide uptake to the mid-femur. This finding represents the most sensitive reflection of intramedullary tumor extension. Transection of the femur at this level would most probably be followed by a stump recurrence. The proper level for femoral transection should be at least 6 cm above the level indicated by the arrow. (B) Rectilinear view of a bone scan from another patient shows the radionuclide marker (arrow) used to identify the proximal limit of tumor uptake. Patient's skin is marked at this level and bone transection during amputation is performed at least 6 cm proximal to this point.

Table 2-6. Guidelines for Level of Amputation of Primary Osteogenic Sarcoma

SITE OF TUMOR	LEVEL OF AMPUTATION
Leg (tibia, fibula)	Above Knee
Thigh (femur)	
Distal to midportion of bone	High above Knee
Proximal to midportion of bone	Modified Hemipelvectomy
Pelvis (pubis, ischium, or ilium)	Hemipelvectomy
Forearm (radius, ulna)	Transhumeral
Arm (humerus)	
Distal	Shoulder Disarticulation
Proxima	Forequarter

stump maturation has usually progressed to the point where measurement for the fitting of a permanent prosthesis is appropriate.

ADJUVANT CHEMOTHERAPY

Adjuvant chemotherapy has remarkably increased overall survival. The bleak 20% survival rate with surgery alone during the 1960s rose to almost 80% with adjuvant treatment regimens in the 1980s.[15–17] Multidrug regimens are now indicated. The timing, mode of delivery, and different combinations of these agents are being investigated at many centers. Both preoperative chemotherapy regimens (by the intravenous or intra-arterial route) and postoperative regimens are being evaluated for their effect on survival. The scientific basis for adjuvant chemotherapy of osteosarcoma is derived from experiments that suggest that micrometastatic disease can be eliminated if the treatment is given when the total body burden of metastatic tumor is sufficiently low.[18] Osteosarcoma is a drug-resistant neoplasm. Results of studies of the response rates of single agents and drugs in combination against macroscopic disease have been disappointing. Few drugs have produced responses in more than 15% of patients, and most responses are limited. Exceptions are the responses observed in trials of adriamycin, cisplatin, high-dose methotrexate with leucovorin rescue, and, more recently, ifosfamide. A steep dose-response relationship may also pertain to the drugs.

Concerns have been raised that adjuvant chemotherapy for osteosarcoma may delay, but not prevent, recurrence. The results of many adjuvant studies suggest that relapse-free survival rates have stable plateaus beyond four years and that recurrence after three years is usual. Most patients surviving three years without evidence of recurrence are probably cured. The favorable impact of postoperative adju-

vant chemotherapy on the natural history of osteosarcoma is incontrovertible. Adjuvant therapy should be a component of treatment for all patients with advanced disease. Selection criteria for patients with early tumors who do not merit adjuvant chemotherapy treatment need to be defined.

INDUCTION (PRESURGICAL) CHEMOTHERAPY

Induction chemotherapy has been used with increasing frequency during the past decade in the management of osteosarcoma. This strategy evolved concurrently with limb-sparing procedures. Initial attempts at limb salvage at the Memorial Sloan-Kettering Cancer Center in 1973 involved the fabrication of customized endoprostheses for select patients undergoing en bloc resection. While the prosthesis was being made, a process requiring up to three months, chemotherapy was administered to prevent tumor progression.[19] Upon histologic evaluation, the response to preoperative chemotherapy by the tumor was found to be a powerful prognostic factor; unfavorable responders were likely to develop distant metastases, despite continued use of chemotherapy after surgery.[20] The prognostic significance of tumor response to preoperative chemotherapy was confirmed in a study conducted by the German Society for Pediatric Oncology.[21] Although the initial impetus for induction chemotherapy was limb salvage, several theoretical advantages of presurgical chemotherapy apply to all patients with osteosarcoma (Table 2–7).

Tailoring Postoperative Chemotherapy

The use of induction chemotherapy to customize the postoperative adjuvant therapy, based on the response of the primary tumor as determined by histologic examination, is called *tailoring*.[22] This strategy was pioneered at the Memorial Hospital in the T-10 protocol.[23] Patients were treated preoperatively with high-dose methotrexate, the BCD (bleomycin, cyclophosphamide, and dactinomycin) combination, and adriamycin. Those with favorable histologic responses received the same agents postoperatively. Patients demonstrating unfavorable (grades I and II) histologic responses were treated on a revised regimen consisting of adriamycin and cisplatin along with the BCD combination (without high-dose methotrexate) postoperatively.

Although only 39% of patients achieved a favorable histologic response to presurgical chemotherapy,

Table 2-7. Considerations for Presurgical and Postsurgical Chemotherapy Regimens

TIMING OF CHEMOTHERAPY	ADVANTAGES	DISADVANTAGES
Preoperative Chemotherapy	Early institution of systemic therapy against micrometastases	High tumor burden (not optimal for first-order kinetics)
	Reduced chance of spontaneous emergence of drug-resistant clones in micrometastases	Increased probability of the selection of drug-resistant cells in primary tumor, which may metastasize
	Reduction in tumor size, increasing the change of limb salvage	Delay in definitive control of bulk disease; increased chance for systemic dissemination
	Provides time for fabrication of customized endoprosthesis	
	Less chance of viable tumor being spread at the time of surgery	Psychological trauma of retaining tumor
	Individual response to chemotherapy allows selection of different risk groups	Risk of local tumor progression with loss of a limb-sparing option
Postsurgical Chemotherapy	Radical removal of bulk tumor decreases tumor burden and increases growth rate of residual disease, making S-phase-specific agents more active and optimizing conditions for first-order kinetics	Delay of systemic therapy for micrometastases
		No preoperative in vivo assay of cytotoxic response
	Decreased probability of selecting a drug-resistant clone in the primary tumor	Possible spread of viable tumor by surgical manipulation

virtually all of the favorable responders were projected to survive free of recurrence.[22] The patients who initially demonstrated an unfavorable histologic response were switched to the cisplatin-containing regimen, and almost 85% were projected to remain relapse-free at three years. Overall, 90% of the patients treated on the T-10 regimen with tailored therapy were projected to remain disease-free at three years. Moreover, a significant difference in outcome could no longer be detected between favorable and unfavorable responders to presurgical chemotherapy, supporting the contention that poor responders were "salvaged" by the administration of alternative chemotherapy postoperatively. The survival of patients on the T-10 protocol is the most favorable reported for the treatment of osteosarcoma.

In a recent study, the Children's Cancer Study Group attempted to duplicate the T-10 regimen in a multi-institutional setting. Results were not as favorable as those initially reported from Memorial Hospital. The overall 61% disease-free survival rate at two years for patients on this study is disappointing, compared with the initial results from Memorial Hospital. The trial tested the strategy of custom-tailoring therapy. The results suggest that patients demonstrating poor response of the primary tumor have poor prognoses and that treatment of poor responders with a salvage regimen does not improve their prognoses. These investigators concluded that active agents (eg, cisplatin) should not be withheld

from the initial therapy of newly diagnosed patients. In conclusion, the value of presurgical chemotherapy, with or without tailoring, in the treatment of osteosarcoma has not been demonstrated conclusively. A study designed to test this question is being conducted by the Pediatric Oncology Group.

INTRA-ARTERIAL CHEMOTHERAPY

Induction (presurgical) chemotherapy may be administered directly into the arterial supply of the tumor to maximize drug delivery.[24] Adriamycin and cisplatin, in particular, have been delivered by intra-arterial infusion to the extremities. Pharmacokinetic studies have shown that intra-arterial chemotherapy produces high local drug concentrations.[23] Dramatic responses in the primary tumors have been observed in a majority of patients, thus facilitating limb salvage surgery. This strategy is discussed in chapter 7. There has been no direct confirmation of whether the responses are superior to those from intravenous administration of the same agents or whether systemic toxicity is less.

MULTI-INSTITUTIONAL OSTEOSARCOMA STUDY

The prognosis for patients with osteosarcoma has improved. This change was largely attributed to the effects of adjuvant chemotherapy. However, Mayo Clinic investigators challenged the apparent contribution of adjuvant chemotherapy, reporting that the prognoses of patients diagnosed and treated with or without adjuvant therapy at that institution had improved over time.[24]

In an effort to resolve the controversy over adjuvant therapy of osteosarcoma, the Multi-Institutional Osteosarcoma Study (MIOS), a randomized controlled trial, was conducted between 1982 and 1984.[17] The objective of this study was to determine if the administration of multiagent adjuvant chemotherapy after surgical removal of the primary tumor would significantly improve the relapse-free survival and survival for patients with nonmetastatic osteosarcoma of the extremity compared with a concurrent control group treated by surgery alone. Patients were randomized to receive intensive multiagent chemotherapy for one year or were assigned to an observation-only control group. The study included 36 randomized patients and 77 additional patients who declined randomization but who accepted therapy according to one of the treatment arms of the study. The event-free survivals of all patients in the control group of this trial, who were treated only with surgery of the primary tumor, matched the historical experience before 1970; more than half of these patients developed metastases within six months of diagnosis, and more than 80% of these patients developed recurrent disease within two years of diagnosis. Disease-free survival from the observation groups of the MIOS are virtually the same as the historical control curves generated at many institutions before the 1970s. Also, the projected disease-free survivals for patients treated with adjuvant chemotherapy in the MIOS was 64% at two years and 60% at four years. Virtually the same results were seen, whether randomized or nonrandomized patients were considered. Among the randomized patients, the disease-free survival advantage for patients treated with immediate adjuvant chemotherapy after surgery is highly significant.

All patients developing recurrent disease on the observation arm of the MIOS were treated aggressively with lung resections and chemotherapy after relapse. This resulted in a remarkable prolongation of survival after relapse and the apparent cure of the substantial proportion of these patients. The overall survival for patients on the MIOS is not yet certain, but with a maximum follow-up of close to five years *no difference in overall survival according to treatment can be demonstrated among the randomized patients.* If randomized and nonrandomized patients are pooled, a trend favoring a survival advantage for patients treated with immediate adjuvant chemo-

therapy is apparent. Comparable results were reported in a similar randomized study conducted at UCLA. Only 20% of patients treated without postoperative adjuvant chemotherapy survived without recurrence, compared with 55% of patients surviving relapse-free in the group receiving postoperative chemotherapy.[27]

REFERENCES

1. Silverberg E, Lubera JA: A review of American Cancer Society estimates of cancer cases and deaths. *J Clin* 1983;33:3–25.
2. Marcove RC: *The Surgery of Tumors of Bone and Cartilage.* New York, Grune & Stratton, 1981.
3. Mirra JM: *Bone Tumors: Diagnosis and Treatment.* Philadelphia, JB Lippincott, 1980.
4. Enneking WF: *Musculoskeletal Tumor Surgery.* New York, Churchill Livingstone, 1983, vol I, pp 1–60.
5. Patterson H, Springfield DS, Enneking WF: *Radiologic Management of Musculoskeletal Tumors.* New York, Springer-Verlag, 1986.
6. Weingard DC, Rosenberg SA: Early lymphatic spread of osteogenic and soft-tissue sarcomas. *Surgery* 1978;84:231–240.
7. Tobias JD, Pratt CB, Parham DM, et al: The significance of calcified regional lymph nodes at the time of diagnosis of osteosarcoma. *Orthopedics* 1985;8:49–52.
8. Jeffree GM, Price CHG, Sissins HA: The metastatic spread of osteosarcoma. *Br J Cancer* 1975;32:87–107.
9. McKeena RJ, Schwinn CP, Soong KY, et al: Sarcomata of the osteogenic series (osteosarcoma, fibrosarcoma, chondrosarcoma, parosteal osteosarcoma and sarcomata) arising in abnormal bone: An analysis of 552 cases. *J Bone Joint Surg AM* 1966;48:1–26.
10. Marcove RC, Mike V, Hajack JV, et al: Osteogenic sarcoma under the age of twenty one. *J Bone Joint Surg Am* 1970;52:411–423.
11. Goldstein H, McNeil BJ, Zufall E, et al: Changing indications for bone scintigraphy in patients with osteosarcoma. *Radiology* 1980;135:177–180.
12. Enneking WF, Kagan A: Intramarrow spread of osteosarcoma, in *Management of Primary Bone and Soft Tissue Tumors.* Chicago, Year Book Medical Publishers, 1976, pp 177–177.
13. Malawer MM, Dunham WF: Skip metastases in osteosarcoma: Recent experience. *J Surg Oncol* 1983;22:236–245.
14. Enneking WF, Spanier SS, Goodman MA: A system for the surgical staging of musculoskeletal sarcoma. *Clin Orthop* 1980;153:106–120.
15. Rosen G, Marcove RC, Caparros B, et al: Primary osteogenic sarcoma. The rationale for preoperative chemotherapy and delayed survey. *Cancer* 1979;43:2163–2177.
16. Cortes EP, Holland JP: Adjuvant chemotherapy for primary osteogenic sarcoma. *Surg Clin North Am* 1981;61:1391–1404.
17. Link MP, Goorin AM, Miser AW, et al: The effect of adjuvant chemotherapy on relapse-free survival in patients with osteosarcoma of the extremity. *N Engl J Med* 1986;314:1600–1606.
18. Schabel FM Jr: The use of tumor growth kinetics in

planning "curative" chemotherapy of advanced solid tumors. *Cancer Res* 1969;29:2385–2388.

19. Rosen G, Murphy ML, Huvos AG, et al: Chemotherapy, en bloc resection, and prosthetic bone replacement in the treatment of osteogenic sarcoma. *Cancer* 1976; 37:1–11.

20. Huvos A, Rosen G, Marcove RC: Primary osteogenic sarcoma. Pathologic aspects in 20 patients after treatment with chemotherapy, en bloc resection and prosthetic bone replacement. *Arch Pathol Lab Med* 1977; 101:14–18.

21. Winkler K, Beron G, Kotz R, et al: Neoadjuvant chemotherapy for osteogenic sarcoma: Results of the cooperative German/Austrian study. *J Clin Oncol* 1984;2:617–624.

22. Provisor A, Nachman J, Krailo M, et al: Treatment of non-metastatic osteogenic sarcoma of the extremities with pre- and post-operative chemotherapy. *Proc Am Soc Clin Oncol* 1987;6:217.

23. Rosen G, Caparros B, Huvos AG, et al: Preoperative chemotherapy for osteogenic sarcoma: Selection of post-operative based on the response of the primary tumor to preoperative chemotherapy. *Cancer* 1982; 49:1221–1230.

24. Jaffe N, Prudich J, Knapp J, et al: Treatment of primary osteosarcoma with intra-arterial and intravenous high-dose methotrexate. *J Clin Oncol* 1983;1:428–431.

25. Jaffe N, Knapp J, Chuang VP, et al: Osteosarcoma: Intra-arterial treatment of the primary tumor with *cis*-diamminedichloroplatinum II (CDP): Angiographic, pathologic and pharmacologic studies. *Cancer* 1983;51:402–407.

26. Taylor WF, Ivins JC, Dahlin DC, et al: Trends and variability in survival from osteosarcoma. *Mayo Clinic Proc* 1978;53:697–700.

27. Eilber F, Guiliano A, Eckardt J, et al: Adjuvant chemotherapy for osteosarcoma: A randomized prospective trial. *J Clin Oncol* 1987;5:21–26.

3

Staging, Pathology, and Radiology of Musculoskeletal Tumors

MARTIN M. MALAWER, M.D.
BARRY M. SHMOOKLER, M.D.

OVERVIEW

An understanding of the basic biology and pathology of bone and soft tissue tumors is essential to an intelligent interpretation of the various staging (imaging) studies, the currently used surgical staging system, and, in general, the terminology used in musculoskeletal oncology. The underlying theme of this chapter is to permit a scientific and pathologic basis for interpretation and clinical decision making in order to arrive at an optimal treatment strategy for a patient with a sarcoma. A detailed description of the clinical, radiographic, and pathologic characteristics is presented for each malignant entity.

NATURAL HISTORY AND BIOLOGY OF BONE AND SOFT TISSUE TUMORS

Tumors arising in bone and soft tissue have characteristic patterns of behavior and growth that distinguish them from other malignant lesions.[1] These patterns, which form the basis of a staging system and present treatment strategies, are described here.[2]

Biology and Growth

Spindle cell sarcomas form a solid lesion that grows centrifugally. The periphery of this lesion is the least mature. In contradistinction to the true capsule that surrounds benign lesions, which is composed of compressed normal cells, the malignant tumor is generally enclosed by a pseudocapsule, which consists of compressed tumor cells, and a fibrovascular zone of reactive tissue with a variable inflammatory component that interdigitates with the normal tissue adjacent and beyond the lesion. The thickness of the reactive zone varies with the degree of malignancy and histogenic type. The histologic hallmark of malignant sarcomas is their potential to break through the pseudocapsule to form satellite lesions, called *skip metastases,* in the bone (Fig. 3–1A).

High-grade sarcomas have a poorly defined reactive zone that may be locally invaded and destroyed by the tumor. In addition, there are tumor nodules in tissue that appears to be normal, ie, not in continuity with the main tumor (Fig. 3–1B). Although low-grade sarcomas regularly interdigitate into the reactive zone, they rarely form tumor nodules beyond this area.

Sarcomas respect anatomic borders. Local anatomy influences the growth by setting natural barriers to extension. In general, bone sarcomas take the path of least resistance. Most benign bone tumors are

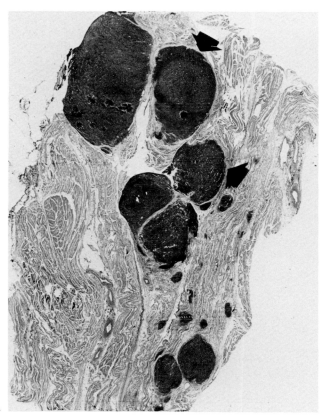
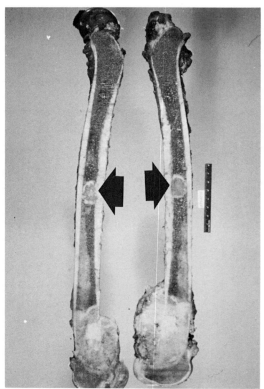

A   B

Figure 3–1.   Skip or "satellite" nodules are characteristic of high-grade bone and soft tissue sarcomas. They are occasionally found in conjunction with low-grade sarcomas. Satellite nodules are foci of a tumor *not* in continuity with the main tumor mass and often occur in the reactive zone ("pseudocapsule") or adjacent normal tissue. **(A)** Multiple satellite nodules (small arrows) associated with a high-grade malignant fibrous histiocytoma (MFH). Note the normal intervening tissue. **(B)** "Skip" metastasis (solid arrows) from an osteosarcoma of the distal femur. This patient was treated by a hip disarticulation. Less than 5% of patients will have skin lesions detected by preoperative staging studies.

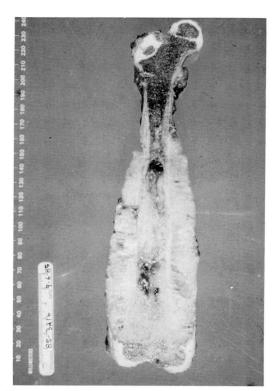

Figure 3–2. Osteosarcoma of the mid-femur and distal femur. Note the large extraosseous component. Most high-grade bone sarcomas are bicompartmental, ie, involving the bone of origin as well as the adjacent soft tissue, and are therefore classified stage IIB (see text).

unicompartmental; they remain confined and may expand the bone in which they arose. Most malignant bone tumors are bicompartmental (Fig. 3–2); they destroy the overlying cortex and go directly into the adjacent soft tissue. Soft tissue tumors may start in one compartment (intracompartmental) or between compartments (extracompartmental). The determination of anatomic compartment involvement has

become more important with the advent of limb preservation surgery.

Patterns of Behavior

Based on biological considerations and natural history, all bone and soft tissue tumors, benign and malignant, may be classified into five categories, each of which shares certain clinical characteristics and radiographic patterns and requires similar surgical procedures. Following are the five general patterns of behavior (Table 3–1)[1]:

1. *Benign latent.* Lesions whose natural history is to grow slowly during normal growth of the individual and then to stop, with a tendency to heal spontaneously. They never become malignant, and heal rapidly if treated by simple curettage.
2. *Benign active.* Lesions whose natural history is progressive growth. Curettage leaves a reactive zone with some tumor.
3. *Benign aggressive.* Lesions that are locally aggressive but do not metastasize. Pathologically there is tumor extension through the capsule into the reactive zone. Local control can be obtained only by removing the lesion with a margin of normal tissue beyond the reactive zone.
4. *Malignant low grade.* Lesions that have a low potential to metastasize. Histologically there is no true capsule but rather a pseudocapsule. Tumor nodules exist within the reactive zone but rarely beyond it. Local control can be accomplished only by removal of all tumor and reactive tissue with a margin of normal bone. These lesions can be treated successfully by surgery alone; systemic therapy is not required.
5. *Malignant high grade.* Lesions whose natural history is to grow rapidly and to metastasize early. Tumor nodules are usually found within and be-

Table 3–1. General Pattern of Behavior of Bone and Soft Tissue Tumors

CLASSIFICATION	BIOLOGICAL CHARACTERISTICS	TYPICAL EXAMPLE	
		Bone	Soft Tissue
Benign Latent	Grows Slowly and Stops Tendency to Heal Spontaneously	Nonossifying Fibroma	Lipoma
Benign Active	Progressive Growth Tendency to Recur	Aneurysmal Bone Cyst	Angliolipoma
Benign Aggressive	Locally Aggressive Tendency to Recur unless Widely Excised Does *not* Metastasize	Giant Cell Tumor	Aggressive Fibromatosis
Malignant Low Grade	Locally Recurrent Small Metastatic Potential (<10%)	Parosteal Osteosarcoma	Myxoid Liposarcoma
Malignant High Grade	Rapid Growth and Early Metastasis	Classical Osteosarcoma	Malignant Fibrous Histiocytoma

yond the reactive zone and at some distance in the normal tissue. Surgery is necessary for local control, and systemic therapy is warranted to prevent metastasis.

Metastasis. Unlike carcinomas, bone and soft tissue sarcomas disseminate almost exclusively through the blood. Soft tissue tumors occasionally (5%–10%) spread through the lymphatic system to regional nodes. Hematogenous spread is manifested by pulmonary involvement in the early stages and by bony involvement in later stages. Bone metastasis occasionally is the first sign of dissemination.

Skip Metastasis. A skip metastasis is a tumor nodule that is located within the same bone as the main tumor but not contiguous to it (see Fig. 3–1). Transarticular skip metastases are located in the joint adjacent to the main tumor.[3] Skip metastases are most often seen with high-grade sarcomas. Skip lesions develop by the embolization of tumor cells within the marrow sinusoids; they are, in effect, local micrometastases that have not passed through the circulation. Soft tissue sarcomas similarly may be associated with noncontinuous tumor nodules away from the main tumor mass. These nodules are responsible for local recurrences that develop in spite of apparently "negative" margins after a resection.

Local Recurrence. Local recurrence is due to inadequate removal and subsequent regrowth of either a benign or malignant lesion. Adequacy of surgical removal is the main determinant of local control. The aggressiveness of the lesion determines the choice of surgical procedure. Ninety-five percent of all local recurrences, regardless of histology, develop within 24 months of surgery.[1,4]

Joint Involvement. Tumor involvement by a bony sarcoma is unusual (Fig. 3–3). Direct tumor extension through the articular surface is rare. Extension into an adjacent joint most commonly occurs following a pathologic fracture with seeding of the joint cavity or by direct pericapsular extension. Occasionally structures that pass through the joint, eg, the cruciate ligaments of the knee, may act as a conduit for tumor growth. Approximately 1% of osteosarcomas will demonstrate transarticular skip lesions. A joint may be directly contaminated by a poorly placed biopsy of an adjacent sarcoma.

STAGING SYSTEM OF MUSCULOSKELETAL TUMORS

In 1980, the Musculoskeletal Tumor Society (MSTS) adopted the Surgical Staging System (SSS) for both bone and soft tissue sarcomas (Table 3–2).[2] The

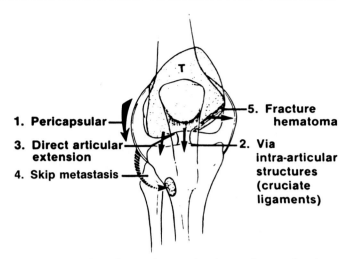

Figure 3–3. The five major mechanisms of tumor involvement of the adjacent joint by a bony sarcoma. Pathologic fracture and direct pericapsular extension are the two most common modes (from Malawer MM et al[5]).

system is based on the fact that mesenchymal sarcomas of bone and soft tissue behave alike, irrespective of histogenic type. The SSS is based on the GTM classification: grade (G), location (T), lymph node involvement, and metastases (M) (Table 3–2). The stage accurately predicts overall survival (Fig. 3–4).

Surgical Grade (G). G represents the histologic grade of a lesion and other clinical data. A low-grade tumor is rate G1. A high-grade tumor is rated G2.

Surgical Site (T). T represents anatomic site, either intracompartmental (T1) or extracompartmen-

Table 3–2. Surgical Staging of Bone Sarcomas*

STAGE	GRADE†	SITE
IA	Low (G1)	Intracompartmental (T1)
IB	Low (G1)	Extracompartmental (T2)
IIA	High (G2)	Intracompartmental (T1)
IIB	High (G2)	Extracompartmental (T2)
III	Any G Regional or Distant Metastasis (M1)	Any (T)

*From Enneking WF et al.[2]
†G = grade: G1 is any low-grade tumor; G2 is any high-grade tumor. T = site: T1 intracompartmental location of tumor; T2 extracompartmental location of tumor.
M = regional or distal metastases: M0 represents no metastases; M1 represents any metastases.

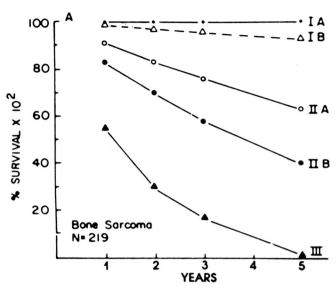

Figure 3–4. Survival by surgical stage (MSTS) of 219 patients with bone sarcomas treated at the University of Florida (see text).

tal (T2). Compartment is defined as "an anatomic structure or space bounded by natural barriers of tumor extension." The clinical significance of T1 lesions is easier to define clinically, surgically, and radiographically than that of T2 lesions, and there is a higher chance of adequate removal by a nonamputative procedure.

Lymph Nodes and Metastases (M). When a bone or soft tissue sarcoma has metastasized through the lymphatic system, the prognosis is extremely poor. Lymphatic spread is a sign of extensive dissemination. Regional lymphatic involvement is equated with distal metastases.

Summary of Staging System. The SSS developed for surgical planning and assessment of bone sarcomas is as follows[2]:

- *Stage IA (G1,T1,M0):* Low-grade intracompartmental lesion without metastasis
- *Stage IB (G1,T2,M0):* Low-grade extracompartmental lesion without metastasis
- *Stage IIA (G2,T1,M0):* High-grade intracompartmental lesion without metastasis
- *Stage IIB (G2,T2,M0):* High-grade extracompartmental lesion without metastasis
- *Stage IIIA (G1 or G2,T1,M1):* Intracompartmental lesion, any grade, with metastasis
- *Stage IIIB (G1 or G2,T2,M1):* Extracompartmental lesion, any grade, with metastasis

If the clinical examination and/or plain radiographs suggest an aggressive or malignant tumor, staging studies should be performed before biopsy. All radiographic studies are influenced by surgical manipulation of the lesion, making interpretation more difficult. Bone scintigraphy, CAT, MRI, and angiography are required to delineate local tumor extent, vascular displacement, and compartmental localization[4,6–8] (Fig. 3–5).

RADIOGRAPHIC EVALUATION

Bone Scans. Bone scintigraphy is useful for evaluation of both bony and soft tissue tumors. It assists in determining metastatic disease, polyostotic involvement, intraosseous extension of tumor, and the relationship of the underlying bone to a primary soft tissue sarcoma.[8]

CAT and MRI. CAT and MRI scans allow accurate determination of intraosseous and extraosseous extension of skeletal neoplasms (Fig. 3–6).[6,7] Both accurately depict the transverse relationship of a tumor. The anatomic compartmental involvement by soft tissue sarcomas is easily determined.[9] Each evaluation must be individualized. To obtain the maximum benefit of image reconstruction, the surgeon should discuss the information desired with the radiologist. Coronal and sagittal sections are useful and are routinely obtained with MRI scans.

Angiography. The technique of arteriography for bone and soft tissue lesions differs from that used for arterial disease (Fig. 3–7). A minimum of two views (biplane) is necessary to determine the relation of the major vessels to the tumor. As experience with limb-sparing procedures has increased, surgeons have become more aware of the need to determine the individual vascular patterns prior to resection. The increasing preoperative use of intra-arterial chemotherapy also has increased the need for accurate angiography.

Biopsy Considerations

If a resection is to be performed, it is crucial that the location of the biopsy be in line with the anticipated incision for the definitive procedure. Extreme care should be taken *before* biopsy not to contaminate potential tissue planes or flaps that will compromise the management of the lesion. To minimize contamination, a needle biopsy of soft tissue masses or of extraosseous components should be attempted *prior* to an incisional biopsy whenever possible.

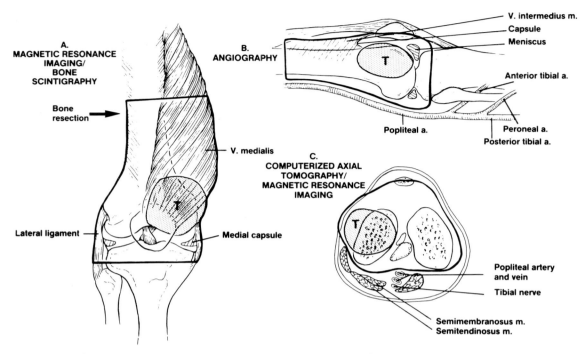

SCHEMATIC RESECTION FOR DISTAL FEMORAL SARCOMAS
(RELATIONSHIP TO PREOPERATIVE EVALUATION)

Figure 3–5.   Schematic relationship of preoperative staging studies for bony sarcomas. Biplane angiography, CAT, MRI, and bone scans are all useful in determining the local extent of a bony and/or soft tissue neoplasm (see text) (from Malawer MM et al).[5]

Needle or core biopsy of bone tumor often provides an adequate specimen for diagnosis.[10,11] Radiographs should be obtained to document the position of the trocar (Fig. 3–8). Core biopsy is preferred if a limb-sparing option exists, since it entails less local contamination than does open biopsy. If a core biopsy proves to be inadequate, a small incisional biopsy is performed. A small incisional or needle biopsy is recommended for all soft tissue tumors.

Frozen-section analyses are performed on all biopsy specimens. Many bone tumors, if the dense fragments of cortical bone are extricated, can be adequately sectioned in the cryostat. The initial purpose of the frozen section is to demonstrate if viable,

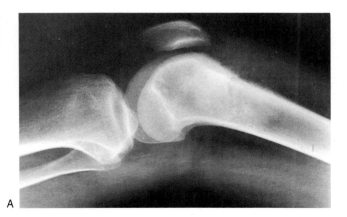
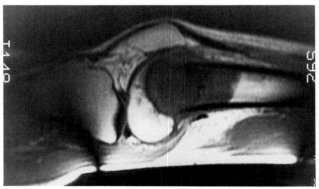

Figure 3–6.   Osteosarcoma of the distal femur. **(A)** Lateral radiograph and **(B)** corresponding sagittal MRI (T1 signal) demonstrating the intraosseous extent (dark area) of tumor.

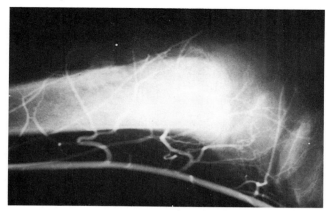

Figure 3–7. Osteosarcoma of the distal femur. Lateral angiogram demonstrating the relationship of the popliteal artery to the tumor. There is no evidence of posterior extension. In general, a limb-sparing procedure is usually feasible if the major vessel is free of tumor involvement.

and therefore diagnosable, tumor has been obtained. If not, additional specimens must be obtained. Furthermore, frozen-section evaluation may suggest that additional tumor tissue with special preparation

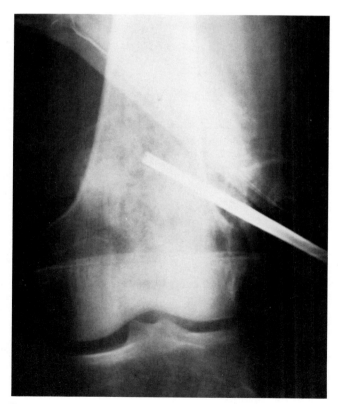

Figure 3–8. Needle biopsy of an osteosarcoma of the distal femur. Needle biopsies are preferred and often will yield a correct diagnosis. Needle biopsies minimize local tissue contamination. An incisional biopsy should only be performed if tissue obtained from a core biopsy is nondiagnostic.

is necessary for specific pathologic studies such as immunohistochemistry, flow cytometry, and electron microscopy.

Classification of Surgical Procedures

A method of classification of surgical procedures based on the surgical plane of dissection (Table 3–3) in relationship to the tumor and the method of accomplishing the removal has recently been developed. This system, summarized below, permits meaningful comparison of various operative procedures and gives surgeons a common language.[2,4]

1. *Intralesional.* An intralesional procedure passes through the pseudocapsule directly into the lesion. A macroscopic tumor is left, and the entire operative field is potentially contaminated.
2. *Marginal.* A marginal procedure is one in which the entire lesion is removed in one piece. The plane of dissection passes through the pseudocapsule or reactive zone around the lesion. When performed for a sarcoma it leaves macroscopic disease.
3. *Wide (intracompartmental).* This is commonly termed en bloc resection. A wide excision includes the entire tumor, the reactive zone, and a cuff of normal tissue. The entire structure of origin of the tumor is not removed. In patients with high-grade sarcomas, this procedure may leave skip nodules.
4. *Radical (extracompartmental).* The entire tumor and the structure of origin of the lesion are removed. The plane of dissection is beyond the limiting fascial or bony borders.

It is important to note that any of these procedures may be accomplished *either* by a local (ie, limb-

Table 3–3. Relationship of Surgical Procedure, Plane of Dissection, and Residual Disease for Musculoskeletal Tumors*

TYPE	PLANE OF DISSECTION	RESULT
Intralesional	Piecemeal Debulking or Curettage	Leaves Macroscopic Disease
Marginal	Shell out en bloc Through Pseudo-capsule or Reactive Zone	May Leave either "Satellite" or "Skip" Lesions
Wide	Intracompartmental en bloc with Cuff of Normal Tissue	May Leave "Skip" Lesions
Radical	Extracompartmental en bloc, Entire Compartment	No Residual

*From Enneking WF et al.[2]

sparing) procedure or by amputation. Thus, an amputation may entail a marginal, wide, or radical excision, depending on the plane through which it passes. An amputation is *not* necessarily an adequate cancer operation, but it is a method of achieving a specific margin. The local anatomy determines how a specific margin is to be obtained. Therefore, the aim of preoperative staging is to assess local tumor extent and relevant local anatomy in order to permit determination of how a desired margin is to be achieved, ie, the feasibility of one surgical procedure *v* another. In general, benign bone tumors are treated adequately by either an intralesional procedure (curettage) or by marginal excision. Malignant tumors require either a wide (intracompartmental) or radical (extracompartmental) removal, be it an amputation or an en bloc procedure. Similarly, benign soft tissue tumors are treated by marginal excision, aggressive tumors by wide excision, and malignant tumors by wide or radical resection.

SOFT TISSUE SARCOMAS

Soft tissue sarcomas (STS) are a heterogeneous group of tumors arising from the supporting extraskeletal tissues of the body, ie, muscle, fascia, connective tissues, fibrous tissues, and fat. They are rare lesions, constituting less than 1% of all cancers. There is a wide morphologic difference among these tumors, probably resulting from the different cells of origin. All soft tissue sarcomas, like bone sarcomas, however, share certain biologic and behavioral characteristics. The clinical, radiographic, and surgical management of most soft tissue sarcomas is identical, regardless of histogenesis. The surgical grading system developed by the Musculoskeletal Tumor Society applies to both bone and soft tissue sarcomas. The various histogenic types and grades are presented in Table 3–4.

Biological Behavior.   The pattern of growth, metastasis, and recurrence of STS is similar to that of spindle cell sarcomas arising in bone. The major distinctions are the tendency to remain intracompartmental and a significant incidence of lymphatic involvement that has been identified in a few of the less common entities such as the epithelioid, synovial, and alveolar soft-part sarcomas.

Pathology and Staging.   Individual grading is at times difficult; in general, however, the extent of pleomorphisms, atypia, mitosis, and necrosis correlates with the degree of malignancy. Notable exceptions are synovial sarcomas, which tend to behave

Table 3-4.   Histologic Types and Grades of Soft Tissue Sarcomas*

HISTOLOGICAL TYPE	GRADE†		
	1	2	3
Well-Differentiated Liposarcoma	X	—	—
Myxoid Liposarcoma	X	—	—
Round Cell Liposarcoma	—	X	X
Pleomorphic Liposarcoma	—	—	X
Fibrosarcoma	—	X	X
Malignant Fibrous Histiocytoma	—	X	X
Inflammatory Malignant Fibrous Histiocytoma	—	X	X
Myxoid Malignant Fibrous Histiocytoma	—	X	—
Dermatofibrosarcoma Protuberans	X	—	—
Malignant Giant Cell Tumor	—	X	X
Leiomyosarcoma	X	X	X
Malignant Hemangiopericytoma	X	X	X
Embryonal Rhabdomyosarcoma	—	—	X
Alveolar Rhabdomyosarcoma	—	—	X
Pleomorphic Rhabdomyosarcoma	—	—	X
Combined Rhabdomyosarcoma	—	—	X
Chondrosarcoma	X	X	X
Mesenchymal Chondrosarcoma	—	—	X
Myxoid Chondrosarcoma	X	X	—
Osteosarcoma	—	—	X
Soft Tissue Sarcoma Resembling Ewing's Sarcoma	—	—	X
Synovial Sarcoma	—	—	X
Epithelioid Sarcoma	—	X	X
Clear Cell Sarcoma	—	X	X
Malignant Superficial Schwannoma	—	X	—
Neurofibrosarcoma	X	X	X
Epithelioid Schwannoma	—	X	X
Malignant Triton Tumor	—	—	X
Angiosarcoma	—	X	X
Alveolar Soft-Part Sarcoma	—	—	X
Malignant Granular Cell Tumor	—	X	X
Kaposi's Sarcoma	—	X	X

*Costa J et al.[12] Reproduced with permission.
†The usual variation in grade is indicated for each recognized common histological type.

like high-grade lesions even in the absence of these findings. The exact histogenesis often cannot be accurately defined, although the grade can be determined. Pathologists may disagree about the specific name, although not about grade (ie, high grade *v* low grade). The surgical stage is determined by grade, location, and the presence or absence of pulmonary or lymphatic metastases.[2]

Pathological Characteristics of Specific Soft Tissue Sarcomas

MALIGNANT FIBROUS HISTIOCYTOMA (MFH)

MFH, first described in 1963, is the most common STS in adults.[13–15] The typical histologic pattern associated with MFH is a storiform or cartwheel appearance of the tumor cells. MFH occurs in adults and most commonly affects the lower extremity. There is a predilection for origin in deep-seated skeletal muscle tissue. The histologic grade is a good prognosticator of metastatic potential. The myxoid variant tends to have a more favorable prognosis than the other subtypes.

Gross Characteristics. The tumors usually present as solitary multinodular masses and reveal well-circumscribed or ill-defined infiltrative borders (Fig. 3–9). The size at the time of diagnosis often correlates with the ease of clinical detection: superficial variants, presenting as dermal or subcutaneous masses, may be but a few centimeters in diameter, whereas those arising in the retroperitoneum often attain a diameter of 15 cm or more. Color and consistency vary considerably and reflect, in part, the cellular composition. The myxoid variant contains a predominance of white-gray, soft mucoid tumor lobules created by the high content of myxoid ground substance. Red-brown areas of hemorrhage and necrosis are not uncommon (Fig. 3–10). Approximately 5% of malignant fibrous histiocytomas undergo extensive hemorrhagic cystification, often leading to a clinical diagnosis of hematoma[14] (Fig. 3–11). In such lesions, thorough sampling for microscopic evaluation is crucial.

Microscopic Characteristics. The currently accepted broad histologic spectrum of MFH encompasses many variants that were formerly considered

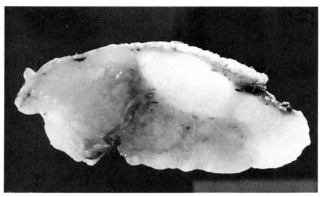

Figure 3–10. A superficial myxoid malignant fibrous histiocytoma (note overlying skin). The light gray translucent areas reflect the high content of myxoid ground substance.

to be distinct clinicopathologic entities. These lesions, which had been named according to the predominant cell type, include fibroxanthosarcoma, malignant fibroxanthoma, inflammatory fibrous histiocytoma, and malignant giant cell tumor of soft parts. The basic neoplastic cellular constituents of all fibrohistiocytic tumors include fibroblasts, histiocyte-like cells, and primitive mesenchymal cells. In addition, there is usually an acute and chronic inflammatory cell component. The proportion of these malignant and reactive cellular elements and the degree of maturation of the neoplastic cells account for the wide variety of histologic patterns. The storiform type, which is the most common variant, is characterized by fascicles of spindle cells that intersect to form a pinwheel or cartwheel (ie, storiform) pattern (Fig. 3–12). Furthermore, this

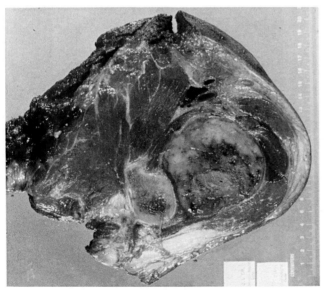

Figure 3–9. Deep-seated malignant fibrous histiocytoma occurring in the thigh of a 58-year-old male. This firm, solitary nodule appears well-circumscribed but revealed multiple infiltrative foci at the microscopic level.

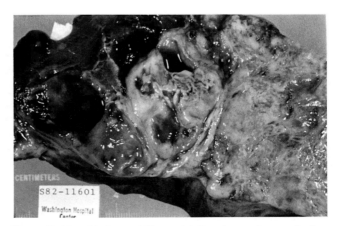

Figure 3–11. Malignant fibrous histiocytoma demonstrating extensive necrosis with formation of hemorrhagic cysts. Fine-needle aspiration of the latter areas can lead to an erroneous benign diagnosis of hematoma.

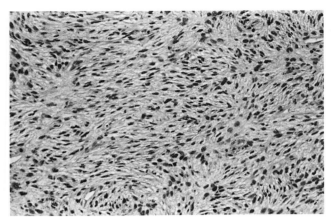

Figure 3–12. The storiform or pinwheel pattern is the hallmark of many fibrohistiocytoma tumors. Note the nuclear hyperchromasia and pleomorphism as well as an atypical mitotic figure.

type can show a considerable degree of pleomorphism with the appearance of atypical and bizarre giant cells, often containing abnormal mitotic figures. Chronic inflammatory cells along with xanthoma cells often permeate the stroma. In the myxoid variant, the tumor cells are dispersed in a richly myxoid matrix (Fig. 3–13). When this change is extensive, the lesion can be mistaken for a benign process, and correct diagnosis depends on the recognition of the cytologic atypia and presence of mitotic figures. The less common giant cell type (malignant giant cell tumor of soft parts) is characterized by abundant bland osteoclast-like giant cells diffusely distributed among the malignant fibrohistiocytic elements.

FIBROSARCOMA

Fibrosarcoma used to be considered the most common soft tissue sarcoma. Following the identification of MFH as a distinct entity and the subsequent assignment of many "pleomorphic fibrosarcomas" to this category, fibrosarcoma has become uncommon. Clinical and histologic difficulties occasionally arise in differentiating low-grade fibrosarcoma from fibromatosis and its variants. The anatomic site, age, and histology must be carefully evaluated.

Gross Characteristics. This neoplasm usually arises from the fascial and aponeurotic structures of the deep soft tissues; superficial variants are rare. The smaller tumors usually present as firm, gray-white, partially to completely circumscribed masses. As the lesions enlarge, a more diffusely infiltrative pattern predominates (Fig. 3–14).

Microscopic Characteristics. The fundamental cell of this neoplasm is the fibroblast, a spindle cell capable of producing collagen fibers. The collagen matrix, appearing as birefringent wavy fibers, can be easily recognized in the better-differentiated fibrosarcomas; moreover, its presence can be confirmed with the application of the Masson trichrome stain. Well-differentiated fibrosarcoma is characterized by intersecting fascicles of relatively uniform spindle cells showing minimal atypical features and sparse mitotic figures. The fascicles often intersect at acute angles to form the typical "herringbone" pattern (Fig. 3–15). In contrast, poorly differentiated fibrosarcoma reveals a barely discernible fascicular arrangement. Furthermore, the smaller cells show increased pleomorphism and nuclear atypia, and often have a high mitotic rate. Necrosis and hemorrhage com-

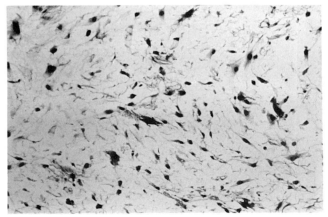

Figure 3–13. The myxoid variant of malignant fibrous histiocytoma reveals a typical spindle and histiocyte-like cells dispersed in a richly mucinous stroma.

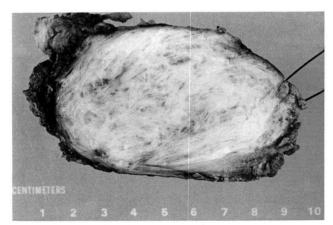

Figure 3–14. Well-differentiated fibrosarcoma of the calf. Note the coarse interlacing pattern and the poorly defined infiltrative margins.

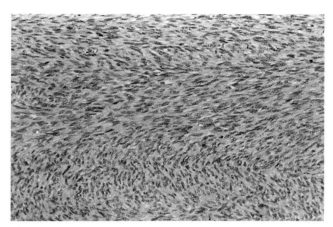

Figure 3–15. Elongated spindle cell fascicles intersecting at acute angles form the characteristic herringbone pattern of fibrosarcoma.

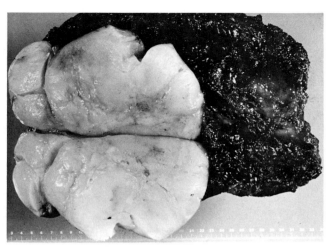

Figure 3–16. Well-differentiated liposarcoma of the thigh. The lesion is well circumscribed, multilobulated, and composed of somewhat firm yellow-white tissue.

monly occur in high-grade fibrosarcomas. In the latter presentation, distinction from malignant fibrous histiocytoma becomes exceedingly difficult.

LIPOSARCOMA

Liposarcoma is the second most common soft tissue sarcoma. It has a wide range of malignant potential directly dependent on the histologic classification of the individual tumor. Accurate determination of this morphologic subtype and, by direct correlation, its grade is essential for appropriate management. Grade I liposarcomas rarely metastasize. Unlike other sarcomas, liposarcomas may be multiple and occur in unusual sites within the same individual. Therefore, careful evaluation of other masses in a patient with a liposarcoma is mandatory. Occasionally, these lesions occur in children. Liposarcomas rarely arise from pre-existing benign lipomas.

Gross Characteristics. Liposarcomas, particularly those arising in the retroperitoneum, can attain enormous size; examples measuring 10 to 15 cm and weighing greater than 25 lb are not unusual. The tumors tend to be well circumscribed and multilobulated. Gross features usually correlate with the histologic composition. For example, well-differentiated liposarcomas, containing variable proportions of relatively mature fat and fibrocollagenous tissue, vary from yellow to white-gray and can be soft, firm, or rubbery (Fig. 3–16). A tumor that is soft, pink-yellow, and reveals a mucinous surface suggests myxoid liposarcoma (Fig. 3–17). The high-grade liposarcomas (round cell and pleomorphic) vary from pink-tan to brown and may disclose extensive hemorrhage and necrosis.

Microscopic Characteristics. A current histologic classification of liposarcoma recognizes four distinct types (Table 3–5). However, regardless of the histologic type, the identification of typical lipoblasts is mandatory to establish the diagnosis of liposarcoma. This diagnostic cell contains one or more round, cytoplasmic fat droplets that form sharp, scalloped indentations on the central or peripheral nucleus (Fig. 3–18).

Well-differentiated liposarcomas often contain a predominance of mature fat cells with only a few, widely scattered lipoblasts. Inadequate sampling can lead to a misdiagnosis of lipoma. In the sclerosing variant of well-differentiated liposarcoma, delicate collagen fibrils that encircle fat cells and lipoblasts make up a prominent part of the matrix. A diagnosis

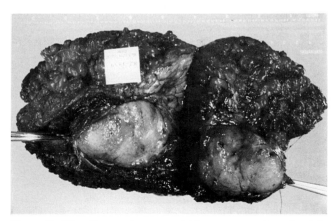

Figure 3–17. On section, myxoid liposarcoma is soft, pink-yellow, and contains abundant mucinous ground substance.

Table 3–5. Histologic Classification of Liposarcoma

Well-Differentiated
    Lipomalike
    Sclerosing
    Inflammatory
    Dedifferentiated
Myxoid
Round Cell
Pleomorphic

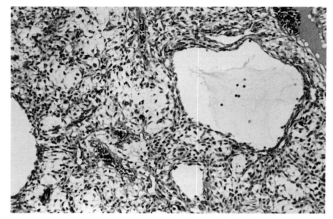

Figure 3–19. The typical features of myxoid liposarcoma include a capillary network associated with mesenchymal cells and lipoblasts. As with this example, microcysts containing a hyaluronic acid matrix commonly occur.

of myxoid liposarcoma, the commonest type, requires the observation of a delicate plexiform capillary network associated with primitive mesenchyme-like cells and a variable number of lipoblasts (Fig. 3–19). The stroma contains a high proportion of myxoid ground substance (hyaluronic acid) that, in areas, may form numerous microcysts. In round cell liposarcoma, the lipoblasts are interspersed within sheets of poorly differentiated round cells. Finally, pleomorphic liposarcoma discloses an admixture of bizarre, often multivacuolated lipoblasts and atypical stromal cells, many of which contain highly abnormal mitotic figures. Areas of hemorrhage and necrosis are common (Fig. 3–20). The presence of lipoblasts distinguishes this high-grade sarcoma from malignant fibrous histiocytoma.

Well-differentiated liposarcoma, after multiple local recurrences, rarely transforms into a high-grade spindle cell sarcoma, often with MFH-like features, the so-called dedifferentiated liposarcoma. This change imparts a high risk of metastasis to the neoplasm.

SYNOVIAL SARCOMA

Synovial sarcoma ranks as the fourth most common soft tissue sarcoma. It characteristically presents a "biphasic" histologic pattern, which refers to the occurrence of both a spindle cell and epithelial cell component. This tumor, however, in spite of its name, does not arise directly from a joint, but rather has a similar distribution as other soft tissue sarcomas. Synovial sarcomas occur in a younger age group than do other sarcomas; 72% of patients in one large study were below the age of 40. There is a propensity for the distal portions of extremities:

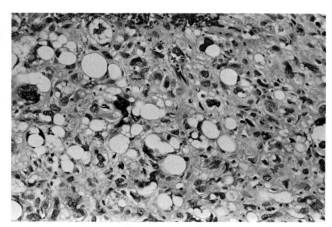

Figure 3–18. This field from a pleomorphic liposarcoma contains several lipoblast variants. Note the monovacuolated signet-ring type and the multivacuolated lipoblast with a central scalloped nucleus.

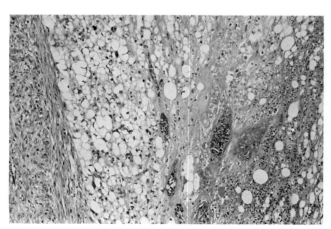

Figure 3–20. Low-power view of pleomorphic liposarcoma demonstrating central area with abundant lipoblasts, one peripheral area containing poorly differentiated spindle cells, and the other side showing tumor necrosis.

hand (5%), ankle (9%), or foot (13%). The plain radiograph often shows small calcifications within a soft tissue mass; this should alert the physician to the diagnosis. Occasionally lymphatic spread occurs (5%–7%). Virtually all synovial sarcomas are high grade.

Gross Characteristics. Typically the tumor presents as a deep-seated, well-circumscribed, multinodular firm mass. Actual contiguity with a synovium-lined space is rare. It is common to find solitary or multiple cysts (Fig. 3–21). The poorly differentiated neoplasms usually present as an ill-defined, infiltrative lesion with a soft, somewhat gelatinous consistency (Fig. 3–22).

Microscopic Characteristics. The classic form of this tumor is a biphasic pattern (Fig. 3–23). This implies the presence of coexisting but distinct cell populations, namely, spindle cells and epithelioid cells. The plump spindle cells, usually the predominant component, form an interlacing fascicular pattern, reminiscent of fibrosarcoma. The arrangement of the epithelioid cells varies from merely solid nests to distinct glandlike structures, When comprising glandular spaces, the constituent cells range from cuboidal to tall columnar: on rare occasions they undergo squamous metaplasia. The application of histochemical stains demonstrates that the glandular lumina contain epithelial-type acid mucins. The neoplasm may contain extensive areas of dense stromal hyalinization, and focal calcification is common. Within the spindle cell portion of the tumor, areas resembling the acutely branching vascular pattern of hemangiopericytoma commonly occur. The presence of extensive areas of calcification, sometimes with modulation to benign osteoid, deserves recognition, as this variant of synovial sarcoma imparts a significantly more favorable prognosis. The exist-

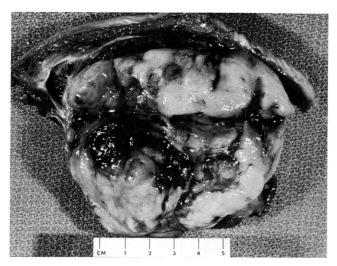

Figure 3–22. Synovial sarcoma arising from the abdominal wall of a 52-year-old male. This high-grade lesion is typified by the confluent geographic areas of hemorrhagic necrosis.

ence of a monophasic spindle cell synovial sarcoma is recognized, although distinction from fibrosarcoma can be exceedingly difficult.

EPITHELIOID SARCOMA

Epithelioid sarcoma was first described in the English literature in 1970.[16] It is an unusually small tumor that is often initially misdiagnosed, both clinically and microscopically, as a benign lesion. It affects the forearm and wrist half the time, and is the most common sarcoma of the hand. This lesion, in contrast to most sarcomas, has a propensity for eventual lymph node involvement. Unlike other sarcomas, it occurs predominantly in adolescents and young adults (average age 26 years). When it arises in

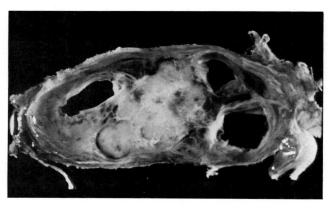

Figure 3–21. Synovial sarcoma showing solid nodular portions adjacent to multiple cystic spaces.

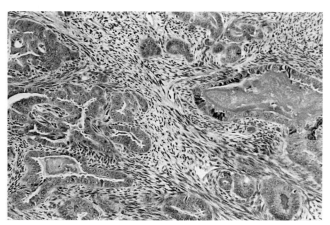

Figure 3–23. The biphasic pattern of synovial sarcoma refers to the presence of glandlike structures within a spindle cell sarcomatous stroma.

the dermis, it often presents as a nodular or ulcerative process.

Gross Characteristics.   Typically, the tumor originates in the deep soft tissues, particularly in relationship to tendons, fascia, and aponeuroses, and presents as a firm, often multinodular mass. Central nodular hemorrhage and/or necrosis is occasionally encountered. Less commonly, the lesion arises within the subcutis or dermis, whereby it presents as a nodular or ulcerative lesion, often simulating benign cutaneous diseases.

Microscopic Characteristics.   The typical low-power picture is that of nodules or granuloma-like collections of epithelioid cells (Fig. 3–24), often disclosing central necrosis. These are large polygonal cells with deeply eosinophilic cytoplasm; the nuclei tend to be angulated and hyperchromatic. Mitotic figures are occasionally seen. This histologic picture, particularly at low power, can be mistaken for necrotizing granuloma or even metastatic squamous cell carcinoma. The predominant epithelioid cells often transform to plump spindle cells. A characteristic feature of this tumor is the tendency for diffuse infiltration of tendinous and fascial structures by small elongated nests of tumor cells, often at a significant distance from the main tumor mass. This aspect of epithelioid sarcoma explains the high rate of local recurrence experienced in inadequately excised lesions.

CLEAR CELL SARCOMA (MALIGNANT MELANOMA OF SOFT PARTS)

Clear cell sarcoma is a small, unusual neoplasm that usually arises in relationship to tendons or aponeu-roses. It occurs most often around the foot and ankle (46%) and in persons between 20 and 40 years of age.[17] The histogenesis is unknown but is considered by some to be related to malignant melanoma. Fifty percent of these lesions contain melanin. However, clear cell sarcoma is not associated with any melanocytic lesions of the skin. Lymphatic as well as hematogenous spread occurs. One must examine the regional lymph nodes carefully. If there is any suggestion of enlargement, a lymph node dissection is recommended. The neoplasm pursues a protracted clinical course; however, due to the high rate of eventual metastasis, long-term prognosis is poor.

Gross Characteristics.   Typically, the neoplasm presents as a solitary or multinodular firm mass attached to tendons or aponeuroses. The tumor infrequently exceeds 6 cm in diameter and varies from white to brown on the cut surface.

Microscopic Characteristics.   The hallmark of this neoplasm is the occurrence of distinct spindle cell fascicles that are separated by well-defined collagenous trabeculae (Fig. 3–25). The uniform spindle cells are often plump and contain pale to faintly eosinophilic cytoplasm. In addition, the cells reveal a vesicular nucleus with a prominent solitary basophilic nucleolus. Frequently, bland-appearing multinucleated giant cells are found within the spindle cells fascicles. Application of special stains discloses that the clear spindle cells contain glycogen (PAS+) and that melanin pigment is present in half of the tumors.

Figure 3–24.   Low-power view of epithelioid sarcoma discloses central necrotic area surrounded by large, atypical, eosinophilic epithelioid cells.

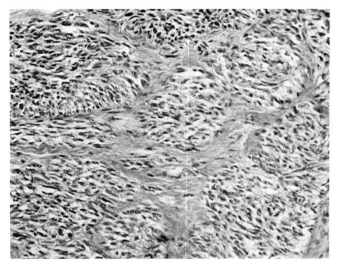

Figure 3–25.   Low-power view of typical clear cell sarcoma reveals fascicles composed of plump spindle cells with clear cytoplasm separated by distant collagenous trabeculae.

MALIGNANT SCHWANNOMA (NEUROFIBROSARCOMA)

Malignant schwannomas are malignant tumors that arise from peripheral nerves. They account for about 10% of all soft tissue sarcomas. A large percentage of tumors (25%–67%) are associated with von Recklinghausen's disease (neurofibromatosis).[16] In general, patients with von Recklinghausen's disease are at high risk (3%–13%) for developing nerve sheath sarcomas, and this risk increases with each decade of life. Unlike other sarcomas, malignant schwannomas often present with neurologic symptoms (pain, paresthesia, and weakness), reflecting their relationship to major peripheral nerves. Malignant schwannomas not associated with neurofibromatosis tend to occur in an older age group. An extremity mass associated with neurologic symptoms must be considered malignant and must be evaluated by the appropriate staging studies.

Gross Characteristics. This neoplasm presents as a fusiform or bulbous enlargement of a large nerve, usually within the deep soft tissues (Fig. 3–26). As the tumor enlarges and infiltrates the adjacent soft tissues, its origin from and relationship to the nerve structure of origin are frequently obscured. On section, the gray-to-white neoplasm varies from firm to soft with areas of necrosis and hemorrhage.

Microscopic Characteristics. Malignant schwannomas occur with a profusion of histologic patterns and variants; however, the fundamental pattern comprises the intersecting spindle cell fascicles, not unlike that observed with fibrosarcoma or leiomyosarcoma. However, the presence of certain additional differential features, coupled with the fascicular arrangement, supports a diagnosis of a malignant nerve sheath tumor. For example, the slender nuclei of the spindle cells tend to be wavy or buckled (Fig. 3–27). Furthermore, a palisading pattern, although not pathognomonic, typifies this entity. In areas, the spindle cells may form a whorled or spiral arrangement. The rarely encountered epithelioid variant may closely resemble malignant melanoma or even carcinoma. Infrequently, heterologous elements, such as osteoid, chondroid, skeletal muscle, or glandular structures, arise within the spindle cell background.

CHARACTERISTICS OF MALIGNANT BONE TUMORS

Osteosarcoma is the most common malignant mesenchymal bone tumor. They usually occur during childhood and adolescence. Other mesenchymal tumors (malignant fibrous histiocytoma, fibrosarcoma, chondrosarcoma) also occur during childhood. This section describes the clinical, radiographic, and pathologic characteristics of the primary bone sarcomas. A detailed discussion of osteosarcomas is presented in chapter 2.

Classic Osteosarcoma

Osteosarcoma (OS) is a high-grade malignant spindle cell tumor arising within a bone. Its distinguishing characteristic is the production of "tumor" osteoid or immature bone directly from a malignant spindle cell stroma.[18–20]

Clinical Characteristics. Osteosarcoma typically occurs during childhood and adolescence. In patients over the age of 40, it is usually associated with

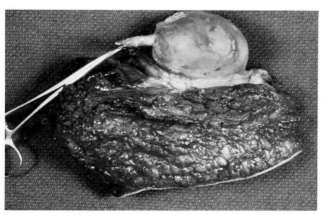

Figure 3–26. Malignant schwannoma from a 46-year-old female with neurofibromatosis. Hemostat is attached to nerve of origin.

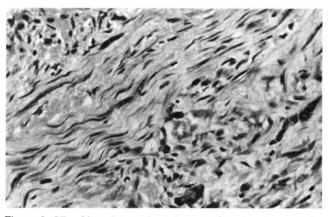

Figure 3–27. Note the marked degree of nuclear hyperchromasia and pleomorphism in the wavy spindle cells of this malignant schwannoma.

a preexistent disease, such as Paget's disease or irradiated bones.[18,21] The most common sites are bones of the knee joint and the proximal humerus. Between 80% and 90% occur in the long tubular bones[18,21]; the axial skeleton is rarely affected. Pain is the most common complaint. Incidence of pathologic fracture is less than 1%, and systemic symptoms are rare. A mass is a common finding.

Radiographic Characteristics. Typical findings are increased intramedullary radiodensity, an area of radiolucency, a pattern of permeative destruction with poorly defined borders, cortical destruction, periosteal elevation, and extraosseous extension with soft tissue ossification.[22] This combination of characteristics is not seen in any other lesions. Osteosarcomas are classified into three broad categories[22]: sclerotic osteosarcoma (32%), osteolytic osteosarcoma (22%), and mixed (46%) (Fig. 3–28). Errors of diagnosis most often occur with pure osteolytic tumors. The differential diagnosis of osteolytic osteosarcoma includes giant cell tumor, aneurysmal bone cyst, fibrosarcoma, and MFH.[23]

Gross Characteristics. This tumor is central in origin, but at the time of diagnosis substantial cortical destruction may have already occurred. Continued tumor growth results in bulky involvement of the adjacent soft tissues. As the neoplasm permeates the cortex, the periosteum may be elevated; this stimulates reactive bone formation and accounts for the radiologic features of Codman's triangle. Longitudinal sectioning of the involved bone often reveals wide extension within the marrow cavity. Rarely, skip areas can be demonstrated. The consistency of the tumor varies greatly and generally reflects the predominant histologic composition. There may be soft necrotic and hemorrhagic foci. Sclerotic and bony regions reflect a preponderance of fibrotic or osteoblastic elements, respectively. Occasionally, a lobulated cartilaginous appearance is observed.

Microscopic Characteristics. The definitive diagnosis of osteosarcoma rests on the identification of a malignant stroma that produces an osteoid matrix. The stroma consists of a haphazard arrangement of pleomorphic cells that contain hyperchromatic, irregular nuclei. Mitotic figures, often atypical, are usually numerous. Deposited between these cells is a delicate, lacelike eosinophilic matrix, assumed to be malignant osteoid (Fig. 3–29). Both malignant and benign osteoblast-like giant cells can be found in the stroma. An abundance of the latter type can create confusion with giant cell tumor of bone.

A predominance of one tissue type in many osteosarcomas has led to a histologic subclassification

of this neoplasm.[24] Thus, osteoblastic osteosarcoma refers to those tumors in which the production of malignant osteoid prevails. The pattern is usually that of a delicate meshwork of osteoid, as noted above (Fig. 3–30), although broader confluent areas can be present. Calcification of the matrix is variable. Alternatively, some tumors reveal a predominance of malignant cartilage production, hence, the term *chondroblastic osteosarcoma*. Even though the malignant cartilaginous elements may be overwhelming, the presence of a malignant osteoid matrix warrants the diagnosis of osteosarcoma.

Yet another variant is characterized by large areas of proliferating fibroblasts, arranged in intersecting fascicles (Fig. 3–31). Such areas are indistinguishable from fibrosarcoma, and thorough sampling may be necessary to identify the malignant osteoid component. The so-called telangiectatic type of osteosarcoma contains multiple, blood-filled cystic and sinusoidal spaces of variable size. Identification of marked cytologic atypia in the septae and in more solid areas rules out the diagnosis of aneurysmal bone cyst.

Chemotherapy Effect on Histology. The advent of several successful chemotherapeutic regimens for osteosarcoma has permitted the examination of multiple posttherapy radical resection specimens.[25] The degree of tumor necrosis is variable and ranges between 0% and 100%. The osteoid or osseous matrix remains without its accompanying cellular component. There may be growth of a reparative type of connective tissue with fibroblastic proliferation and clusters of small vessels. The spindle cells may reveal a degree of cytologic atypia.

Variants of Osteosarcoma

There are 11 recognizable variants of the classical osteosarcoma.[19] Parosteal and periosteal osteosarcomas are the most common variants of the classical osteosarcoma occurring in the extremities. In contrast to classical osteosarcoma, which arises within a bone, parosteal and periosteal osteosarcomas arise on the surface of the bone (Table 3–6).[26]

PAROSTEAL OSTEOSARCOMA (POS)

POS is a distinct variant (4%) of conventional osteosarcoma.[27] It arises from the cortex of a bone and generally occurs in an older age group. It has a better prognosis than classical osteosarcoma.

Clinical Characteristics. Females are more commonly affected than males. Characteristically the

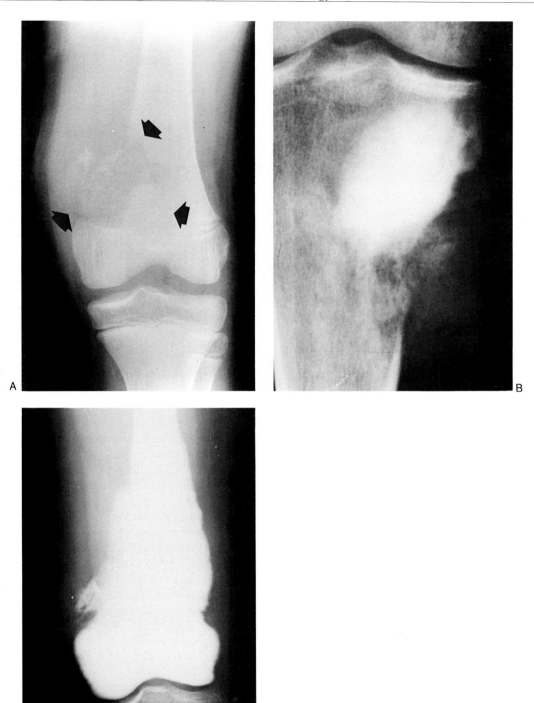

Figure 3–28. The three radiographic types of osteosarcoma. (**A**) Osteolytic (solid arrows indicate tumor), (**B**) mixed, osteolytic, and osteoblastic, and (**C**) sclerosing type. There is no prognostic difference in survival based on radiographic type.[5]

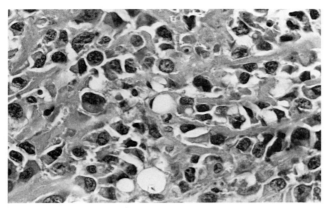

Figure 3–29.   Markedly atypical and bizarre stromal cells set in an eosinophilic osteoid matrix. This feature is the hallmark of malignant bone matrix forming neoplasms.

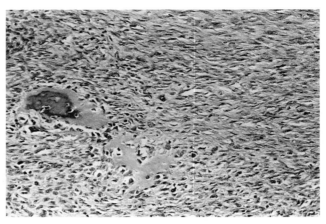

Figure 3–31.   A few islands of malignant osteoid can be found in this fibroblastic variant of osteosarcoma.

distal posterior femur is involved; the proximal humerus and proximal tibia are the next most frequent sites. POS is a slow metastasizing tumor with a high rate of survival; overall survival ranges from 75% to 85%.[27,28] The natural history is progressive enlargement and late metastasis. POS clinically presents as a mass and occasionally is associated with pain.

Radiographic Findings.   Roentgenograms characteristically show a large, dense, lobulated mass broadly attached to the underlying bone without involvement of the medullary canal (Fig. 3–32). If present long enough, the tumor may encircle the entire bone. The periphery of the lesion is characteristically less mature than the base. Despite careful evaluation, intramedullary extension is difficult to determine from the plain radiographs.[27] In addition, tumors with high-grade foci do not usually alter the roentgenographic appearance.[28]

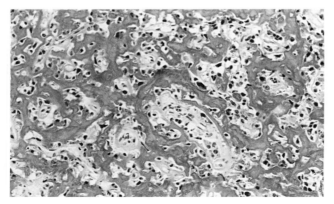

Figure 3–30.   Osteoblastic type of osteosarcoma can show a lacelike network of osteoid lined by malignant stromal cells.

Diagnosis and Grading.   The diagnosis is difficult and must include evaluation of the radiographs, age of the patient, and location of the tumor. Differential diagnoses are osteochondroma, myositis ossificans, and conventional osteosarcoma. Cortical tumors of the posterior femur should always be suspected of malignancy.

POS are graded as grade I (low grade), grade II (intermediate), and grade III (high grade). The majority are grade I. The survival rate of grade III tumors is similar to that of conventional osteosarcoma.

Gross Characteristics.   The tumor arises from the cortical surface and presents as a protuberant multinodular firm mass. The surface of the lesion may be covered in part by a cartilaginous cap, resembling an osteochondroma, whereas other areas may infiltrate adjacent soft tissue. The tumor usually encircles, partially or even completely, the shaft of the underlying bone (Fig. 3–33). In contrast to the osteochondroma, the medullary canal of the bone is not contiguous with that of the neoplasm.

Microscopic Characteristics.   This neoplasm is generally of low grade. In grade I POS, irregularly formed osteoid trabeculae, usually of woven bone, are surrounded by a spindle cell stroma containing widely spaced, bland-appearing spindle cells (Fig. 3–34). There may be foci of atypical chondroid differentiation. Infrequently, one encounters a more cellular stroma with appreciable atypia and mitotic activity, grade II or III tumors. A grading system has been proposed that is based on features of the fibrous and chondroid components,[29] with the likelihood of intramedullary involvement ("backgrowth") in the

Table 3-6.   Radiographic and Clinical Differential of Classical, Parosteal, and Periosteal Osteosarcoma

TYPE OF TUMOR	COMMON ANATOMICAL SITE	LOCATION	RADIOGRAPHIC APPEARANCE	HISTOLOGY	METASTASES
Classical	Distal Femur Proximal Tibia	Intramedullary	Destructive, Osteoblastic/Osteolytic	High Grade (fibroblastic, chondroblastic, and osteoblastic)	Early
Parosteal	Posterior Distal Femur	Cortical	Dense, Homogeneous New Bone	"Mature" Bone and Fibroblastic Stroma, Low Grade	Late
Periosteal	Proximal Tibia and Humerus	Cortical	"Scooped-out" Lesion with Calcification	Chondroblastic High Grade	Intermediate

From Malawer et al.[26]

higher grades. This, in turn, correlates well with the occurrence of distant metastasis.

Treatment.   Wide excision of the tumor is the treatment of choice. Parosteal osteosarcomas are often amenable to limb preservation due to their distal location, low grade, and lack of local invasiveness. The major surgical decision usually is whether to remove the entire end of the bone and the adjacent joint or to perform a wide excision with preservation of the joint. If the medullary canal is involved, the joint usually cannot be preserved. A second factor mitigating against joint preservation is extensive cortical involvement. Small lesions can be resected with joint preservation. Resection and reconstruction techniques are similar to those described for conventional osteosarcoma.

PERIOSTEAL OSTEOSARCOMA

Periosteal osteosarcoma is a rare cortical variant of osteosarcoma that arises superficially on the cortex, most often on the tibia shaft.[30] Radiographically, it is a small radiolucent lesion with some evidence of bone spiculation. The cortex is characteristically intact with a scooped-out appearance and a Codman's triangle (Fig. 3–35). Periosteal osteosarcomas are one third as frequent as the parosteal variant. Treatment is similar to that of other high-grade lesions. En bloc resection should be performed when feasible.

Gross Characteristics.   Like parosteal osteosarcoma, this lesion arises from the periosteal (cortical) surface. It projects as a well-circumscribed lobulated mass into the overlying soft tissues. On section, the tumor reveals a dominant chondroid consistency.

Microscopic Characteristics.   The features are essentially those of an intermediate-grade chondroblastic osteosarcoma. The cartilaginous lobules can contain markedly atypical chondrocytes. At the periphery of the lobule is situated a cellular spindle cell component, wherein a fine intercellular osteoid matrix is produced. Areas of malignant osteoid and

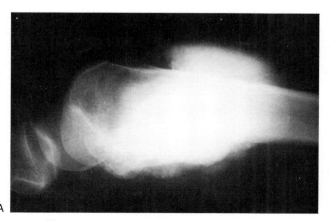
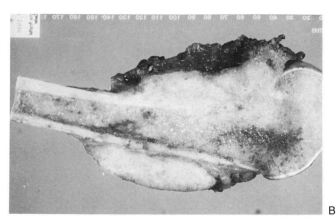

A   B

Figure 3–32.   Parosteal osteosarcoma of the distal femur. (**A**) Plain radiograph demonstrating a radiodense, lobular, relatively mature bony lesion. (**B**) The corresponding gross specimen demonstrating the tumor is confined to the cortical surface of the bone. Occasionally, there may be backgrowth into the medullary canal. Further preoperative evaluation with a CT scan would have better documented the cortical nature of the tumor. Parosteal osteosarcomas represent about 4% of all osteosarcomas and tend to be of a low histologic grade.

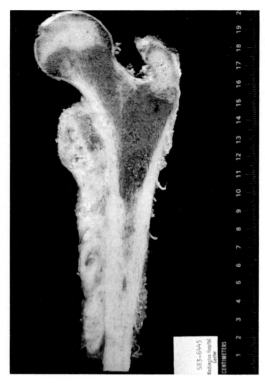

Figure 3–33. Parosteal osteosarcoma of proximal femur. This extramedullary tumor partially encircles the diaphysis and neck of the bone.

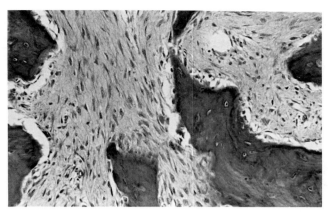

Figure 3–34. Relatively bland spindle cells dispersed in a dense collagen matrix that fills the space between trabeculae of immature bone. This picture is characteristic of parosteal osteosarcoma, grade I.

chondroid can be seen to infiltrate the cortical bone at the base of the neoplasm.

SMALL-CELL OSTEOSARCOMA

Small-cell osteosarcoma is a rare variant of osteosarcoma. The cells are round rather than spindle-shaped. There is definite evidence of osteoid production, thus the inclusion of this entity as an

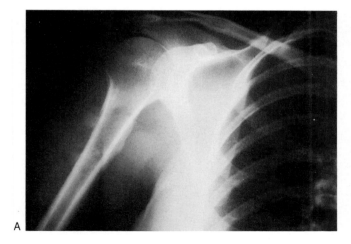

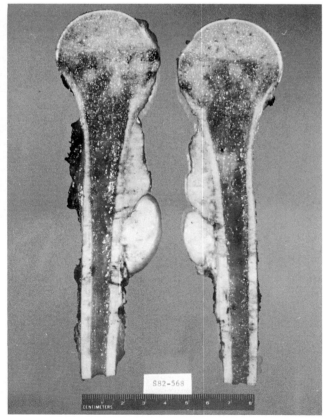

Figure 3–35. Periosteal osteosarcoma of the proximal humerus. **(A)** Plain radiograph showing the typical "scooped-out" appearance of the lesion arising from the cortex. **(B)** Gross specimen showing a lobular-appearing mass not involving the medullary canal. Histologically, periosteal osteosarcoma is mainly chondroblastic (accounting for the radiolucent appearance) with only a small amount of malignant osteoid. They represent about 1% of all osteosarcomas.

osteosarcoma. The recommendations for treatment vary. Radiation and chemotherapy are used at some institutions; others choose primary surgical ablation with preoperative and/or postoperative chemotherapy. Too few cases have been reported to make definitive recommendations.

Microscopic Characteristics. The tumor consists of nests and sheets of small round cells separated by fibrous septae, a pattern reminiscent of Ewing's sarcoma (Fig. 3–36). Occasionally, transition to spindled cells is noted. The cells have well-defined borders and a distinct rim of cytoplasm. The round nuclei disclose a delicate chromatin pattern. The presence of a characteristic delicate lacelike osteoid matrix, often surrounding individual or small nests of cells, confirms the diagnosis of osteosarcoma (Fig. 3–37).

Chondrosarcoma

Chondrosarcoma is the second most common primary malignant spindle cell tumor of bone.[18] Chondrosarcoma is a heterogeneous group of tumors whose basic neoplastic tissue is cartilaginous without evidence of primary osteoid formation. There are five types of chondrosarcoma: central, peripheral, mesenchymal, dedifferentiated, and clear cell.[18,20,24,31] The classic chondrosarcomas are central (arising within a bone) (Fig. 3–38) or peripheral (arising from the surface of a bone) (Fig. 3–39). The other three are variants and have distinct histologic and clinical characteristics. Their characteristics are summarized in Table 3–7.

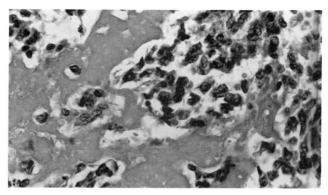

Figure 3–37. A different field from the same case illustrated in Figure 3–36, which demonstrates the deposition of osteoid matrix by the tumor cells. This points to a diagnosis of small-cell osteosarcoma.

Both central and peripheral chondrosarcomas can arise either as primary tumors or as tumors secondary to underlying neoplasm. Seventy-six percent of primary chondrosarcomas arise centrally.[18,31,32] Secondary chondrosarcomas most often arise from benign cartilage tumors.

CENTRAL AND PERIPHERAL CHONDROSARCOMAS

Clinical Characteristics. Half of all chondrosarcomas occur in persons above the age of 40.[9,18] The most common sites are the pelvis, femur, and shoulder girdle.[9,33] Pelvic chondrosarcomas are often large and present with referred pain to the back or thigh, sciatica secondary to sacral plexus irritation, urinary symptoms from bladder neck involvement, unilateral edema due to iliac vein obstruction, or as a

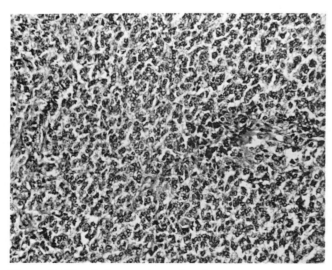

Figure 3–36. A focus of small-cell osteosarcoma where sheets of small round poorly differentiated cells lack evidence of matrix production.

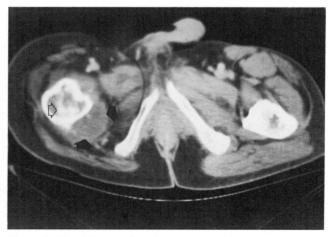

Figure 3–38. Primary chondrosarcoma of the proximal femur. Note the extraosseous extension (arrow) and the intramedullary calcification. This patient had multiple enchondromatosis.

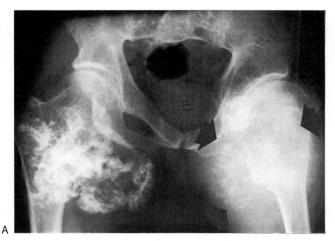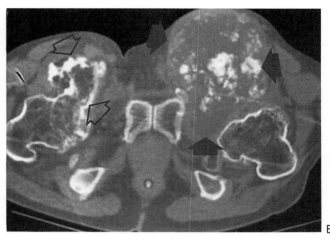

A   B

Figure 3–39. Secondary chondrosarcomas arising from the left proximal femur in a patient with multiple hereditary enchondromatosis. **(A)** Plain radiograph showing a large, benign-appearing osteochondroma arising from the right proximal femur and a large, poorly demarcated cartilage tumor from the left. **(B)** CAT dramatically demonstrates the different radiographic characteristics of the large benign (right, open arrow) osteochondroma from the secondary chondrosarcoma (left, solid arrow). Note the malignant tumor has completely replaced the original osteochondroma, and a large, centrally calcified mass (solid arrows) almost fungating through the skin is present. This patient required a modified hemipelvectomy and remains free of disease at five years.

painless abdominal mass. Conversely, central chondrosarcomas present with dull pain.

Radiographic Diagnosis and Evaluation. Central chondrosarcomas have two distinct radiologic patterns.[34] One is a small, well-defined lytic lesion with a narrow zone of transition and surrounding sclerosis with faint calcification. This is the most common malignant bone tumor that may appear radiographically benign. The second type has no sclerotic border and is difficult to localize. The key sign of malignancy is endosteal scalloping.

Correlation of the clinical, radiographic, and histologic data is essential for accurate diagnosis and evaluation of the aggressiveness of cartilage tumor. In general, proximal or axial location, skeletal maturity, and pain point toward malignancy, even though the cartilage may appear benign.

Table 3-7. Classification and General Characteristics of Chondrosarcomas

TYPE	SIZE, LOCATION, GRADE	PRIMARY* OR SECONDARY†
Central	Intramedullary Moderate to High Grade Small Extraosseous Component Little Calcification	Usually Primary
Peripheral	Cortical Usually Low Grade, Myxomatous Large Soft Tissue Component Heavily Calcified	Usually Secondary
Mesenchymal	Intramedullary High Grade, May Respond to Radiotherapy Small Round Cells	Primary
Dedifferentiated	High-Grade Anaplastic (osteosarcoma, MFH) in Association with Recognizable Low-Grade Chondrosarcoma	Primary
Clear Cell Chondrosarcoma	Low Grade Appears as a Chondroblastoma Locally Recurrent	Primary

*76% of primary chondrosarcomas are central.
†Usually from benign cartilage tumors, ex. osteochondromas.

Grading and Prognosis. Chondrosarcomas are graded I, II, and III; the majority are grades I or II.[9,18,33] The metastatic rate of moderate grade *v* high grade ranges from 15% to 40% *v* 75%.[18,31,32]

In general, peripheral chondrosarcomas are a lower grade than central lesions. Ten-year survival rates among those with peripheral lesions were 77% *v* 32% among those with central lesions.[35] Secondary chondrosarcomas arising from osteochondromas also have a low malignant potential; 85% are grade I.

Gross Characteristics. Primary intraosseous (central) chondrosarcoma is an expansile lesion that causes cortical destruction (Fig. 3–40). Subsequent extension into soft tissue often ensues. Chondrosarcoma arising from a rib or from the pelvis may protrude, as a smooth-surfaced multinodular mass, into the pleural cavity or pelvic retroperitoneum, respectively (Fig. 3–41). Typically, the tumor consists of fused, variably sized nodules that, on cut section, are composed of a white-gray hyaline tissue. Areas of calcification and even ossification are common. There may be focal myxoid areas. The nodules occasionally contain degenerative cysts of varying sizes.

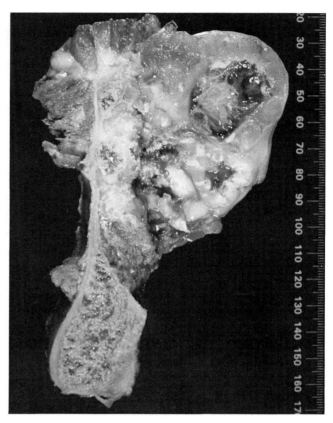

Figure 3–41. Chondrosarcoma, grade II, arising in the pelvis and protruding into the pelvic cavity. The multinodular mass reveals areas of secondary calcification and cystic degeneration.

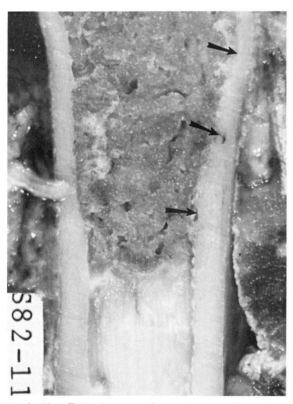

Figure 3–40. This closeup of an intramedullary chondrosarcoma discloses its lobular architecture and its translucent hyaline-like tissue. Note the characteristic endosteal erosions (arrows).

Microscopic Characteristics. The histologic spectrum and the ease of diagnosis of chondrosarcoma vary tremendously. High-grade examples can be easily identified as such. In contrast, certain low-grade tumors are exceedingly difficult to distinguish from chondroma or enchondroma. When this diagnostic dilemma arises, correlation of the histologic features with both the clinical setting and the radiographic changes is therefore of utmost importance in avoiding serious diagnostic error. The grade of malignant cartilaginous tumors correlates with clinical behavior. Grade I tumors are characterized by a slightly increased number of chondrocytes set in a lobular chondroid matrix, occasionally with focal myxoid changes. The cells contain hyperchromatic nuclei, occasionally binucleate forms, and show minimal variation in size (Fig. 3–42). Areas of markedly increased cellularity with more prominent pleomorphism and significant nuclear atypia define a grade II lesion (Fig. 3–43). Binuclear forms are more common in this group. Grade III chondrosarcomas, which are relatively uncommon, disclose still greater

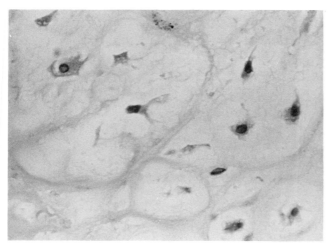

Figure 3–42. The presence of chondrocytes with central hyperchromatic nuclei is typical of chondrosarcoma, grade I. Binucleate forms are not uncommon. The matrix may vary from chondroid to myxoid.

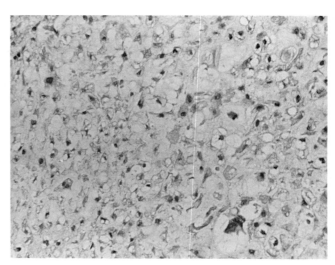

Figure 3–44. Still greater cellularity with the addition of pleomorphic forms and of significant mitotic activity is the hallmark of chondrosarcoma, grade III.

cellularity, often with spindle cell areas, and reveal prominent mitotic activity. Chondrocytes may contain large, bizarre nuclei (Fig. 3–44). Areas of myxoid change are common.

Calcification and enchondral ossification can be observed in tumors of all grades. However, the presence of unequivocal malignant osteoid production, even in the face of chondrosarcomatous areas, dictates that the tumor be classified as osteosarcoma.

Treatment. The treatment of chondrosarcoma is surgical removal. Guidelines of resection for high-grade chondrosarcomas are similar to those for osteosarcomas. The shoulder and pelvic girdle are the most common sites for chondrosarcoma. These sites, combined with the fact that these tumors tend to be low grade, make these tumors amenable to limb-sparing procedure.

Variants of Chondrosarcoma

CLEAR CELL CHONDROSARCOMA

Clear cell chondrosarcoma, the rarest form of chondrosarcoma, is a slowly growing, locally recurrent tumor resembling a chondroblastoma, but has some malignant potential.[36] It generally occurs in adults. The most difficult clinical problem is early recognition; it is often confused with chondroblastoma. Metastases occur only after multiple local recurrences. Primary treatment is wide excision. Systemic therapy is not required.

Gross Characteristics. The neoplasm commonly presents as a solid expansile mass with focal cystic change.

Microscopic Characteristics. The diagnostic picture consists of sheets of vague lobules composed of distinct round clear cells with a central nucleus (Fig. 3–45). Occasional mitoses are observed. Variably sized foci that are typical of chondrosarcoma frequently occur. In addition, minor areas indistinguishable from other primary bone lesions can obscure the underlying clear cell neoplasm. Foci resembling aneurysmal bone cyst, osteosarcoma, osteoblastoma, chondroblastoma, and giant cell tumor have been identified.[37]

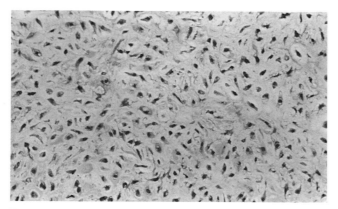

Figure 3–43. Increased cellularity, large irregular nuclei, and preponderance of a myxoid stroma all indicate that this is a chondrosarcoma, grade II.

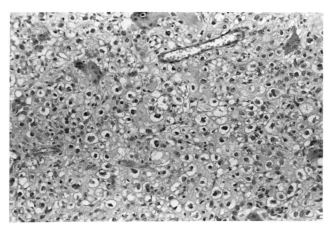

Figure 3–45. Sheets of round cells with clear cytoplasm and central nuclei point to a diagnosis of clear cell chondrosarcoma. Multinucleated giant cells, very rare in the usual chondrosarcoma, are common in this entity.

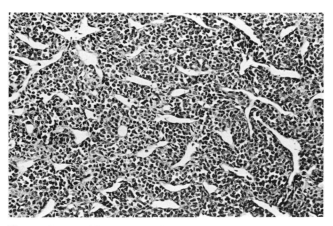

Figure 3–46. Mesenchymal chondrosarcoma contains a clearly distinguishable component of poorly differentiated cells set in a prominent pericytomatous stroma.

MESENCHYMAL CHONDROSARCOMA

Mesenchymal chondrosarcoma is a rare, aggressive variant of chondrosarcoma characterized by a biphasic histologic pattern, ie, small compact cells intermixed with islands of cartilaginous matrix.[38] These have a predilection for flat bones; long tubular bones are rarely affected. They tend to occur in the younger age group and have high rate of metastatic potential. The ten-year survival rate is 28%. This entity responds favorably to radiotherapy. Radiotherapy is recommended if the tumor cannot be completely removed.[38]

Gross Characteristics. The firm white-gray tumor usually contains hard calcified or ossified areas. Prominent cartilaginous features are unusual.

Microscopic Characteristics. The hallmark of this neoplasm is the juxtaposition of foci of poorly differentiated round cells with islands of relatively mature chondroid tissue. The small, round to slightly spindled cells are arranged in broad sheets and typically form a hemagiopericytoma-like pattern (Fig. 3–46). Scattered islands of chondroid, which can be focally calcified or ossified, arise abruptly among the sheets of round cells (Fig. 3–47).

DEDIFFERENTIATED CHONDROSARCOMA

Chondrosarcomas may dedifferentiate (10%) into a fibrosarcoma, a malignant fibrous histiocytoma, or an osteosarcoma.[31,39] They occur in older individuals and are highly fatal. Surgical treatment is similar to that described for other high-grade sarcomas.

Gross Characteristics. The central region of the tumor is identical to that of ordinary chondrosarcoma and is characterized by distinctly lobulated gray-white translucent tissue. Calcified foci are commonly found within this zone. Peripheral to this chondroid portion, but contiguous to it, is a firm-to-soft, often focally necrotic component that, after eroding the cortical bone, often extends into the adjacent soft tissue (Fig. 3–48).

Microscopic Characteristics. Two distinct components, correlating with the gross findings, are identified. The central portion shows features of a low-grade chondrosarcoma (grades I and II), identical to that described elsewhere in this chapter. At the periphery of the lobules arises an anaplastic high-grade infiltrative sarcoma that can present features

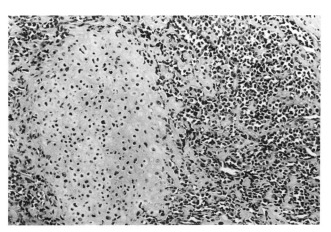

Figure 3–47. Islands of cartilage are formed throughout the small-cell stroma.

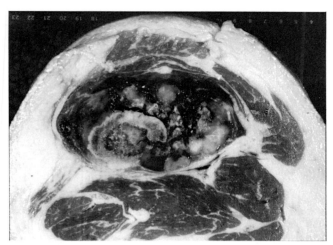

Figure 3–48. This dedifferentiated chondrosarcoma of the mid-femur contains an intramedullary chondroid component. The tumor erodes through the cortex and extends into the soft tissues as a high-grade pleomorphic sarcoma.

of malignant fibrous histiocytoma, osteosarcoma, or fibrosarcoma.

Giant Cell Tumor of Bone (GCT)

GCT is an aggressive, locally recurrent tumor with a low metastatic potential.[9,35,40–43] Giant cell sarcoma of bone refers to a de novo, malignant GCT, not to the tumor that arises from the transformation of a GCT previously thought to be benign. These two lesions are separate clinical entities.

Clinical Characteristics. GCTs occur slightly more often in females than in males. Eighty percent of giant cell tumors in the long bones occur after skeletal maturity; 75% of these develop around the knee joint. An effusion or pathologic fracture, uncommon with other sarcomas, is common with GCTs. GCTs occasionally occur in the vertebrae and the sacrum.

Natural History. Although GCTs are rarely malignant de novo (2%–8%),[44] they may undergo transformation and demonstrate malignant potential histologically and clinically after multiple local recurrences.[35,41] Between 8% and 22% of known GCTs become malignant following local recurrence.[35,40,41,44] This rate decreases to less than 10% if patients who have undergone radiotherapy are excluded. Approximately 40% of malignant GCTs are malignant at the first recurrence.[41] The remainder become malignant by the second and third recurrences; thus, each recurrence increases the risk of malignant transfor-

mation. Primary malignant GCT generally has a better prognosis than does secondary malignant transformation of typical GCT, especially if the transformation occurs after radiation therapy. Local recurrence of a GCT is determined by the adequacy of surgical removal, not by the histologic grade.

Radiographic and Clinical Evaluation. Giant cell tumors (GCT) are eccentric lytic lesions without matrix production (Fig. 3–49). They have poorly defined borders with a wide area of transition. They are juxtaepiphyseal with a metaphyseal component. Periosteal elevation is rare; soft tissue extension is common.

Gross Characteristics. The typical lesion presents as a large expansile mass in the region of the epiphysis. Cortical destruction of the overlying cortical bone is not uncommon. The periphery of the tumor is often partially surrounded by a thin, delicate rim of reactive bone (Fig. 3–50). The soft, somewhat gelatinous tumor tissue varies from gray-tan to red-brown. (Areas of hemorrhage with hemosiderin deposition account for the latter color.) Small, cystlike foci frequently occur; however, occasionally the cystic degeneration can become so extensive that the tumor resembles an aneurysmal bone cyst (Fig. 3–51). Firm fibrous or osteoid tissue can form at a site of pathologic fracture.

Microscopic Characteristics. The typical giant cell tumor comprises two basic cell types (Fig. 3–52). The stroma consists of polygonal to somewhat spindled cells containing central round nuclei (Fig. 3–53). Mitotic figures, sometimes numerous, are often noted, but they are not atypical. Scattered diffusely throughout the stroma are benign osteoclast-like giant cells. Small foci of osteoid matrix, produced by the benign stroma cells, can be observed; however, chondroid matrix never occurs. Extensive hemorrhage, pathologic fracture, or previous surgery can alter significantly the usual histologic picture of giant cell tumor so that it simulates sarcoma. These events must be recognized at the time of histologic interpretation in order to prevent diagnostic errors. Cystic areas with surrounding hemosiderin pigment and xanthoma cells correspond to the grossly observed cysts.

Grading. The grading of giant cell tumors into three groups in order to reliably predict clinical behavior, as originally proposed, has been generally abandoned. Recognition of the overtly malignant type (grade III), as will be described below, is valid; however, low-grade lesions (grade I or II) have been shown to metastasize.[24,45]

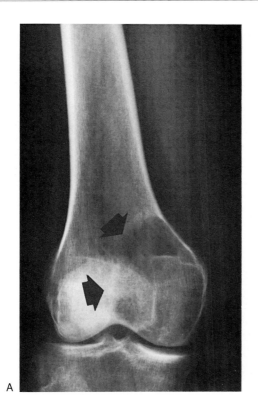

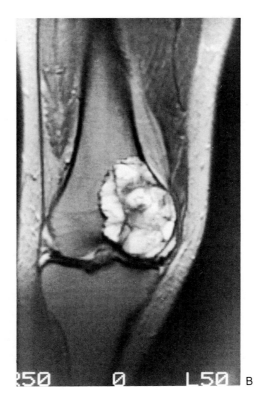

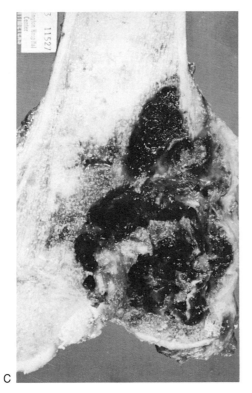

Figure 3–49.   Giant cell tumor of the distal femur. (A) Plain radiograph demonstrating a typical eccentric, osteolytic lesion with a thinned cortex without periosteal elevation. Note there is no evidence of matrix formation. (B) Corresponding MRI showing a heterogeneous pattern. (C) Gross specimen showing hemorrhage with an expanded but intact periosteum. The major clinical differential is an osteolytic osteosarcoma, MFH of bone, or a primary bony fibrosarcoma.

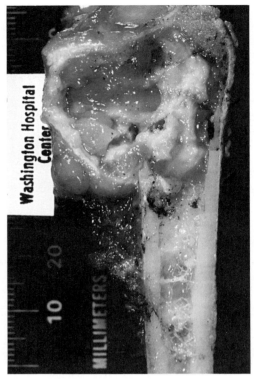

Figure 3–50.   Giant cell tumor arising in epiphyseal region of distal radius. This is an expansile destructive lesion surrounded by a rim of reactive bone.

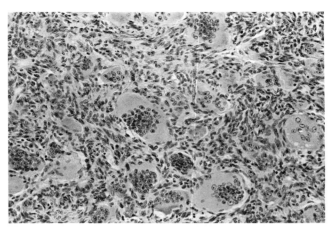

Figure 3–52.   In giant cell tumor, abundant multinucleated giant cells are diffusely distributed throughout a bland-appearing stroma.

A malignant GCT contains areas of unequivocal sarcomatous transformation, usually typical fibrosarcoma or osteosarcoma. The sarcomatous component is devoid of GCT features, thus, it is only by the recognition of foci of residual benign GCT or by the confirmation of preexisting benign GCT that an accurate diagnosis of malignant GCT can be established.

Treatment.   Treatment of bone GCT is surgical removal. Resection is curative in 90% of these cases.[40,41] In contrast, curettage, with or without bone grafts, has a recurrence rate of 40% to 75%.[35,40–42] Though en bloc excision offers reliable results, routine resection is not recommended.[46] Primary resection of a joint has a significant morbidity. Under certain situations it is reasonable to perform a curettage. In general, curettage does not rule out a later curative resection. Curettage should be performed with a mechanical burr. This simple maneuver probably reduces local recurrence to about 15%

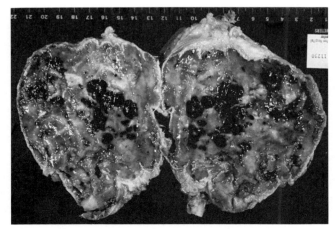

Figure 3–51.   Bisected proximal fibula markedly expanded by a giant cell tumor. There is a circumferential rim of reactive bone; also areas with coalescent hemorrhagic cysts are reminiscent of aneurysmal bone cyst.

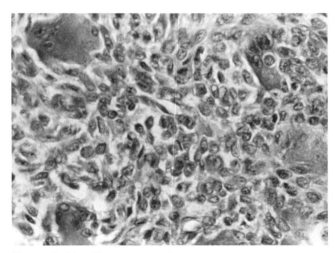

Figure 3–53.   The stroma of giant cell tumor consists of polygonal to plump spindle cells.

to 20%. Amputation is reserved for massive recurrence, malignant transformation, or infection. Due to the risk of malignant transformation, lack of effectiveness, and pathologic fracture, radiation is used only for surgically inaccessible sites.

Malignant Fibrous Histiocytoma (MFH)

Clinical Characteristics. MFH is a high-grade bone tumor histologically similar to its soft tissue counterpart.[47–49] It is a disease of adulthood. The most common sites are the metaphyseal ends of long bones, especially around the knee. Pathologic fracture is common. MFH disseminates rapidly. Lymphatic involvement, although rare for other bone sarcomas, has been reported.

Radiographic Characteristics. MFH is an osteolytic lesion associated with marked cortical disruption, minimal cortical or periosteal reaction, and no evidence of matrix formation.[47] The extent of the tumor routinely exceeds plain radiographic signs. MFH may be multicentric (10%) and associated with bone infarcts (10%).[48]

Gross Characteristics. The features are nonspecific and vary greatly. Firm, fibrouslike areas can alternate with soft necrotic foci. Some lesions are relatively homogeneous white-gray, whereas others are more variegated with ill-defined brown-red and yellow regions (Fig. 3–54).

Microscopic Characteristics. As does its soft tissue counterpart, primary malignant fibrous histiocytoma of bone reveals a remarkably broad histologic spectrum. Plump histiocyte-like cells and spindled fibroblastic cells, in variable proportion, are the chief elements. The storiform or pinwheel pattern, in which the fibroblasts radiate from a central focus, typifies this lesion. The histiocyte-like cells can form sheets or transform into markedly bizarre, often multinucleated, cells with atypical mitotic figures (Fig. 3–55). The spindle cell component may predominate, forming areas resembling fibrosarcoma. Chronic inflammatory cells and occasional osteoblast-like giant cells are usually scattered throughout the stroma. Small foci of osteoid matrix production by tumor cells can be observed. Metastatic pleomorphic carcinoma, particularly from the kidney, can closely, if not identically, mimic malignant fibrous histiocytoma; such a possibility must be included in the differential diagnosis. At the histologic level, routine histochemistry and immunohistochemistry

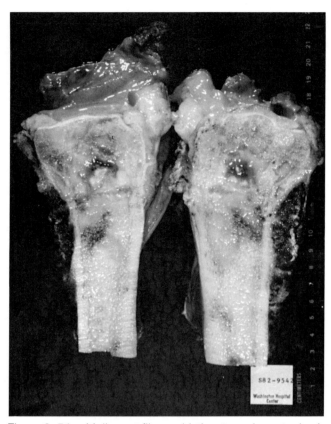

Figure 3–54. Malignant fibrous histiocytoma in metaphysis of the tibia. This high-grade neoplasm reveals areas of necrosis and cyst formation.

procedures can readily contribute to the solution of this problem.

Treatment. Treatment is similar to that of other high-grade sarcomas.

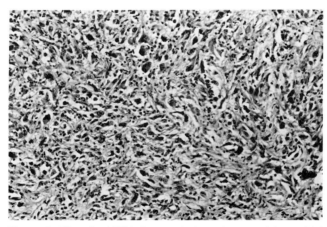

Figure 3–55. An MFH demonstrates pleomorphic and bizarre tumor cells admixed with spindle cells and inflammatory cell infiltrates.

Fibrosarcoma of Bone

Clinical Characteristics. This is a rare entity characterized by interlacing fascicles of spindle cells (herringbone pattern) without any evidence of tumor bone or osteoid formation. Fibrosarcoma occurs in middle age. The long bones are most affected. Fibrosarcomas occasionally arise secondarily in conjunction with an underlying disease such as fibrous dysplasia, Paget's disease, bone infarcts, osteomyelitis, postirradiation bone, and giant cell tumor. Fibrosarcoma may be either central or cortical (termed *periosteal*). The histologic grade is a good prognosticator of metastatic potential. Overall survival rate is 27% and 52% for central and peripheral lesions, respectively. Late metastases do occur, and 10- and 15-year survival rates vary. In general, periosteal tumors have a better prognosis than do central lesions.

Radiographic Features. Fibrosarcoma is a radiolucent lesion that shows minimal periosteal and cortical reaction. The radiographic appearance closely correlates with the histologic grade of the tumor. Low-grade tumors are well-defined, whereas high-grade lesions demonstrate indistinct margins and bone destruction similar to osteolytic osteosarcomas. Plain radiographs often underestimate the extent of the lesion. Pathologic fracture is common (30%).

Gross Characteristics. The presentation correlates reasonably well with the histologic grade. Low-grade lesions tend to be firm and white-gray and may appear encapsulated. With the higher-grade tumors, the tissue becomes soft, somewhat myxoid, and even necrotic. Transgression of the cortex with soft tissue extension is not uncommon.

Microscopic Characteristics. The hallmark of this neoplasm is the formation of fascicles of elongated spindle cells containing tapered nuclei. The fascicles often intersect at acute angles, forming the so-called herringbone pattern (Fig. 3–56). Intercellular collagen production may be abundant, especially in the low-grade examples. In contrast, high-grade fibrosarcoma is characterized by more pleomorphic spindle cells with atypical nuclear features. Mitotic activity is brisk. Collagen production may not be discernible. Differentiation of a grade I fibrosarcoma from a desmoplastic fibroma is frequently difficult.

Staging and Treatment. Staging and treatment are similar to other spindle cell sarcomas. Low-grade central and peripheral variants are treated by en bloc resection.

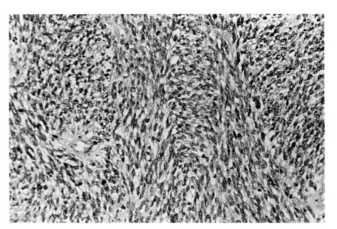

Figure 3–56. Acutely intersecting spindle cell fascicles form the herringbone pattern, a characteristic feature of fibrosarcoma. The nuclear atypia and hyperchromasia, mitotic activity, and absence of discernible collagen production all indicate that this is a high-grade tumor.

Secondary Tumors

Secondary tumors are neoplasms arising from an underlying pathologic process or from another tumor (Table 3–8). Though rare, this diverse group of lesions requires separate consideration. In general, the management of each tumor is similar to that of its primary counterpart.

PAGET'S SARCOMA

Sarcomas arising in a bone affected with Paget's disease have been termed *Paget's sarcoma*. These tumors develop with equal frequency in Paget's patients of all ages. Histologically, osteosarcoma is the most common; fibrosarcoma, chondrosarcomas, and MFH also have been described. The anatomic distribution is similar to that of uncomplicated Paget's disease. The femur, pelvis, and humerus are most

Table 3–8. Secondary Tumors

PRIMARY DISEASE	SECONDARY TUMOR
Osteochondroma	Peripheral Chondrosarcoma
Enchondroma	Central Chondrosarcoma
Fibrous Dysplasia	MFH, Fibrosarcoma
Paget's Disease	Paget's Sarcoma (usually osteosarcoma)
	Giant Cell Tumor (rare)
Irradiated Tissue	Radiation-Induced Sarcoma of the Bone* or Soft Tissue (osteosarcoma, MFH, fibrosarcoma)

*Approximately 200 cases. Average latent period is 10 to 12 years; range 4 to 30 years.

often involved. Increasing pain is the chief presenting complaint.

The diagnosis may be difficult due to the presence of the underlying Paget's disease. Radiographic studies may show an area of increased destruction, with or without increasing sclerosis. Periosteal elevation may not be present. Paget's sarcoma often presents with a pathologic fracture. Any patient with Paget's disease with increasing pain, a soft tissue mass, and/or pathologic fracture must be carefully evaluated for a secondary sarcoma. Prognosis is poor. There have been few long-term survivors among patients who receive surgery alone. Adjuvant chemotherapy is warranted following surgical removal.

RADIATION-INDUCED SARCOMA

Sarcomas rarely arise in previously irradiated bone. Approximately 200 cases have been reported. The average latent period is 10 to 12 years with a range of 4 to 30 years.[9] Criteria for diagnosis of a radiation-induced sarcoma are

1. Histologically proven sarcoma
2. Tumor arising in documented previously radiated field
3. Asymptomatic latent period (minimum of three to four years)

Surgical management is similar to other high-grade sarcomas. Overall survival ranges from 25% to 35%.

REFERENCES

1. Enneking WF: *Musculoskeletal Tumor Surgery.* New York, Churchill Livingstone, 1983, vol I, pp 1–60.
2. Enneking WF, Spanier SS, Goodman MA: A system for the surgical staging of musculoskeletal sarcoma. *Clin Orthop* 1980;153:106–120.
3. Enneking WF, Kagan A: Intramarrow spread of osteosarcoma, in *Management of Primary Bone and Soft Tissue Tumors.* Chicago, Yearbook Medical Publishers, 1976, pp 171–177.
4. Enneking WF, Spanier SS, Malawer MM: The effect of the anatomic setting on the results of surgical procedure for soft parts sarcoma of the thigh. *Cancer* 1981;47:1005–1022.
5. Malawer MM, Link M, Donaldson S: Bone sarcomas, pp 1418–1468. In DeVita VT Jr, Helman S, Rosenberg SA (eds): *Principles and Practice of Oncology,* ed 3. Philadelphia, JB Lippincott, 1989, Chap 41.
6. deSantos LA, Bernardino ME, Murry JA: Computed tomography in the evaluation of osteosarcoma: Experience with 25 cases. *AJR* 1979;132:535–540.
7. Destouet JM, Gilula LA, Murphy W: Computed tomography of long bone osteosarcoma. *Radiology* 1979; 131:439–445.
8. McKillop JH, Etcubanas E, Goris ML: The indications for and limitations of bone scintigraphy in osteogenic sarcoma: A review of 55 patients. *Cancer* 1981;48: 1133–1138.
9. Huvos AG: *Bone Tumors. Diagnosis, Treatment and Prognosis.* Philadelphia, WB Saunders, 1979.
10. Moore TM, Meyers MH, Patzakis MJ, et al: Closed biopsy of musculoskeletal lesions. *J Bone Joint Surg Am* 1979;61:375–380.
11. Schajowicz F, Derqui JC: Puncture biopsy in lesions of the locomotor system. Review and results in 4050 cases, including 941 vertebral punctures. *Cancer* 1968;21:5331–5487.
12. Costa J, Wesley RA, Glatstein E, et al: The grading of soft tissue sarcomas. Results of a clinicohistopathologic correlation in a series of 163 cases. *Cancer* 1984;53: 530–541.
13. Soule EH, Enriquez P: Atypical fibrous histiocytoma, malignant fibrous histiocytoma and epithelioid sarcoma. A comparative study of 65 tumors. *Cancer* 1972;30(1):128–143.
14. Weiss SW, Enzinger FM: Malignant fibrous histiocytoma. An analysis of 200 cases. *Cancer* 1978;41:2250.
15. Weiss SW, Enzinger FM: Myxoid variant of malignant fibrous histiocytoma. *Cancer* 1977;39:1672.
16. Enzinger FM, Weiss SW: *Soft Tissue Tumors.* St Louis, CV Mosby Co, 1983.
17. Huvos AG, Rosen G, Dabska M, et al: Mesenchymal chondrosarcoma: A clinicopathologic analysis of 35 patients with emphasis on treatment. *Cancer* 1983; 51:1230–1237.
18. Dahlin DC: *Bone Tumors: General Aspects and Data on 6,221 Cases,* ed 3, Springfield, Il, Charles C Thomas, 1978.
19. Dahlin DC, Unni KK: Osteosarcoma of bone and its important recognizable varieties. *Am J Surg Path* 1977;1(1):61–72.
20. Jaffe HL: *Tumors and Tumorous Conditions of the Bone and Joints.* Philadelphia, Lea & Febiger, 1958.
21. Dahlin DC, Coventry MB: Osteosarcoma, a study of 600 cases. *J Bone Joint Surg* 1967;49A:101–110.
22. Wilner D: Osteogenic sarcoma (osteosarcoma), in Wilner D (ed): *Radiology of Bone Tumors and Allied Disorders.* Philadelphia, WB Saunders, 1982, pp 1897–2095.
23. deSantos LA, Edeiken B: Purely lytic osteosarcoma. *Skel Radiol* 1982;9:1–7.
24. Lichtenstein L: *Bone Tumors,* ed 4. St Louis, CV Mosby Co, 1972.
25. Huvos AG, Rosen G, Marcove RC. Primary osteogenic sarcoma. Pathologic aspects in 20 patients after treatment with chemotherapy, en bloc resection and prosthetic bone replacement. *Arch Path Lab Med* 1977;101:14–18.
26. Malawer MM, Abelson HT, Suit HD: Sarcomas of bone, in DeVita VT, Hellman S, Rosenberg SA (eds): *Cancer, Principles and Practice of Oncology,* ed 2. Philadelphia, JB Lippincott, 1985, pp 1293–1343.
27. Ahuja SC, Villacin AB, Smith J, et al: Juxtacortical (parosteal) osteogenic sarcoma. *J Bone Joint Surg Am* 1977;59:532–547.
28. Unni KK, Dahlin DC, Beaubout SW, et al: Parosteal osteogenic sarcoma. *Cancer* 1976;37:2466–2475.
29. Companacci M, Picci P, Gherlinzona F, et al: *J Bone Surg* 1984;66B:313–321.
30. Unni KK, Dahlin DC, Beaubout SW: Periosteal osteogenic sarcoma. *Cancer* 1976;37:2476–2485.
31. Shives TS, Wold LE, Dahlin DC, et al: Chondrosarcoma and its variants, in Sim FH (ed): *Diagnosis and*

Treatment of Bone Tumors: A Team Approach. Mayo Clinic Monograph, Thorofare, NJ, Slack Inc, 1983, pp 211–217.

32. Pritchard DJ, Lunke RJ, Taylor WF, et al: Chondrosarcoma: A clinicopathologic statistical analysis. *Cancer* 1980;45:149–157.

33. Marcove RC, Mike V, Hutter RVP, et al: Chondrosarcoma of the pelvis and upper end of femur. *J Bone Joint Surg Am* 1972;54:561–572.

34. Edeiken J: Bone tumors and tumor-like conditions, in Edeiken J (ed): *Roentgen Diagnosis of Diseases of Bone,* ed 3. Baltimore, Williams & Wilkins, 1981, pp 30–414.

35. Johnson EW Jr, Dahlin DC: Treatment of giant cell tumor of bone. *J Bone Joint Surg Am* 1959;41:895–904.

36. Unni KK, Dahlin DC, Beaubout JW, et al: Chondrosarcoma: Clear-cell variant. A report of 16 cases. *J Bone Joint Surg Am* 1976;57:676–683.

37. Bjornsson J, Unni KK, Dahlin DC, et al: Clear cell chondrosarcoma of bone. Observations in 47 cases. *Am J Surg Pathol* 1984;8:223–230.

38. Harwood AR, Krajbich JI, Fornasier VL: Mesenchymal chondrosarcoma: A report of 17 cases. *Clin Orthop* 1981;158:144–148.

39. Marcove RC: Chondrosarcoma: Diagnosis and treatment. *Orthop Clin NA* 1977;8:811–819.

40. Dahlin DC, Cupps RE, Johnson EW Jr: Giant cell tumor: A study of 195 cases. *Cancer* 1970;25:1061–1070.

41. Hutter VP, Worcester JN Jr, Francis KC, et al: Benign and malignant giant cell tumor of bone. A clinicopathological analysis of the natural history of the disease. *Cancer* 1962;15:653–690.

42. Goldenberg RR, Campbell CJ, Bongfiglio M: Giant cell tumor of bone. An analysis of two hundred and eighteen cases. *J Bone Joint Surg Am* 1970;52:619–664.

43. Uehlinger E: Primary malignancy, secondary malignancy and semimalignancy of bone tumors, in Grundman E (ed): *Malignant Bone Tumors.* New York, Springer-Verlag, 1976, pp 109–119.

44. Nascimento AG, Huvos AC, Marcove RC: Primary malignant giant cell tumor of bone. A study of eight cases and review of the literature. *Cancer* 1979;44: 1393–1402.

45. Rock MG, Pritchard DJ, Unni KK: Metastases from histologically benign giant-cell tumor of bone. *J Bone Joint Surg* 1984;66A:269–274.

46. Campanacci M, Giunti A, Olmi R: Giant-cell tumors of bone: A study of 209 cases with long-term follow-up in 130. *Ital J Orthop Traumatol* 1977;1:249–277.

47. Huvos AG: Primary malignant fibrous histiocytoma of bone. Clinicopathologic study of 18 patients. *NY State J Med* 1976;76:552–559.

48. McCarthy EF, Matsuno T, Dorfman HD: Malignant fibrous histiocytoma of bone: A study of 35 cases. *Human Path* 1979;10:57–70.

49. Spanier SS, Enneking WF, Enriquez P: Primary malignant fibrous histiocytoma of bone. *Cancer* 1975; 36:2084–2098.

4

Rehabilitation of Patients with Extremity Sarcoma

MARSHA H. LAMPERT, R.P.T.
PAUL H. SUGARBAKER, M.D.

OVERVIEW

Rehabilitation is a process that should begin prior to treatment intervention and continue for the rest of the patient's life. The combined efforts of many health care professionals in the physical medicine and rehabilitation department serve to provide information to the patient concerning the level of function that is expected following treatment. Patients who have limb-sparing procedures, with or without adjunctive radiation therapy and chemotherapy, are evaluated and treated in order to preserve range of motion, control lymphedema, remediate pain, maintain or improve strength. They are instructed in safe ambulation and provided with recommendations for assistive devices that will allow for maximum independence in activities of daily living, on the job, in the school, or in the home. If an amputation is the treatment of choice, the patient is evaluated and an appropriate prosthesis is prescribed. Some prostheses are functional and others serve largely to improve the patient's appearance; both are useful to optimize quality of life. These patients should also be provided with advice concerning necessary equipment that would ensure independence.

Planning and implementing effective physical rehabilitation requires close collaboration between that staff and the oncologic surgeon, radiation therapist, and physician. Reassurance that other patients have coped successfully with this clinical situation must be reinforced. Rehabilitation is a process that combines the efforts of many health professionals (including occupational and physical therapists, physiatrists, psychologists, vocational counselors, and others) to help patients achieve their maximal potential for function. We define function in the broadest sense, which includes physical, psychosocial, vocational, or educational activity.

For the patient to attain maximal function, the rehabilitation team must restore lost function, using prosthetics, orthotics, or adaptive aids, or maintain a level of function by prescribing exercise programs and educating patients about the impact that treatment will have on their physical ability as well as on their disease. A comprehensive rehabilitation program must evaluate each patient to select appropriate rehabilitation interventions that maximize the quality of survival. The following elements must be considered in planning treatment strategies: the general health of the patient; the extent of surgery and the likely postoperative course; the patient's stage in life and his or her life's goals; and the availability of rehabilitation services.

REHABILITATION FOR AMPUTATIONS

The initial phase of rehabilitation is preoperative. For example, the rehabilitation team should discuss with the surgeon the level of amputation and the technique used to fashion the stump. For all amputative procedures there should be a minimum of redundant tissue on the stump. If there is too much tissue around the residual bone, prosthetic fitting and function are difficult. On the other hand, if skin flaps are pulled too tightly, bony prominences may be covered inadequately. This causes stump skin to be abraded when a prosthesis is worn. Many of these problems can be avoided by meticulous surgical technique. Pain may result from neuroma formation. A painful neuroma develops if nerves are divided at points that are apt to receive pressure while a prosthesis is being used. Thick scars and skin grafts are not as able to withstand the trauma imposed upon stump surface when a prosthesis is used and often can be avoided by careful planning of the surgical incision. The growing child is also presented with the possibility of bony overgrowth of periosteum osteophytes. Bevelling of the periosteum may help prevent this.

Next, the rehabilitation team provides the patient with a preoperative orientation to amputation. This occurs after the patient and the patient's family have been apprised of the likelihood of amputation by the responsible surgeon. A child is always oriented in the presence of and with the consent of an adult family member or guardian. The orientation consists of a walk through the rehabilitation department, where other amputees are often being trained. The postoperative time course is discussed in terms of when patients will be out of bed, sitting, and walking as well as the possibility of returning to a productive job or to school. Next follows a brief introduction to stump wrapping, fitting for a prosthesis, and alerting patients to the possibility of stump and phantom limb pain. A prosthesis may be viewed at this time by the patient.

Frequently, many questions about body appearance and function follow the preoperative orientation. Examples include: Can I walk without crutches? Will I be able to have children? Will I be able to swim? All questions are answered honestly. Pictures of former patients that demonstrate a variety of activities have been found useful.

A successfully rehabilitated amputee can help dispel a prospective amputee's anxiety about the approaching surgery and the consequences of a lost limb by sharing his or her experiences in regard to the surgery and its aftereffects. The development of this kind of relationship has proven to be beneficial and is recommended whenever possible.

Finally, in the preoperative phase, patients who are about to undergo lower-extremity amputation are instructed in a non-weight-bearing gait on straightaway and stairs. This instruction alerts the patient to the importance of protecting a potentially fragile bone when balance is good and pain is likely to be less, and trains them for the immediate postoperative period. A back evaluation and posture assessment are made. Evaluation is made for general strength and stamina, personal hygiene habits, pain history, vocational and avocational status, and family role. For the patient undergoing a forequarter amputation, a shoulder mold using a thermoplastic material is made at this time, provided there is no significant distortion of the shoulder. Questions for the potential upper-extremity amputee pertaining to self-care and one-handed techniques are addressed.

In preparation for surgery, the bed should be equipped with an overhead trapeze to encourage independence in bed mobility (especially if movement is associated with pain) and to maintain upper-extremity strength. The telephone, nurses' call button, and bedside table should be placed on the patient's nonoperative side to ensure easy accessibility.

RIGID DRESSINGS

Members from the rehabilitation department (occupational and physical therapists) should be trained in rigid-dressing application. They are called to the operating room at the time when initial closure of the wound begins. The soft dressing over the suture line should be moist. Preferences range from use of petroleum-impregnated gauze or an antibiotic ointment over dry gauze or telfa. This minimizes friction within the cast when mobility begins. Using too moist a dressing, however, may result in the formation of water blisters and increased discomfort. With an organized team, fabricating a rigid dressing should add no more than 30 minutes to the operating room time. The patient should remain anesthetized during the procedure to avoid inadvertent trauma to the stump or other motion that would impair fabrication movements.

For all ablative procedures that have a stump (above elbow, below elbow, above knee or below knee), rigid dressings applied immediately following surgery are recommended. This rigid dressing is used to protect the stump, control edema and pain, shape the stump, and hasten wound healing. The hard protective shell allows for early mobilization and earlier independence for the patient, with less fear of inadvertent trauma. It should not be used if there is compromised circulation or known infection.

Critical details must be respected for either upper or lower extremities. Suspensions for the cast must be adjustable to permit tightening for increased security as postoperative swelling decreases and the cast becomes loose. Padding should be placed over bony prominences, as in a below-knee amputation to minimize pain over the cut bone on motion. The closed suction drainage system should not be sewn to the skin so that after three days or so it may be withdrawn without necessitating cast removal. Indications for an emergency cast removal should be decided upon before this procedure is initiated, and honored by all those attending the patient. These factors should include (1) localized pain within the rigid dressing and not just a complaint of generalized pain over the entire operative area, (2) a spike in fever with no obvious source accountable, (3) bloody staining through the plaster, and (4) any unusual odor emanating from the rigid dressing. Use of a rigid dressing for hip disarticulation, hemipelvectomy, or forequarter amputations in the immediate postoperative period is rarely done.

PREPARATORY PROSTHESIS

Upper Extremity

The initial rigid dressing becomes increasingly loose within the first week following surgery. Because this area is not a weight-bearing one, a new cast with a terminal device can be made in the rehabilitation department as early as four days postoperative. Concurrent with prosthetic fabrication, an ongoing program of range of motion and strengthening of residual musculature is introduced. At the first cast change, the skin sutures are not usually removed, although some that appear unusually tight may be taken out. Old blood is removed from the incision with a 3% peroxide solution.

The terminal device used in a preparatory upper-extremity prosthesis is usually a hook with a voluntary opening. Abduction of the contralateral shoulder girdle, which tightens a cable running the length of the suspension harness to the rigid dressing, allows for opening the terminal device. The patient can be trained to control the tension in order to hold objects of varying size and weights. Interfaces of one-ply cotton stockinette stump socks are used as these dressings become loose. It is not unusual to utilize several temporary preparatory prostheses as healing and shaping occur.

At night to allow maximal comfort during sleep the stump is wrapped using an ace bandage, or preferably a commercial stump shrinker sock. This procedure shapes and molds the residual limb in preparation for the permanent prosthetic prescription. The shaping of a standard below-elbow or above-elbow amputation stump occurs much more rapidly than with lower-extremity amputations. Less swelling and faster healing from a greater vascularity translates into quicker stump maturation. The permanent prosthesis for the patient with an upper-extremity sarcoma can usually be measured at six to eight weeks following amputation. The best results occur when the amputee is fitted as early as possible and trained in the use of the prosthesis.

Lower Extremity

Temporary prosthesis for the above-knee or below-knee amputee (BKA) can be fabricated in the rehabilitation department at any time between 10 and 14 days postoperative (Fig. 4–1). At this time, coordination can be made with the attending surgeon for suture removal or incision inspection. A silesian belt for the above-knee amputee (AKA) or supracondylar cuff for the BKA are the only means necessary for suspension. In the AKA a universal joint, allowing for flexion and extension of the knee, is attached to an aluminum pylon and a SACH (solid ankle cushion heel) foot. The BKA needs a rigid dressing and a

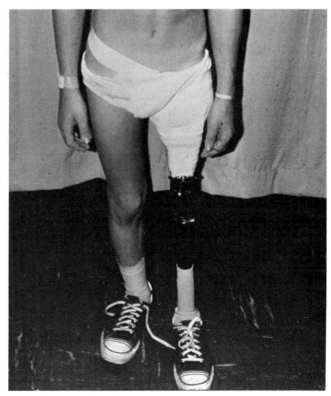

Figure 4–1. Temporary prosthesis for the short above-knee amputation.

much shorter pylon with a SACH foot. Weight-bearing and dynamic alignment are carried out when the plaster is dry (24 hours). The cast can be detached from the mechanical joints and should remain on the individual whether he or she is walking or not.

Ace wrapping for shaping should be done each evening. As with the upper extremity, several changes of the rigid dressing may be needed until the shaping and edema are sufficiently stabilized to allow for measurement of the permanent prosthesis.

The rehabilitation program for the lower-extremity amputee should include an exercise program to maintain or restore full range of motion and strength in joints necessary for ambulation and for efficient operation of the prosthesis. The therapist should be aware of the common problems (ie, hip or knee flexion contractures) that occur with specific amputations. Individualized programs to combat these are developed. Concern should also be given for muscle coordination, edema control, and relief of painful symptoms. Phantom pain and sensation are usually appreciated intermittently, although they are more intensely perceived at night. The more active the amputee, the less these discomforting sensations interfere with his or her functioning.

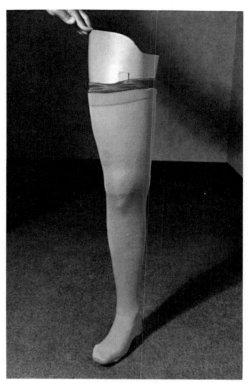

Figure 4–2. Above-knee endoskeletal prosthesis.

PERMANENT PROSTHESIS

Artificial limbs should be as lightweight as possible and still be able to withstand heavy loads. They may be fabricated out of plastic laminate, thermoplastic materials, or soft foam placed over a load-carrying central aluminum pylon. These are referred to as exoskeletal (the hard plastic or crustacean limb) or endoskeletal (the soft foam, cosmetic-appearing limb) (Fig. 4–2). Use of a prosthesis is generally good if the limb is comfortable and it performs a desired task as well as being cosmetically acceptable. Training and limb compliance are made more difficult if there are unacceptable auditory noises made such as escaping air, slapping of the foot on the floor, or the click of an elbow locking. Energy expenditure and fatigue factors are high in the training process.

The lower-extremity prosthesis is a better substitute for the lost extremity than the upper-extremity prosthesis. Walking is a cyclical repetitive activity occurring in two planes, whereas the upper extremity functions in three planes. The final prescription requires consideration of the patient's as well as the physician's goals. Communication between physical and occupational therapist, prosthetist, and doctor is essential in order to prescribe a limb with components that will meet the amputee's needs. Prostheses cannot be adjusted to weight fluctuations. Obesity

may do more to limit the mobility of an amputee than anything else. With less exercise, weight control may be more difficult. Often the course of chemotherapy causes decreased energy levels, thus causing decreased motivation to exercise. From the beginning, the patient and his or her family must be cautioned against excessive weight changes. With nutritional guidance at the time of discharge, obesity may be preventable.

Upper-Extremity Prescription Components

The more distal the amputation, the simpler is the prosthetic prescription. The length of residual limb, age of patient, and activity level determine the type of upper-extremity prosthesis necessary to meet functional needs.

For patients with a below-elbow (BE) amputation, the terminal device (hook or hand) derives energy from the residual limb through its muscular contraction on surface electrodes within the socket or via a cable connected to the chest or shoulder harness that becomes tight as the contralateral scapular abducts. Terminal devices replace hand functions. They may be hooks that give lateral prehension or cosmetic hands with palmar prehension. Hooks made of steel for durability or aluminum for lightness are used for manual occupations requiring dexterity. These may be utility or heavy-duty work devices.

Hands may be interchangeable with hooks. Hands are essentially more cosmetic and tend to act as a stabilizer (Fig. 4–3). Latex gloves are applied to hands for a more realistic appearance and need to be changed often because they are easily soiled or stained. Wrist units attach the terminal device to the rest of the prosthesis and provide supination and pronation. The hand is passively moved by the sound extremity. This unit allows for alternative terminal devices.

Below-elbow residual limbs are referred to as *long* if greater than 55% of the forearm remains, *short* if from 35% to 55% remains, and *very short* if there is less than 35% remaining. The range of pronation and supination decreases with the length of the stump. With 60% of the forearm amputated, the motion is lost.

The fit of the prosthesis must be snug; rigid hinges connect the socket to the triceps cuff about the upper arm for shorter residual BE limbs. These may also require a figure 8 harness over the shoulder or chest, with a crossover to the contralateral upper extremity.

A Muenster-type socket may be fitted around the humeral condyles without additional suspensions for medium-length residual limbs.

Above-elbow (AE) amputations often require a lock at the elbow joint in order to activate the terminal device. The elbow lock may be actively engaged through a cable system that becomes tense with shoulder depression and arm extension or passively locked by using the sound hand on an external device.

A new and sophisticated prosthesis called a myo-electric prosthesis for the upper extremity has been developed for the individual who can demonstrate motivation and has very good cognitive and motor skills (Fig. 4–4). The patient needs a good sense of control of his or her muscles and must be able to learn to use surface electrodes to control the terminal device. This item is readily accepted by the amputee. The price averages four to five times that of a conventional prosthesis. Length of stump is critical. A BE stump should be 6 in. distal to the antecubital fossa or 6 cm proximal to the ulnar styloid. An AE residual limb should be 6 in. below the floor of the axilla or 6 cm proximal to the medial epicondyle of the humerus. There must be room at the elbow for mechanical advantage of remaining musculature and to allow for enough room to house the components. The shoulder disarticulation patient may be fitted with a myoelectric prosthesis but is still functionally limited in some bimanual activities. Training in the use of an upper-extremity prosthesis is frustrating and requires several sessions in order to learn the care and fine uses of the limb.

Forequarter Amputation

Forequarter amputees are usually ambulatory 24 hours after surgery and are provided with self-care aids (plateguard, rocker-knife, and a piece of removable plastic that provides a nonskid surface). It is necessary to instruct and encourage neck range of motion and head positioning as soon as the patient is allowed out of bed. The shoulder cosmesis, which was fabricated preoperatively, should be modified for comfort and fit and given to the individual at the time of suture removal. A cosmetic shoulder has no

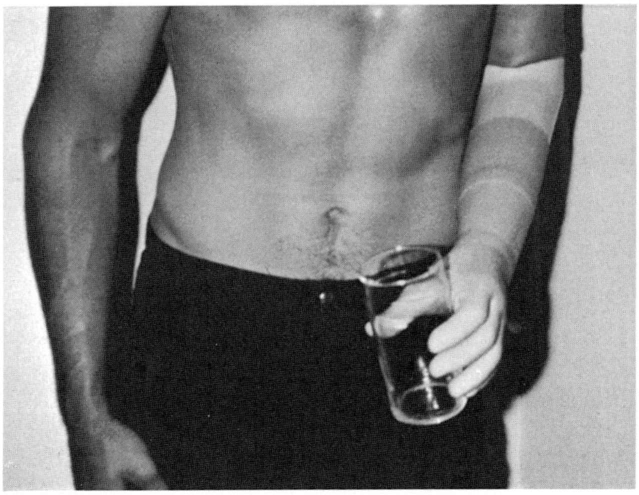

Figure 4–3. Below-elbow prosthesis with cosmetic hand.

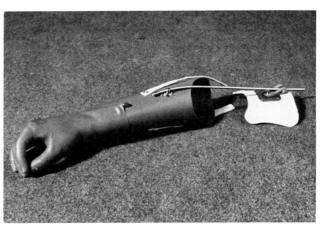

Figure 4–4. Below-elbow myoelectric prosthesis with triceps cuff.

movable parts but has a twofold function: (1) It provides symmetry for the shoulder girdle and permits almost normal posture for the head and neck (Fig. 4–5); (2) and it provides a shelf upon which to rest a bra strap and heavier outer clothing (Fig. 4–6).

Because the function of the forequarter prosthesis is very limited, for most patients a cosmetic soft shoulder or an endoskeletal non-cable-driven unit is recommended. The decision about providing a prosthetic device for the forequarter amputee is usually

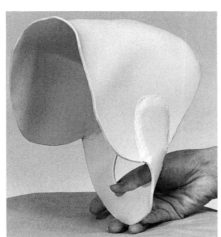
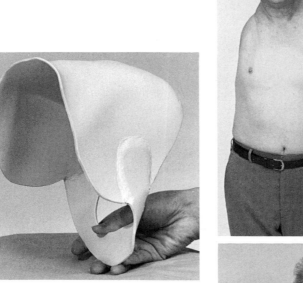
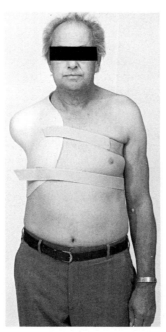
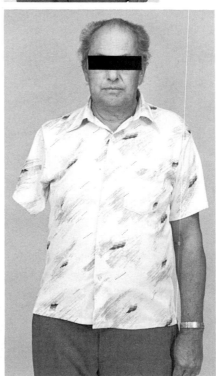

Figure 4–5.   Shoulder cosmesis used following forequarter amputation (*Top left*). The shoulder cosmesis is fabricated over the shoulder before surgery. If this is not possible, a mold is taken from another person with similar contours. The remaining photographs illustrate that the cosmesis lends balance to the upper trunk and results in a more normal body image.

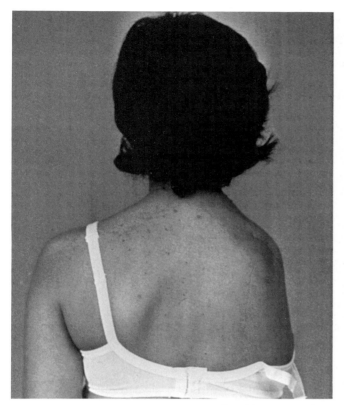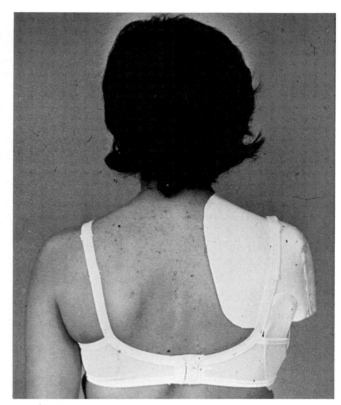

Figure 4–6. Shoulder cosmesis provides a shelf to support the bra strap.

delayed until several months after surgery, when chemotherapy and radiation therapy are completed and the patient has determined what his functional needs are. The final prescription is based on specific patient needs. Most patients will want a cosmetic soft unit with a terminal device that looks like a hand. Requests made for units that are functional may serve as a stabilizer. Very rarely an individual will request a true operational functional unit. They are available with cables and manual locks to position the elbow or with myoelectrically driven terminal devices and a mechanical elbow (Fig. 4–7). Fabrication is considerably more protracted for the functional forequarter prosthesis, and training may take weeks to learn to control elbow and hand together. Prior to release of the prosthesis, patients must be instructed in the need to observe their skin under the limb, and they must be educated about prosthetic maintenance. If there are any signs of abrasion, prosthetic use should be avoided and mechanical adjustments made. Clothing modifications may be required, such as stitching additional fabric onto a bathing suit for women to ensure modesty. Participation in sports activities should be encouraged. Water activities, snow skiing, and hiking are reasonable leisure pursuits. Returning to work or school is ex-

pected as soon as the medical condition allows. The individual who was employed as a physical laborer probably will require a change of occupation and job retraining. Referral to a professional vocational counselor should be made promptly. Frequently, clerical positions are resumed with only modifications at the job site. Resumption of a "normal" lifestyle with a minimum of time interruption is the goal of rehabilitation. This goal can be met only with the cooperation and motivation of the patient and all members of the medical team.

Lower-Extremity Prescription Components

The minimum length of tibia in a BKA for function is 1½ in. For good prosthetic fit the amputation should be close to the upper to middle third of the shank to allow full use of the knee. A patellar tendon-bearing (PTB) prosthesis allows for intimate fitting with a flexible distal thigh cuff for suspension (Fig. 4–8). Soft liners may be used to protect the bony surfaces. A PTB with additional height over the patella and femoral condyles (supracondylar suprapatellar) is suspended by the placement of a removable medial

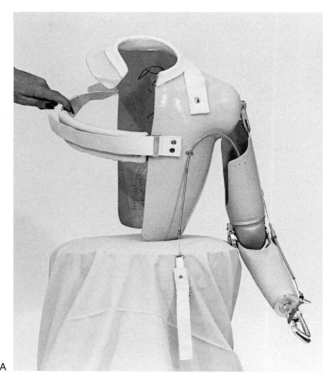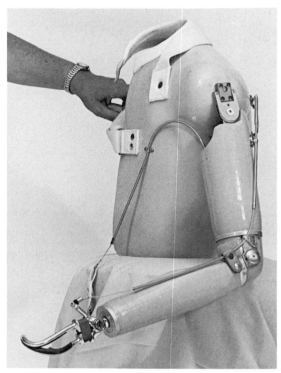

A

B

Figure 4–7. (A) The functional forequarter prosthesis (front view) has cable-driven controls for elbow placement and manipulation of the terminal device. (B) Side view of the forequarter prosthesis.

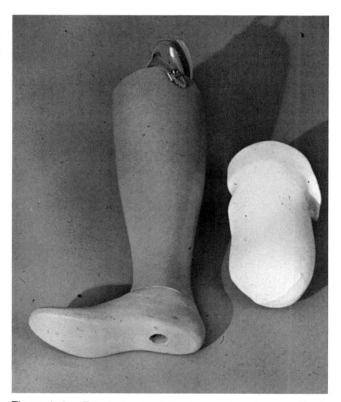

Figure 4–8. Exoskeletal patellar tendon-bearing prosthesis with soft liner, suspended by a supracondylar cuff.

wedge that holds the limb in the socket or a rubber sleeve. For additional stability, a thigh corset may be added to the BKA prosthesis.

Prosthetic feet have recently undergone revolutionary changes that allow the lower-extremity amputee to become more active and functional in sports and on the job. The foot acts to support and propel the body and must be flexible and rigid simultaneously. Standard feet are still available such as the SACH, which simulates plantar flexion through heel wedges of varying elasticity. This is a low-cost component but is heavier than the newer feet. A SAFE (stationary ankle flexible endoskeleton) foot has a flexible heel to help the foot accommodate to uneven surfaces, thus reducing stresses on the stump. Multi-axis or single-axis feet allow for even greater mobility and stability, but have mechanical parts prone to breakdown.

The newer, or energy-storing, feet include the Seattle Foot with a flexible plastic keel that provides a force during push-off. This acts similarly to a diving board and is good for jogging. The Sten Foot has a keel extending from heel to toe with rubber plugs acting like bumpers. It offers stability but is not very responsive for fast starts. A Carbon Copy Two Foot is a solid ankle like the SACH but is lighter weight and is good for all lower-extremity amputations. A Flex Foot is fabricated out of graphite, but requires a distance of at least 5 in. from the distal residual limb to the floor for fitting of the BK amputee. This component is covered by a cosmetic foam sleeve. The Flex Foot is very responsive and good for geriatrics because it is less tiring. Volleyball players claim that there is low inertia (Fig. 4–9).

Above-knee amputees require sockets that may be held on by suction and are shaped in a quadrilateral configuration with intimate contact over the residual limb. Special valves are used to allow for donning and removal by breaking the air pressure seal. Strong thigh musculature is needed to use this socket. A prosthetic sock may be added if there is more redundant tissue or a short limb to allow for close, but not suction-fit. A lightweight belt, silesian belt, or a more substantial pelvic band may be used to suspend the prosthesis and minimize rotation at the hip.

Newer concepts in socket design attempt to fit the AKA residual limb in its more normal dynamic alignment, allowing for adduction of the femur and restoring the normal pelvic femoral angle. These sockets are reported to be more comfortable than the quadrilateral socket. The following are all modifications of the natural-fitting concepts: natural shape natural alignment (NSNA), continued adducted trochanteric controlled alignment method (CATCAM), and others.

Knee mobility may be obtained by a single-axis constant-friction unit that does not allow for changes in cadence. Hydraulic or pneumatic knee units are used to provide automatic control in swing and stance phases of walking. These knee units allow for changing speeds and stride lengths.

HIP DISARTICULATION AND HEMIPELVECTOMY REHABILITATION

Patients undergoing hip disarticulation or hemipelvectomy usually begin ambulation when skin flaps have started to heal and closed suction drainage is minimal. The process begins with tilt table standing and advances to parallel bars, walker, and crutches. When balance and strength on flat surfaces have been demonstrated, stairs and ramps are attempted. Eventually, arising from the floor and negotiating doors is taught.

When the medical condition permits and the flap integrity is ensured, the patient is permitted to sit in a chair. The hip disarticulation patient may need a soft cushion for comfort, but the hemipelvectomy patient always needs a wedge-shaped cushion under the

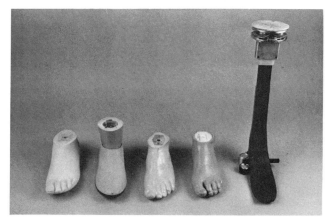

Figure 4–9. Optional foot components left to right: SACH, single-axis, Carbon Copy Two, Seattle, Flex Foot.

operative side to level the pelvis, to prevent early onset of scoliosis and back pain, and to provide sitting comfort. After suction drains are removed, stump wrapping begins in order to shape the stump and control edema. Occasionally an elastic girdle brief is suggested with one leg opening sewn closed. Stump wrapping is the responsibility of the patient, but often a family member is also instructed for reinforcement. The amputee should be wrapped all the time except while bathing.

Bathroom safety is addressed, and patients with hip disarticulation or hemipelvectomy are encouraged to use a bathtub seat, grab bars, and other equipment to prevent an accidental fall.

The staff of the department of rehabilitation medicine usually introduces the topic of providing an artificial limb or prosthesis just prior to discharge from the hospital. The patient who has had a hip disarticulation or hemipelvectomy is discharged when the surgeon determines that he or she is medically ready and his or her ambulation and self-care skills are adequate. The average is 14 days postoperatively.

Nutritional guidance is imperative with this group of high-level amputees because they tend to be more sedentary than most. Exercise is difficult and requires a great deal of energy. Rapid weight gain can be debilitating.

At approximately eight weeks after amputation, the hip disarticulation or hemipelvectomy patient's stump should be firm and not tender, the suture line well healed, weight stable, and urinary continence achieved. It is time to consider prescribing a prosthesis. The staff must be confident that the patient is fully informed about the potential benefits and shortcomings of the prosthesis and that it is the patient who wants the limb, not a well-intentioned family or staff member.

The final prosthetic prescription is based on clinical judgment of the patient's needs and personal habits. The exoskeletal, wood-laminated hip disarticulation and hemipelvectomy prosthesis weighs approximately 11 lbs. (Fig. 4–10). The endoskeletal foam-covered prosthesis weighs about 9 lbs. (Fig. 4–11). The exoskeletal unit is usually prescribed for children and adults who are particularly active or who are likely to pull or snag the cover of an endoskeletal unit. Women usually prefer the soft cover because it is more cosmetic and can be worn with skirts and dresses, presenting a positive and complete body image. The knee component most frequently prescribed is a single-axis knee, but occasionally we use a knee unit that increases extension (safety knee); a hydralic unit, which may be used for particularly strong ambulators, is not often recommended because of its added weight. The foot component we select is usually single-axis, although occasionally a SACH foot or an energy-storing foot is chosen.

The first step in furnishing a prosthesis is making a cast of the pelvis. From the cast a positive plaster mold is made upon which a socket is fabricated and a limb is attached. Within ten days an interim fitting can be completed and a dynamic evaluation of alignment can be made. If all looks well aligned, the limb can be finished and delivered to the patient within about five more days. Pregnancy limits use of the hip disarticulation or hemipelvectomy prosthesis after about the fifth month. Extension straps may be added to allow for some increased girth.

Patients usually require three to five days of gait training following delivery of the limb. During the training period, hygiene and stump care are reviewed, and instruction about keeping the stump dry and inspecting it for rash, blisters, and erythema is reinforced. Just prior to releasing the prosthetic unit, the patients are educated about prosthetic maintenance and the need for routine follow-up in rehabilitation. This is particularly true for children whose growth will necessitate adjustments in the prosthesis length and careful examination of the back in order to detect and treat scoliosis. Patients should be cautioned about the need to inspect the stump and to discontinue using the prosthesis if the skin is

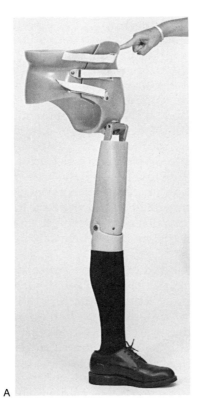

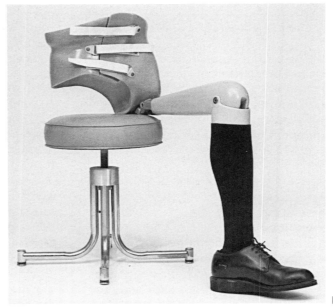

A

B

Figure 4–10. Left hemipelvectomy or hip disarticulation exoskeletal prosthesis. This device is made of wood laminate; it is prescribed for very active patients because of its durability. (A) Weight is distributed along the lower thoracic area and circumferentially along the body surfaces in contact with the jacket. The knee is fully extended while bearing weight. Components are generally single-axis knee and SACH foot. Patients who are discharged with this prosthesis must use a crutch or cane on the contralateral side. (B) The buttock region should be symmetrical with the remaining side for balance sitting posture.

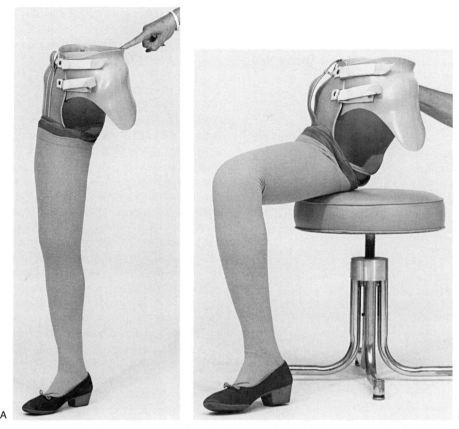

A   B

Figure 4–11.   Right hemipelvectomy or hip disarticulation endoskeletal foam prosthesis. This device is used for more sedentary persons. **(A)** Note the cosmetic thigh and leg that match the contours of the sound extremity. Components are generally the same as exoskeletal prosthesis. **(B)** Right endoskeletal prosthesis shown in a sitting position.

abraded. Usually, return to near-normal function occurs after several months of regular prosthetic use. During this time, conditioning occurs, stamina improves, and the patient is less diaphoretic and more comfortable in the prosthesis. Clothing should fit easily over bulky sockets and allow the prosthesis to be easily donned and removed. Adaptations will need to be made for bathing suits (eg, stitching closed the leg opening on the side of the amputation) for modesty.

Usually, the hip disarticulation or hemipelvectomy patient is not as active as the BKA or AKA because of the greater energy required to ambulate. In both hemipelvectomy and hip disarticulation patients there is a greater energy expenditure when ambulating than in two-limbed individuals (80% to 125% more). Most of the higher-level amputees walk faster on crutches than they do on a prosthesis and consume less oxygen. It is often difficult to convince this amputee of the benefits of wearing a prosthesis. In the event of compromised pulmonary function or other medical conditions (eg, chronic back pain) that

would not allow for additional energy expenditure, a custom-made sitting jacket may be recommended for the high-level amputee (Fig. 4–12). This prosthesis stabilizes the remaining pelvis and equalizes the sitting surface. The patient may wear this prosthesis when seated or when walking with crutches. The younger amputee tends to adapt more easily, use the prosthesis more often, and participate more in all activities.

Many individuals who have suffered amputations as a result of cancer are otherwise able-bodied and sports-oriented. The lower-extremity amputee is especially encouraged to attain physical fitness through athletics. Many national organizations have developed in response to the needs of this population. There are several special prostheses available, eg., one that could be used at the beach with a drainage hole to allow for removal of sand and water.

Amputees can be encouraged to participate in several sports including baseball (pitcher and infield). A substitute runner may be used after the amputee reaches first base. Bicycling may be done

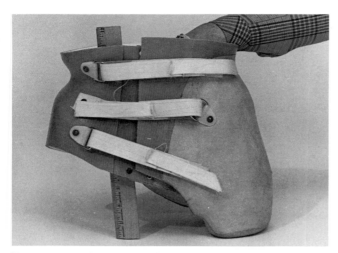

Figure 4–12.   Sitting jacket for hemipelvectomy or hip disarticulation patient. This prosthesis stabilizes the remaining pelvis and equalizes the sitting surfaces. The hemipelvectomy patient wears it when seated or while walking with crutches. It is useful for the aged amputee who may have markedly reduced ambulation because of other medical conditions. The younger amputee who desires the added mobility of crutch walking also may prefer this, and it permits more comfortable sitting.

with the heel placed on the pedal or with use of a toe clip. Some amputees with good balance prefer riding a bicycle without their prosthesis. Bowling can be done from a stationary position. The amputee can garden from a seated position, and can golf by using a limited follow-through on a stroke. Hiking may require additional suspensions on a prosthesis. Ice skating and skiing using outrigger skates and poles are also popular, and there are many other activities that can be tried. Motivation is the prime factor to getting out and resuming a normal life-style. Pain is usually the greatest deterrent to participation. Those who were athletic before surgery usually have strategies to relieve pain that worked for them before, and can easily call upon after their amputations.

Skin care and pressure areas in limbs must be treated prophylactically to minimize problems. Friction within a limb may be prevented by using several commercially available preparations. Bio-occlusive, Tegaderm, and Acuderm may be left in place four to five days before removal. Second Skin is a gel placed on the skin to decrease friction between the skin and moving surfaces. Spenco skin care pad comes in varying thicknesses and is reusable, although it cannot be used with suction sockets. Op Site is a transparent dressing that can be placed over a sensitive area.

LIMB-SPARING PROCEDURES

Wide Local Excision and Radiation Therapy

The criteria for wide local excision or limb-sparing procedures are that (1) the tumor must be totally resectable, without sacrifice of major vessels and nerves, or (2) reconstruction utilizing bone grafts or an endoprosthesis must provide limb function equal or superior to the function of a prosthesis. It should be remembered that a limb-sparing procedure is more complex than an amputation. The duration of surgery is longer, infection and pain may be more common, and the physical rehabilitation process may be more intense. The presumed psychological advantage of limb sparing versus amputation has yet to be established. When the prognosis of a soft tissue sarcoma treated by amputation or by a limb conserving approach are similar, ultimate treatment decisions may be determined by functional or quality-of-life issues. There are rare times when, in spite of all sound advice, the patient will adamantly refuse an amputation on the basis of psychological, social or cosmetic reasons and receive a limb-sparing procedure.

The impact of therapies should be discussed with the patient as part of the decision-making process. Wound and limb problems are often predictable and preventable, and may be reversible when a physical rehabilitation program is included in the patient care package. The extent of surgery and tumor size at presentation contribute to more tissue injury in the high-grade sarcoma. The larger the tumor, the greater the volume of radiation that will be needed for treatment. Patients receiving radiation tend to have decreased joint motion, increased edema, and less muscle strength than patients not receiving radiation.

Studies show that chemotherapy does not impose much physical disability on the limb-spared individual, but it does accelerate skin changes seen from radiation therapy. Also, if the patient is a young child, it is important to consider leg-length discrepancies. Epiphyseal plates, particularly in the tibia, may be dramatically disturbed when irradiated. If radiation is given at the ankle, there will also be differences in shoe sizes. Scoliosis may also be a secondary effect of unequal leg lengths.

If a wide excision of a sarcoma is to be followed by radiation therapy, the department of rehabilitation must be involved prior to surgery. Unfortunately, the extent of tumor invasion rather than functional considerations must dictate the extent of muscle group excision or excision of individual muscle bundles. However, presurgical discussion of a planned surgical approach gives the rehabilitation department some idea of the extent of resection, so they can advise the patient regarding postoperative function.

Throughout the course of radiation therapy the goal of the rehabilitation department is to preserve range of motion, to control lymphedema, and to reduce pain. Often, if the muscular excision has been extensive, strengthening will be required before a reasonable functional result is achieved. With the sacrifice of major nerves, appropriate orthotic devices may be necessary.

Even long after the radiation therapy is completed, the rehabilitation department must continue to follow the patient and repeatedly assess the functional capacity of the patient at periodic intervals. Months after completion of therapy, especially if healing is imperfect, contractures may progress to the point that function is lost. Undoubtedly, the most important feature that will ensure optimal function after wide excision and high-dose radiation therapy is continuous physical therapy while the radiation therapy is progressing and frequent follow-up in the first 18 months after treatment.

Delicate areas, such as hands and feet, especially the plantar surface, are still considered risk areas for limb salvage because of the difficulty in the application of adjuvant radiation therapy to such uneven, thin surfaces. With sophisticated equipment and trained personnel, radiation has been successfully applied to these areas.

The following section will describe the physical rehabilitation process for patients who received radiation therapy (XRT) with limb-sparing surgery and several procedures that do not require this adjuvant treatment.

Late Sequelae of Radiation Therapy to the Extremity

We must be aware that as a result of the efforts to save a limb there may be a price to pay. The following problems may be encountered.

1. *Fractures:* Radiation affects the wholesomeness of bone, making it osteoporotic and fragile. The patient must be cautioned about risk-taking situations such as skydiving and football. Encourage the patient to swim, golf, play tennis, or work on construction. If there is a fracture due to cellular and vascular necrosis, healing of the bone is significantly delayed.

2. *Edema:* This may be minimized by advising the individual to elevate his or her leg when possible and to use intermittent compression machines if the swelling is severe, as well as elastic support garments.

3. *Pain:* A trial of transcutaneous electric nerve simulation (TENS) may be successful. Strong or addictive analgesics destroy the quality of life. With a TENS unit one may allow the patient to at least exert some control over the treatment and recovery, in conjunction with milder pain medications.

4. *Wound healing:* Problems can result in open wounds, which are prone to infection for up to two years. Advise the patient on keeping the area clean and protecting it with light dressings. Fistulae may occur and carry infection to deeper structures. Skin care for the affected extremity should continue for at least two years. Light applications of moisturizers, such as commercial preparations of vitamin E cream, aloe, or baby cream, should be carried out. These may be used during radiation therapy only with permission of the radiologist. Scented products have a higher volume of alcohol, which is drying and thus defeats the purpose of using a lubricant. Deep massage during application can delay or prevent a hard, woody extremity.

5. *Deformity:* Deformities or defects can be remedied by externally filling the areas with heat-moldable thermoplastic materials to ensure an intact positive body image.

6. *Muscle fibrosis:* This is sometimes unavoidable, resulting in contractures that occur long after supervised physical therapy has ended. A 5-minute workout each day may allay a major problem. Chronic changes occur in the supportive tissues and may be irreversible. These changes can be fibrosis, bone necrosis, endarteritis, decreased elasticity, obstruction of lymphatic channels, all of which can cause severe edema, pain, and decreased function.

Upper Extremity

The upper-extremity wide excisions and limb salvage have not imposed a great problem within the rehabilitation process especially in terms of pain, edema, or limitation of strength or motion. It is still important to understand and instruct the individual in order to gain maximum use of the extremity. Our major input is to those individuals who have had nerve resections and limb salvage procedures.

The tumors found in the upper extremity are generally smaller than those found in the lower extremity, which allow for more conservative or limited surgery. Rarely are whole muscle groups removed. If any muscles or nerves are resected close to the wrist or hand, it could render the hand insensate. Then the procedure of choice would be an amputation.

Postoperatively, the morbidity in the upper extremity is less than that of the lower. Suction drainage is less prolonged, wound infection is less frequent, and radiation is better tolerated most of the time. The anatomic location of the tumor and the volume to be treated determine the reaction.

The rehabilitation department and its interdisciplinary services of occupational and physical therapy and physical medicine have much to offer patients undergoing a Tikhoff-Linberg procedure. These patients are likely to retain hand function and some elbow function but lose shoulder function. The outcome is clearly superior to a forequarter or shoulder disarticulation procedure. Further, the Tikhoff-Linberg procedure is minimally disfiguring and is associated with only mild to moderate pain and edema. In our experience, the patient's acceptance of the procedure and its outcome has been good.

The rehabilitation process begins with a patient orientation program. Often, the patient is shown pictures of patients who have undergone the procedure, demonstrating what they can do postoperatively and what limitations in function are likely. Next, a shoulder mold is fashioned, using the involved shoulder, provided that its contours are not distorted. A heat-moldable material is used for this. The cosmetic shoulder helps preserve the symmetry and appearance of the shoulder contour and can support a bra strap or heavy overcoat. This cosmesis is the same as that provided following forequarter amputation. In patients where the deformity following surgery is minimal, a commercially available shoulder pad may suffice (Fig. 4–13). The use of these devices is optional. Other clothing options for women would be to purchase blouses with asymmetrical (off-center) closures and use of decorative scarves to mask the body contour.

On the first postoperative day an arm sling is provided for support and to restrict abduction. The motion restriction should be maintained until the incision is healed (usually about two weeks). Edema, when present, should be controlled with an elasticized glove or elastic stockinette. At the same time,

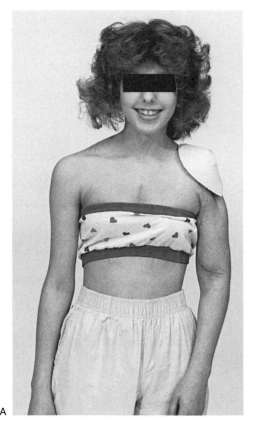
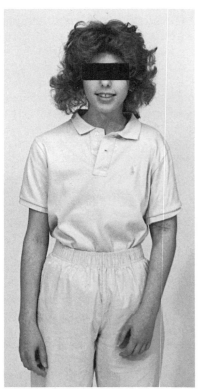

A

B

Figure 4–13.   Shoulder pad used as a cosmesis following the Tikhoff-Linberg procedure. A rather disfiguring loss of contour of the shoulder occurs with this procedure. Although functional results are excellent, the cosmesis result may be disappointing. (**A**) A simple, commercially available shoulder pad may be used to fill out the shoulder. (**B**) The cosmetic results with this shoulder pad can be excellent.

active, maximal hand movement is begun to preserve strength, range of motion, and to help mobilize edema through the pumping action of muscles.

Teaching the patient to be aware of proper head and neck positioning and cervical range of motion is initiated during the first postoperative days (or when the patient first becomes ambulatory).

When permission is given to begin motion, usually at two weeks postoperatively, active and assistive elbow motion within the confines of the sling are started. At about three weeks, the sling is removed for passive shoulder range of motion and wrist pronation and supination. The sling is discontinued after the suture line is healed, but is used intermittently for upright activities in which arm support increases comfort.

It is well known that joint immobilization for less than two weeks results in capsular adhesions that are easily overcome. Longer periods of immobilization often result in a fixed contracture; hence they should be avoided. Once the arm is out of the sling, full elbow range of motion (flexion, extension, pronation, and supination) should be performed for several minutes daily. Passive shoulder range of motion (flexion, abduction, and external and internal rotation) and pendulum exercises should be done for several minutes daily with the help of a family member or health professional. We recommend the use of bathroom safety equipment, grab bars, and tub seats to enhance safety for these patients.

Normal daily activities are encouraged. We recommend that not more than 20 lb be lifted with the arm that has received the Tikhoff-Linberg procedure. Modified tennis and even rowing can be done following completed rehabilitation. Pain and shoulder or arm dysfunction have not been significant management problems. Pain is often controlled with minimal analgesia.

Partial or total scapulectomies are procedures performed when tumors involve the scapula or the surrounding soft tissue. Removal of all or part of the scapula, including the glenoid fossa, may be necessary. If the glenoid complex is left intact, upper-extremity function may be close to normal. Removal of the glenoid creates restrictions of arm movement, often actively beyond 90°. Pain and complaints of fatigue at the end of the day are not uncommon. Recommendation of TENS and a sling for temporary support may be adequate because dependency increases the chance of edema.

The deltoid muscle mass forms the roundness of the shoulder and moves the upper extremity at the glenohumeral joint.

Following a partial resection, the arm is usually held in a sling until drainage subsides. Active range of

motion at the shoulder is not initiated until the sutures are removed, although external rotation can be started with the arm held at the side. Full elbow motions can be done. At the time the staples or sutures are removed, active and resistive motion can be performed. No chronic residual problems have been observed.

Vital structures adjacent to soft tissue sarcomas of the axilla are often difficult to determine. It may be impossible to discern the proximity to the brachial plexus unless the patient has neurological signs. The tumor's proximity to the humerus is difficult to identify despite sophisticated scanning devices. There may be a need to sacrifice adjacent musculature, such as the long head of the triceps from its origin or the latissimus dorsi as it approaches the axilla posteriorly. Generally, if deeper structures are involved, surgery for cure cannot be done except by a forequarter amputation or Tikhoff-Linberg procedure.

After a sarcoma excision in the axilla the arm is held in a sling until drainage subsides. This may be for more than two weeks since this area is intimately associated with major lymphatic channels. If radiation is prescribed, the desire to get the patient in a position of a "salute" or at least 100° abduction/flexion and 75° external rotation is essential. It is probably one of the most difficult postures to assume without discomfort following surgery. Use of TENS to decrease pectoral muscle spasm, which is a great inhibitor to full shoulder range of motion and other modalities is suggested. The patient assumes this position while radiation is being given to minimize radiation exposure to the breast and upper arm. Twice a day physical therapy treatment may be needed. Once the shoulder can be moved about 90°, there is generally no problem until the area becomes sensitive to radiation.

Skin breakdown is not uncommon and delays the delivery of radiation treatment. The arm again is positioned by the side. Suggest to your patient to wear all-cotton T shirts for absorbency. No deodorants or body creams are allowed unless recommended by the radiation therapist.

Recovery of arm motion becomes easier during the second and third time radiation therapy is resumed, but throughout the course of treatment the program repeats itself.

Chronic lymphedema is common. An elastic stockinette or a customized sleeve may be adequate to control the swelling. If lymphedema is severe, the use of an intermittent compression machine is recommended.

If the brachioradialis muscle must be excised, the elbow should be protected in a splint until closed suction drainage slows and healing is underway. Once this has occurred, active range of motion to the elbow is progressed as tolerated.

If radiation must be applied to the antecubital fossa, the tendons of the biceps, and brachialis muscles may become fixed. The brachial artery and the median nerve may become enclosed in scar tissue. Damage to any or all of these can cause secondary problems such as an insensate nonfunctioning hand, at the very worst, or a weak elbow.

With a soft tissue sarcoma adjacent to the head of the radius and radial nerve, the elbow is left vulnerable over the surgical area. A protective device can be made from thermoplastic material, or else a commercial elbow protector should be provided (Fig. 4–14). Emphasis in rehabilitation is on maintaining a functional position during elbow and finger range of motion.

A dynamic splint should be fabricated with wrist and fingers stabilized in a functional position so that finger flexors and interossei can function well in grasping. After there is complete recovery from surgery and radiation, tendon transfers may be attempted using the flexor carpe radialis and thumb stabilizers.

Trunk

Retroperitoneal tumors are difficult to excise and often recur due to the problems in attaining negative surgical margins. Physical therapy is usually re-

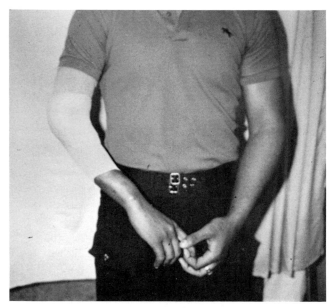

Figure 4–14. Commercial elbow protector used following resection of the radial head and radial nerve.

quested in conjunction with adjuvant radiation therapy. It is not unusual for the femoral nerve to be within the radiation field, resulting in the need to protect and support the quadriceps muscles. Edema is a secondary complication if the inguinal nodes lie within the field. Use of support stockings is recommended along with elevation of the lower extremities throughout the day.

A buttockectomy is performed when there is en bloc resection of the gluteus maximum muscle. The surgeon must be careful not to damage the sciatic nerve intraoperatively. Closure of the incision may be tenuous if large amounts of skin are removed. The patient may complain of difficulty in stair climbing, pain along the incision, and altered body image. Radiation that includes the buttock will disrupt normal sexual functioning and bowel habits.

The physical therapist may encourage strengthening of other hip girdle muscles and provide seat cushions. A custom buttock cosmesis may be fabricated out of thermoplastic material to resemble the contralateral buttock. This is secured with Velcro to the undergarments. Seat cushions or wedges may be needed for comfortable sitting and symmetric weight bearing on the buttocks.

An internal hemipelvectomy may be indicated with a diagnosis of soft tissue sarcoma in the upper thigh and/or buttock or a low grade sarcoma of the pelvic bones. The sacrum is transected through the neural foramina with resection of the hemipelvis, proximal femur, and, occasionally, the bladder, rectum or genitalia. In cases of an intrapelvic tumor, the peritoneal cavity will be entered. Stabilization of the pelvis and femur requires prolonged bed rest with skeletal traction to allow for fusion and maintenance of as much leg length as possible. Shoe lifts are imperative as soon as bed restrictions are removed, which is usually between three and six weeks postoperative. Partial weight bearing is allowed on crutches until a fibrous union of the remaining pelvis or ilium and femur occurs. This process may take up to six months. Strengthening of the distal muscles and upper extremities is important through repetitive active exercise against gravity. Sensation generally remains intact with few complaints of pain. Variations of this procedure are common, and a close relationship is necessary between the therapist and surgeon to monitor progress. At six months, the patient can walk on all levels with only a cane and/or shoe lift to equalize pelvic height in the event of a leg length discrepancy.

If the sciatic nerve is sacrificed, there will be motor loss combined with leg anesthesia, promoting a tendency for skin to ulcerate with trauma. An ankle-foot orthosis (AFO) will be necessary to assist with foot clearance. Following initial treatments, an ankle fusion or a posterior tibialis transfer may be recommended. The patient must be educated as to proper foot care, shoeing, and orthotic application.

Lower Extremity

The thigh is probably one of the most difficult anatomic areas in which to attain a high level of local tumor control without significant morbidity, and it is an area most likely, historically, to develop a soft tissue sarcoma. Tumors discovered in the lower extremity are generally large because they are masked by bulky muscle tissue. The morbidity involved in irradiating the upper medial thigh and groin is potentially severe. Because of radiation scatter, sexual dysfunction is probable. Chronic lymphedema following irradiation of the lymph node complex in the groin is frequently observed. Hip joint dysfunction and pain are not usually symptoms but may be late findings.

For most wide local excisions of the thigh there is prolonged serosanguinous drainage. When the drainage has decreased or the suction tubing has been removed, ambulation and active exercises can begin in earnest. Commercial immobilizers may be used to protect the lower extremity from poor positioning, but also prevent wounds from being inadvertently overstretched, particularly when the incisions cross a joint.

A large soft tissue sarcoma within the anterior thigh group may require an excision from origin to insertion of the whole quadriceps muscle. This procedure is reserved for high-grade tumors. Lower grades may be adequately excised by removal of some portion of the quadriceps.

Radiation treatment is not usually required with a formal muscle group excision because it would have to include two joint spaces and be a most morbid procedure. Also, if the patellar tendon is irradiated with 6,000 rads or more, tendon breakdown would occur over time.

At approximately two weeks postoperative, a dual-channel aluminum AFO is provided that blocks out dorsiflexion and allows only 5° plantar flexion. Use of a cane is encouraged on precarious terrain. Continued use of the AFO should be expected. The knee can be extended by locking in hyperextension and by increasing the lordotic curve. We had seen patients who discarded the brace and fell, fracturing patella, femur, and shoulder.

Some patients are uncomfortable with the cosmetic appearance of the thigh. To enhance body image, an orthosis or cosmesis can be fabricated out of pelite to simulate the contours of the sound extremity and allow for the wearing of contemporary fashions. This is suspended by ace wrap or held in place with pantyhose.

For patients with soft tissue sarcoma of the medial thigh, an adductor muscle group excision is required. This procedure is usually followed by radiation and chemotherapy. A frequent complication following this procedure is prolonged drainage through the suction catheters. The patient may require bed rest for long periods of time, sometimes longer than two weeks with the obvious resultant sequelae. The lymph nodes are not specifically removed as in a groin dissection, but the medial thigh contains major lymphatic channels that are sacrificed with the specimen.

Initially all motion of the extremity is kept at a minimum. Loose elastic wrapping can be done to help protect the incision. Isometric contractions of the quadriceps seem to increase drainage when done as part of an exercise program following surgery to this area and should not be recommended.

Weight bearing, when allowed, is tolerated, but a cane may be necessary for balance. Custom-measured elastic stockings or commercial support stockings should be applied for all upright activities. Rarely are there complaints of motor dysfunction, but edema and pain are common. Patients should be educated about the importance of leg elevation and avoiding prolonged sitting. Techniques of basic skin care including caution when shaving the legs should also be reviewed.

When there is removal of a tumor from the posterior thigh, tight wound closure may compromise skin in the area of the popliteal fossa. If adjuvant radiation and chemotherapy are required, the incision may open and remain a problem for the first year following treatments despite active participation in PT. The PT is usually interrupted and resumed spasmodically as complete wound healing progresses.

The patient remains in bed, frequently in a knee immobilizer, until drainage subsides. The patient should be taught quadriceps isometrics and ankle motions. When the incision appears to be healing well, range of motion can be started. Initiation of knee flexion may be difficult, but this motion can be accomplished especially in the side lying position.

Functionally there are little physical complaints except for stiffness following prolonged sitting and an unsteadiness when running.

Chronic problems that may occur long after medical treatments have been completed are knee flexion and plantar flexion contractures. Programs should include whirlpool and debridement for slow-healing wounds, serial casting for contractures, and a review of exercises. A woman should be discouraged from wearing too high a heel on her shoes.

Lateral thigh excisions frequently render the individual with a significant cosmetic and physical deficit, although not so limiting as to prevent normal work or social habits.

Bony tumors involving the proximal tibia or distal femur result in limb salvage procedures with use of the kinematic rotating hinged knee joint or a distal femoral replacement. The incision is long and lateral to the patella. Removal of the distal femur or proximal tibia along with the joint capsule ligaments and muscle is necessary. The endoprosthesis maintains skeletal continuity and near-normal function of the knee. There is an inherent lack of knee stability. Problems with the growing child and use of this knee joint are resolved by the use of an expanding or telescoping device.

The patient is placed in a bulky dressing and knee immobilizer in the operating room. Because methyl methacrylate is used to hold the endoprosthesis in place, the dressing is only for control of swelling and comfort. Physical therapy can be started as early as day one for quadriceps sets, especially for those with only a femoral replacement. Patients with a proximal tibial prosthesis only are restricted from vigorous quadriceps function and knee flexion to protect the attachment of the patella tendon. Usually these patients are started on gentle active flexion and extension strengthening four weeks postoperatively.

Some patients with the kinematic rotating hinged knee joint might be placed on continuous passive motion machines immediately. This has not been found to be more beneficial than an active program.

There is a potential for many complications, such as wound infections, edema, and temporary peroneal nerve palsies caused by overstretching during surgery. Full active range of motion is expected as well as full weight bearing. The rehabilitation process begins with quadriceps muscle sets and progresses until the patient has the ability to walk on a cane.

The leg muscles are compartmentalized but not so definitively as those in the thigh. There is an anterior, posterior, and small lateral compartment; the interosseus membrane between the tibia and fibula separates the anterior and posterior regions. The anterior compartment is actually more anterolateral and contains muscles that act as dorsiflexors of the foot. If surgical excision is necessary, the patient should be placed in a posterior leg/ankle splint early postoperatively to prevent a heel cord contracture and overstretching the incision. It is placed over the surgical dressing as additional protection to the wound and kept in place while the patient is in bed. The patient is requested to use the splint for extended periods of time even after discharge. For ambulation, an aluminum double-upright AFO with dorsiflexion assist is provided.

The simple plastic posterior leaf AFO does not offer sufficient medial-lateral stability, although this may be worn until the permanent AFO is received. Edema may be observed. Use of a knee-high support stocking and low-heeled shoes or high-quartered sneakers is recommended. The patient must be educated about proper foot care. It is not unusual for the peroneal nerve and the peroneus longus muscle to be partially or totally sacrificed. They act to evert the foot. The physical therapy treatment usually is heel cord stretching and maintenance with fitting of a custom-made ankle stabilizer, air splint, or aluminum AFO.

The gastrocnemius muscle spans two joints. It joins with the soleus to form the Achilles tendon, which inserts on the calcaneus. These muscles flex the knee or plantar flex the ankle. They comprise the posterior compartment. If radiation is necessary following surgery in the posterior compartment the knee joint should be spared. Radiation fields are generally directed laterally to spare the skin behind the knee as well as that of the Achilles tendon. Skin over the popliteal area is at high risk to break down during treatment.

The lower extremity is secured in a long leg immobilizer with a posterior splint on the foot. This is applied in the operating room to facilitate ease in transferring the patient without disturbing the wound or suction catheters. After two weeks the physical therapist may be allowed to remove the splints and start on gentle range of motion to the knee. Partial weight bearing can also be initiated with the knee splint in place. The contralateral shoe may have to be temporarily raised to allow for clearance during swing through phase. As healing is ensured, increased weight bearing is allowed. The shoe on the involved foot may have to be modified to include a rocker bottom to make for easier push-off. An AFO may have to be added to maintain a neutral ankle. Heel cord stretching should be done daily.

If the posterior tibial nerve is excised, sensation is interrupted along the lateral sole of the foot. There does not seem to be any additional problems. If radiation causes small fractures at the calcaneus, an ankle stabilizer (hindfood orthosis) would be sufficient to hold the foot.

When soft tissue tumors cannot be easily excised and the complications from adjuvant radiation are apt to render the foot nonfunctional, excision of one or several rays may result in satisfactory foot function. An orthotic must be fabricated to act as a shoe filler and ankle stabilizer. Modifications may be necessary to the external sole of the shoe, such as a rocker bottom to enhance push-off or a lateral flare can be added to the outer heel to increase stability at heel strike. If these changes are not made, there may be resultant problems of recurring sprained/strained ankles with internal bleeding, metatarsal bone displacement, and painful limited ambulation. Concurrently, with recovery from surgery, an exercise program for strengthening ankle musculature and heel cord stretching should be initiated.

It is important to remember that many patients with soft tissue sarcomas are ideal candidates for physical therapy. There may be functional limitations as a direct result of their disease or as a result of the treatment. The barrier to optimal rehabilitation has been a failure in the past to identify these problems. The obligation of any rehabilitation service is to allow the patients to achieve their fullest possible physical, psychological, social, vocational, and educational potentials.

BONE METASTASES

Nearly 80% of all patients with bone metastasis have primary tumors in the breast, lung, or prostate gland. The most common symptom is pain, especially on weight bearing or by nerve entrapment. Treatment goals are to relieve pain and increase ambulation. Localized radiation therapy may offer partial or complete remediation of pain whether from bone or from neurologic impairment as a result of tumor. As follow-up treatment, instruction of partial weight-bearing ambulation using crutches and application of slings on non-weight-bearing bones should be done either postoperatively or concurrent with radiation therapy. In patients with vertebral metastases spinal orthoses may be used to minimize any untoward motions and pain and to prevent further destruction of spinal vertebrae. Safety in activities of daily living must also be reviewed.

REFERENCES

1. Burgess EM: Surgery as related to prosthetics and orthotics. *Bull Prosthet Res* 1974;10:15–21.
2. Chang AE, Steinberg SM, Culnane M, et al: Functional and psychosocial effects of multimodality limb-sparing therapy in patients with soft tissue sarcoma. *J Clin Oncol* 1989;7(9):1217–1228.
3. Dalsey R, Gomez W, Seitz W Jr, et al: Myoelectric prosthetic replacement in the upper extremity amputee. *Ortho Rev* 1988;18(6):697–702.
4. Delisa JA, Miller RM, Melnick RR, et al: Rehabilitation of the cancer patient, in DeVita VT, Hellman S, Rosenberg SA (eds): *Principles and Practice of Oncology*, Philadelphia, JB Lippincott, 1983, chap. 46.
5. Deitz JH Jr: *Rehabilitation Oncology*, New York, John Wiley & Sons, 1981, pp 46–57.
6. Lampert MH, Gerber LH, Glatstein R, et al: Functional outcome of patients undergoing wide local excision and radiation therapy for soft tissue sarcoma. *Arch Phys Med Rehabil* 1984;65 (August) 477–480.
7. Lindberg RD, Martin RG, Romsdahl MM: Surgery and postoperative radio-therapy in the treatment of soft tissue sarcomas in adults. *A J Roentgenol Rad Ther Nucl Med* 1975;123:123–129.
8. Michael J: Energy storing feet: A clinical comparison. *Clin Ortho* 1987;11(3):134–168.
9. Nowroozi, Salvanelli M, Gerber LH: Energy expenditure in hip disarticulation and hemipelvectomy amputees. *Arch Phys Med Rehab* 1983;64:300–303.
10. Riley R: The amputee athlete, *Clin Ortho* 1987;3(3):109–113.

5

Phantom Limb Pain

KIM J. BURCHIEL, M.D.

OVERVIEW

When a limb is amputated either surgically or traumatically, most patients will report the perception of a phantom that replaces the lost extremity.[1] This phantom sensation is also commonly felt after complete local anesthetic blockade of the arm or leg. The phantom sensation is not simply a loss of a portion of the body image but typically a strikingly vivid perception. As the phenomenon has been better understood, a variety of treatment options have become available. Reduction of the incidence and severity of the condition is possible.

INTRODUCTION

After amputation, the incidence of unpleasant phantom sensations has been stated to be in the range of 0.5% to 10%.[1-8] More recent analyses indicate that this may be a substantial underestimate of the problem. In fact, phantom pains are present immediately after limb loss in up to 86% of cases and may persist in 60% two years after amputation.[9] Surprisingly, one of the factors that may account for this discrepancy is the observation that when the study population is a group of patients seeking treatment to relieve their pain, the rate of phantom pain decreases. Another explanation may be that phantom pain is an extremely variable phenomenon. Only about 20% of patients report daily attacks of pain, and so it may be underreported.[10] The conclusion is that phantom pain is probably a much more common entity than commonly represented in the literature.

Typically, after amputation the phantom may be perceived as distorted, grotesque or in an abnormal posture which in an intact limb would be painful. Patients can report sensations of painful telescoping of the phantom limb, uncontrollable movements of the extremity, that the nails of the phantom are being painfully driven into the palm, and burning or throbbing pains in the missing body part.

In the minority of cases, the sensation of a phantom fades with time and is never perceived as painful. In fact, the limb may seem to foreshorten as the sensations disappear. However, long-term follow-up studies of amputees indicate that the overwhelming majority of patients experience phantom pain of some degree after amputation. Carlen et al[11] found that 67% of young soldiers having traumatic amputation had pain in the phantom during the first months. Sherman and colleagues found that painful phantom sensations occurred in 78% of patients an average of 26 years after amputation.[12] In this study about half reported that the pain had decreased somewhat with time, while the other half reported no change or an increase in pain. Interestingly, this patient group received a total of 40 different treatments, but only 1% indicated lasting benefits from therapy.

In another study, Jensen and his associates found that the incidence of phantom pain eight days, six months, and two years after amputation was 72%, 65%, and 59%, respectively. In their group, within the first half year after limb amputation, phantom pain was significantly more frequent in patients with long-lasting preamputation limb pain and in patients with pain in the limb immediately prior to amputation. Both the localization and character of phantom pain changed within the first half year, but no further

change occurred later in the course. The incidence of stump pain at the same intervals was 57%, 22%, and 21%, respectively. They suggested that preoperative limb pain plays a role in phantom pain immediately after amputation, but probably not in the late persistent phantom pain.[10]

In addition to the presence of preamputation pain, other factors may influence the development of a painful phantom. Shukla et al[9] found that phantom pain developed in every case when the upper right (dominant) arm was amputated, while it occurred in only 75% of those who lost left upper extremities. Laterality differences were not evident following amputation of the legs. Lower-extremity amputees tended to experience the phantom pain earlier than those that lost upper extremities. On the other hand, Jensen et al[10] found that neither the age nor sex of the patient, the cause, or side of the amputation was related to development of phantom pain. However, they did find that phantom pain was more common in those patients with concurrent stump pain.

Phantom pain tends to become more complex with time, and in most cases the pain becomes distinctly different from the postoperative pain at the surgical site.[9,10] Fatigue, anxiety, exposure to cold, and weather changes may aggravate the condition. For some patients, seemingly benign activities such as yawning, defecation, or micturition can cause exacerbation. These observations suggest that sympathetic activation may play a role in such pain syndromes. Stump pains also seem to assume greater importance in the pattern of pain in these patients over time. Neuromas which inevitably develop in the stump can become quite mechanosensitive. Pressure on them may produce severe, lancinating (knifelike) pain. The phantom pains themselves also evolve over the first six months or so, after which the pattern becomes more stable. Pains that can be categorized as *interoceptive* (knifelike or sticking) are initially described early on, but these tend to change to more *exteroceptive* (burning or squeezing) sensations located in the distal phantom over time.[8]

PATHOPHYSIOLOGY

The pathophysiologic mechanisms underlying phantom pain are not generally agreed upon. Peripheral, segmental (spinal cord), and supraspinal mechanisms have been proposed.[8,13-15] Some authors have suggested that phantom pain is a "reminiscence" of pain existing in the limb prior to amputation, leading to the hypothesis that the phantom pain is, in effect, an "engram," or memory trace of the pain in some cerebral structures.[13,14]

Loss of sensory input to the CNS is termed *deafferentation*. We know that damage to peripheral nerves sets in motion a complex series of events. The completely transected primary afferent (sensory) neuron undergoes a sequence of physiologic changes, including slowing of conduction velocity proximal to the injury. The cell soma located in the dorsal root ganglion (DRG) swells and begins to synthesize axon membrane and intracellular proteins as part of the regenerative effort, a process identified histologically as chromatolysis. Central degeneration of the central projection of the DRG neuron (dorsal root) occurs in a small percentage of cells (transganglionic degeneration), and degeneration is even seen in higher-order neurons in the dorsal horn and other suprasegmental nuclei of the somatosensory pathways (transsynaptic degeneration).

Even as the regenerating peripheral nerve prepares to sprout distally, profound reorganization of the central somatosensory nervous system occurs. The net result of this is a rapid shift in sensory receptive fields, and changes in modality and response characteristics of central sensory neurons.[16]

Thus, deafferentation affects many levels of the nervous system, and is, to a certain extent, a process that normally does not lead to chronic pain. An example of how the CNS successfully deals with deafferentation is the loss of deciduous teeth. Although this process probably produces the same type of degenerative and reorganizational changes seen in other nerve lesions, "phantom" tooth pain is not a recognized clinical entity! How the system goes awry and generates phantom pain is still very much a matter of speculation. Two possible explanations will be discussed.

The first possibility is that the phantom pain is simply a function of pathophysiologic abnormalities that are solely at the level of the peripheral nerve/neuroma. It has been well established that injured axons and their parent DRG somata generate spontaneous electrical discharges, and that they are both abnormally mechanosensitive and chemosensitive.[17] These properties may explain some types of mechanosensitive stump pains, but it is unlikely that alone they could account for the highly structured stereotyped pains that conform to the somatotopic projection of a phantom limb. Furthermore, painful phantom sensations are relatively common after avulsive injuries of the brachial or lumbosacral plexus. In these cases the nerve roots are avulsed from the spinal cord, and therefore it is impossible for peripheral abnormalities to mediate the syndrome. On the other hand, in nonavulsive injuries, peripheral pathophysiologic abnormalities may participate in the genesis of the syndrome, and the establishment of the central pain engram.

The second general hypothesis is that phantom pain is indeed a "central" pain, not dependent on peripheral input, but set in motion by the deafferenting lesion. This model is consistent with the clinical observation that nerve root avulsion injuries produce phantom pain. A substantial amount of data also indicate that profound physiologic and functional abnormalities occur in higher-order neurons of the sensory pathway following deafferentation. Several lines of theoretical consideration have been put forth to explain the pathophysiology of the seemingly paradoxical clinical circumstance of severe, unremitting, distressing pain in an otherwise missing body part.

The often-discussed, and as often incorrectly implied as proven, mechanism of phantom pain is that deafferentation of dorsal horn nociceptive transmission neurons produces a kind of denervation hypersensitivity of the cell. The analogy has been to the case of skeletal muscle, where denervation produces hypersensitivity to acetylcholine, and spontaneous myofibrillar activity (fibrillations and fasciculations). This state of deafferentation hyperactivity has also been compared to an epileptic-like phenomenon.[18] Whether this type of denervation supersensitivity occurs after *neuronal* deafferentation remains in question. Studies of the dorsal horn in experimental animals after dorsal rhizotomy and other deafferenting lesions have both shown hyperactivity and spontaneous discharges[19–22] and no hyperactivity.[23]

An alternative view is that after deafferentation, the dorsal horn nociceptive neurons are released from "powerful central inhibitory systems." Some experimental evidence does seem to indicate that descending inhibition is diminished after dorsal horn deafferentation.[24,25] It has also been shown that receptive fields for dorsal horn neurons remaining after injury manifest dramatic shifts in their receptive fields and response characteristics.[16,19] This may imply either a change in descending control, plasticity, or even sprouting at the segmental level. How these observations might relate to the genesis of a clinical pain syndrome is unclear.

Lastly, it has been stated that deafferentation leads to a fundamental change in the neurochemical milieu of the dorsal horn. In experimental preparations there is gliosis in Lissauer's tract and the substantia gelatinosa, as well as loss of substantia gelatinosa interneurons and somatostatin terminals. It appears that following injury levels of enkephalin, substance P and somatostatin all decrease. The possibility is that there is either a denervation supersensitivity to substance P, or an "imbalance" of somatostatin/enkephalin.[26]

Thus, although it is likely that phantom pain is organized at the level of the central nervous system, it is not clear what role, if any, the various physiologic and biochemical abnormalities have in the production of the pain. This open question leads us to the third and final part of this chapter, a discussion of therapy for phantom limb pain. It is likely that by analyzing effective treatments we can gain further insights into the pathophysiologic mechanisms of phantom pain.

TREATMENT

Ideally, medical or surgical therapy should alleviate the pathology that accompanies a particular disorder. It should be specific and produce no attendant morbidity or mortality. We are severely limited in our understanding of the pathophysiology of phantom limb pain, and, primarily for this reason, treatment of this disorder has been largely empirical.

Deafferentation pain is typically intractable to conventional therapy. The pain is notoriously refractory to opiates, possibly because in many cases, the neural substrate that would normally possess opioid receptors has been damaged or destroyed by the deafferenting process. Nonopioid analgesics and nonsteroidal anti-inflammatory agents have little to no effect on this type of pain.

Available pharmacologic options can be broadly categorized in two groups: (1) anticonvulsants, such as phenytoin or carbamazepine, and (2) antidepressants, such as amitriptyline or doxepin. A general rule is that pains that are described as fleeting, lancinating, radiating, or electrical in quality will best respond to anticonvulsant therapy, particularly to carbamazepine.[27] Pains that are constant or burning in character will be better treated by the antidepressants. Because of the distressing quality of deafferentation pain, and the general tendency of "central pains" to increase with stress, anxiolytic agents may also be useful. The use of these anxiolytic or other major psychotropic drugs must be approached with great caution, since they may produce behavioral and cognitive impairment, psychologic dependence, and profound withdrawal effects.

Transcutaneous neurostimulation is rarely effective in these cases since the analgesic potential of this technique depends on intact sensation in the area of pain. This is, of course, not the situation in patients with deafferentation. Psychological counseling, relaxation techniques, biofeedback, or a formal "pain clinic program" in the outpatient or inpatient setting may be of some palliative benefit.

Overall, the best nonsurgical therapy for deafferentation pain has been only marginally effective.[14,28] This fact must be considered when we judge the indications and results of dorsal root entry zone (DREZ) lesions and other surgery for these conditions.

The procedure of selective posterior rhizotomy (SPR) as envisioned by Sindou[29] involves destruction of the lateral dorsal root and the medial portion of Lissauer's tract (LT). It consists of microsurgical incision and bipolar coagulation performed ventrolaterally at the entrance of the rootlets into the dorsolateral sulcus, along the spinal cord segments elected to be operated on. The lesion, which penetrates the lateral part of the DREZ and the medial part of LT, extends down to the apex of the dorsal horn. The lesions are 2 mm deep and made at a 45° angle (Figure 5–1). Although autopsy confirmation is lacking, these lesions are presumed to (1) preferentially destroy the pain pathway; that is, the lateral dorsal root that contains nociceptive A delta and C fibers, the medial part of LT that contains the excitatory nociceptive primary afferent collateral fibers, and possibly the superficial laminae of the dorsal horn; and (2) preserve, at least partially, the inhibitory structures of the DREZ, namely the lemniscal fibers reaching the dorsal column, as well as their recurrent collaterals to the substantia gelatinosa (SG) and the inhibitory intersegmental fibers of the lateral LT.[30]

Selective destruction of the superficial laminae of the dorsal horn was first described by Nashold[31] (Fig. 5–2). Early on, the technique involved the use of an RF electrode without temperature control. Thermocoupled temperature monitoring electrodes have become available for the DREZ operation only in the past several years. Recent reports of DREZ lesions made by CO_2 laser have also indicated that the damage to tracts in proximity to the DREZ can be largely avoided by a discrete laser lesion.[32–35]

It is not yet clear which laminae of the dorsal horn need to be destroyed to maximally alleviate the pain. Available autopsy data[34] would indicate that the deeper layers (IV–VI), are coagulated by DREZ lesion. Nevertheless, the intent of the operation is to disrupt at least the first five layers of Rexed (2 mm depth).[18]

DREZ lesions have a limited, but definite, role in the management of postamputation pain. Saris et al[35] have reported a series of 22 cases with limb amputations of various causes, and either phantom pain, stump pain, or both. Follow-up was six months to four years. Only eight patients had pain relief, no patient with stump pain alone had relief, and only two of seven patients with stump and phantom pain were improved. However, good results were obtained in six of nine (67%) patients with phantom pain alone, and five of six (83%) patients with traumatic amputations associated with root avulsion.

Using RF DREZ lesions, Young[36] has likewise

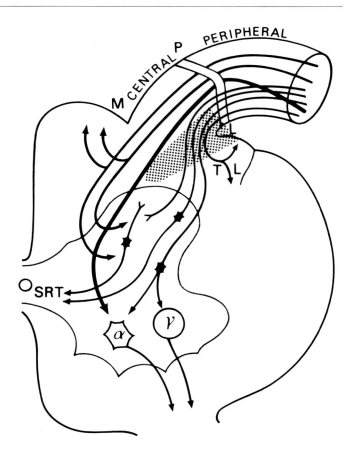

Figure 5–1. Fiber organization of the dorsal root at its entry zone into spinal cord and the selective posterior rhizotomy (SPR) technique. Each rootlet has both a peripheral and central component. The junction between the two constitutes the pial ring (P). Peripherally the fibers have no organization. Near the pial ring, the small fibers are situated on the rootlet surface, predominantly on its lateral side. In its central component these small fibers group laterally (3) to enter Lissauer's tract and the posterior horn. The large fibers are situated centrally for the myotactic fibers and medially for the lemniscal (proprioceptive and cutaneous) ones. Selective posterior rhizotomy affects the shaded triangle. Posterior rootlet projections to the spinal cord. The small fibers terminate on the spinoreticulothalamic (SRT) cells, which they activate, and by polysynaptic arcs on the gamma and alpha motoneurons of the anterior horn. The short collateral of the large fibers (of cutaneous or proprioceptive origin) terminate on and inhibit the SRT cells (modified from Sindou and Daher[30]).

obtained good results in 67% of a group of postamputation pain patients. In a small series of patients, Dieckmann and Veras[37] have also found that phantom pain after amputation is reduced in 80% of cases after DREZ lesion. Sindou and Daher[30] found that

SPR also relieved either stump or stump and phantom pain in three of four cases (75%) after follow-up of 2 to 14 years.

Thus, DREZ lesions may be used for postamputation pain, but at present it appears they are most

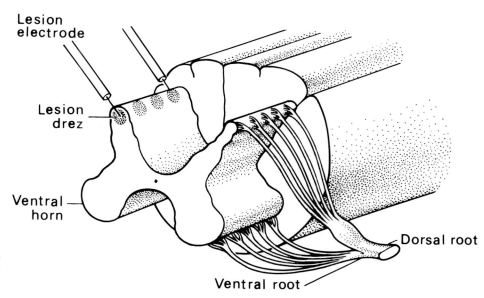

Figure 5–2. Schematic drawing showing the dorsal root entry zone and the region for DREZ lesions (modified from Nashold[18]).

useful in cases where phantom rather than stump pain, possibly due to neuromata, predominates.

Stump pain that is mechanical in origin, particularly pain associated with Tinel's phenomena in the stump, may respond to treatment of associated neuromas. The temptation is to remove these neuromas, and sometimes mere excision of a neuroma with development of a subsequent neuroma at a site not subject to repeated mechanical stimulation will suffice to relieve the pain. However, neuroma resection must be approached with trepidation since this may also produce further denervation and increased pain. Therefore, only in selected cases neuromas may be excised and the nerve reimplanted into muscle or bone marrow to facilitate regeneration without neuroma formation.

CONCLUSIONS

Phantom pain most likely has its origins in the central nervous system's response to complete loss of sensory input from all or part of a limb. The pain is difficult to treat medically or surgically, but recent advances in surgical neuroablative techniques directed at the dorsal horn and root entry zone show promise. Improvement in the recognition and early treatment of phantom limb pain may help to reduce its incidence and severity.

REFERENCES

1. Melzack R, Wall PD: *The Challenge of Pain.* New York, Basic Books, 1983.
2. Abramson AS, Feibel A: The phantom phenomenon: Its use and disuse. *Bull NY Acad Med* 1981;57:99–112.
3. Browder J, Gallagher JP: Dorsal cordotomy for painful phantom limbs. *Ann Surg* 1948;128:456–469.
4. Cronholm B: Phantom limb in amputees. *Acta Psychiat Neurol Scand* 1951;72(suppl):1–310.
5. Ewalt JR, Randall GC, Morris H: The phantom limb. *Psychosom. Med* 1947;9:118–123.
6. Henderson, WR, Smyth GE: Phantom limbs. *J Neurol Neurosurg Psychiat* 1948;11:88–112.
7. Herrmann LG, Gibbs, EW: Phantom limb pain. *Am J Surg* 1945;67:168–180.
8. Jensen TS, Rasmussen P: Amputation, in Wall, PD, Melzack R (eds): *Textbook of Pain.* Edinburg, Churchill Livingstone, 1984, pp 402–412.
9. Shukla GD, Sahu SC, Tripathi RP, et al: Phantom limb: A phenomenological study. *Br J Psychiatr* 1982;141:54–58.
10. Jensen TS, Krebs B, Nielsen J, et al: Immediate and long-term phantom limb pain in amputees: Incidence, clinical characteristics and relationship to pre-amputation limb pain. *Pain* 1985;21:267–278.
11. Carlen PL, Wall PD, Nadvorna H, et al: Phantom limbs and related phenomena in recent traumatic amputations. *Neurology (Minneap)* 1978;28:211–217.
12. Sherman RA, Sherman CJ, Parker L: Chronic phantom and stump pain among American veterans: Results of a survey. *Pain* 1984;18:83–95.
13. Melzack R: Phantom limb pain. Implications for treatment of pathological pain. *Anesthesiology* 1971;35:409–419.
14. Melzack R, Loeser JD: Phantom body pain in paraplegia: Evidence for a central "pattern generating mechanism" for pain. *Pain* 1979;4:195–210.
15. Wall PD: On the origin of pain associated with amputation, in Siegfried J, Zimmerman M (eds): *Phantom and Stump Pain*, Springer, Berlin, 1981, pp 2–14.
16. Devor M, Wall PD: Reorganization of spinal cord sensory map after peripheral nerve injury. *Nature* 1978;276:75–76.
17. Wall PD, Gutnick M: Ongoing activity in peripheral nerves. The physiology and pharmacology of impulses originating in a neuroma. *Exp Neurol* 1974;43:580–593.
18. Nashold BS Jr, Higgins AC, Blumenkopf B: Dorsal root entry zone lesions for pain relief, in Wall PD, Melzack R (eds): *Pain.* Edinburgh, Churchill Livingstone, 1984, pp 2433–2437.
19. Basbaum AI, Wall PD: Chronic changes in the response of cells in adult cat dorsal horn following partial deafferentation: The appearance of responding cells in a previously nonresponsive region. *Brain Res* 1976;116:181–204.
20. Brinkus HB, Zimmerman M: Characteristics of spinal dorsal horn neurons after partial chronic deafferentation by dorsal root transection. *Pain* 1983;15:221–236.
21. Kjerulf TD, Loeser JD: Neuronal hyperactivity following deafferentation of the lateral cuneate nucleus. *Exp Neurol* 1973;39:70–85.
22. Loeser JD, Ward AA Jr: Some effects of deafferentation on neurons of the cat spinal cord. *Arch Neurol* 1967;17:629–636.
23. Pubols LM, Goldberger ME: Recovery of function in dorsal horn following partial deafferentation. *J Neurophysiol* 1980;43:102–118.
24. Ovelmen-Levitt J, Johnson B, Bedenbaugh P, et al: Dorsal root rhizotomy and avulsion in the cat: A comparison of long term effects on dorsal horn neuronal activity. 1984;15:921–927.
25. Teasdale RD, Stravraky GW: Responses of deafferented spinal neurons to corticospinal impulses. *J Neurophysiol* 1953;16:367–373.
26. Blumenkopf B: Neuropharmacology of the dorsal root entry zone. *Neurosurgery* 1984;15:900–903.
27. Swerdlow M: The treatment of shooting pain. *Postgrad Med J* 1980;56:159–161.
28. Pagni CA: Central pain and painful anesthesia: Pathophysiology and treatment of sensory deprivation syndromes due to central and peripheral nervous system lesions. *Prog Neurol Surg* 1976;8:132–257.
29. Sindou M: *Etude de la jonction radiculo-medullaire posterieure: la radicellotomie posterieure selective dans la chirurgie de la douleur,* these. Lyon, p 182.
30. Sindou M, Daher A: Spinal cord ablation procedures for pain, in Dubner R, Gebhart GF, Bone MR (eds): *Proceedings of the Fifth World Congress on Pain.* Amsterdam, Elsevier, 1988, pp 477–495.
31. Nashold BS Jr, Urban B, Zorub DS: Phantom relief by focal destruction of substantia gelatinosa of Rolando. *Adv Pain Res Ther* 1976;1:959–963.
32. Levy WJ, Nutkiewicz A, Ditmore QM, et al: Laser-

induced dorsal root entry zone lesions for pain control. *J Neurosurg* 1983;59:884–886.

33. Powers SK, Adams JE, Edwards SB, et al: Pain relief from dorsal root entry zone lesions made with argon and carbon dioxide microsurgical lasers. *J Neurosurg* 1984;61:841–847.

34. Iacono RP, Aguirre ML, Nashold BS Jr: Anatomic examination of human DREZ lesions. *Appl Neurophysiol* 1988;51:225–229.

35. Saris SC, Iacono RP, Nashold BS Jr: Dorsal root entry zone lesions for post-amputation pain. *J Neurosurg* 1985;62:72–76.

36. Young RF: Radio frequency and laser drez lesions. *J Neurosurg* 1990;72:715–720.

37. Dieckman G, Veras G: High frequency coagulation of dorsal root entry zone in patients with deafferantation pain. *Acta Neurochir*, Suppl. 1984 33:445–450.

6

Combined Wide Local Excision Plus High-Dose Radiation for Sarcoma

PAUL H. SUGARBAKER, M.D.
JULIANA SIMMONS, M.D.

OVERVIEW

Wide local excision plus radiation therapy is the most common plan for treating soft tissue sarcoma. For head, neck, and truncal sarcomas it is the treatment option routinely employed. For extremity sarcoma, wide excision plus radiation therapy is one of several treatments available. Routine examinations needed to evaluate the primary tumor include a careful physical examination, plain radiographs, and a bone scan. Computed axial tomography, arteriography, and venography are frequently needed to decide if wide local excision can adequately remove the primary tumor without exposing the tumor capsule during its excision and without spillage of malignant cells. The surgeon should strive to achieve a 2- to 3 cm margin of normal tissue surrounding the tumor specimen. To ensure this margin, the procedure begins with the construction of skin flaps to the lateral extent of the dissection. This is determined by palpation of the tumor mass through surrounding soft tissue. Repeatedly during the dissection the lateral and deep margins of excision are reevaluated to determine their adequacy. The surgeon is guided in this dissection by the extent of tumor rather than by anatomic landmarks. The margins of the dissection are marked by metal clips to help plan the field of radiation. Following examination of the specimen by the pathologist, skin flaps are closed over generous suction drainage after the incision is securely healed. High-dose radiation therapy is applied over a wide field that includes a large portion of the muscle group.

INDICATIONS FOR TREATMENT BY WIDE LOCAL EXCISION PLUS RADIATION THERAPY

Wide local excision plus radiation therapy is the treatment of choice for nearly all head, neck, and truncal sarcomas. Few other treatment plans are suitable. Local excision plus high-dose radiation was reported by Suite and co-workers to give a high incidence of local control with maintenance of a useful extremity.[1-3] Recent studies by Rosenberg and colleagues support the reliability of this option for treating extremity soft tissue sarcoma.[4] This treatment modality has become the one most frequently employed and is applicable to a wide variety of tumors in many different locations. Unless amputation is indicated, it is usually employed for tumors in the lower extremity below the knee joint and for upper extremity tumors. A wide excision of anterior tibial muscles, or gastrocnemius plus soleus muscle, rarely achieves the generous negative margins required of a compartmental excision so that radiation is needed postoperatively. If the tumor is present over the ankle, knee, or hip joint, merely obtaining negative margins of excision may be extremely difficult, and a compartmental excision is out of the question. In sarcomas of the hand or foot, the location of the tumor demands that high-dose radiation therapy be delivered. The hand is not traumatized nearly so repetitively as the foot, so that radiation therapy for hand sarcomas is usually well tolerated.

Another major indication for wide local excision plus radiation therapy as a treatment modality involves those sarcomas that occur between muscular compartments or at the limits of a muscle compartment. For example, tumors that occur along the superficial femoral artery, between the quadriceps and adductor muscle groups, cannot be treated adequately by a compartmental excision. However, a sarcoma in these difficult anatomic locations can usually be removed with a narrow rim of normal muscle and fibrous tissue. Then a wide margin of muscle around the resection site is irradiated to a total dose of 6,000 rads.

MARGINS OF EXCISION

In order for this treatment modality to succeed, the primary sarcoma cannot be excised through its pseudocapsule. If this is done, microscopic and gross deposits of tumor will remain following the excision. Rosenberg and colleagues have shown clearly that even a microscopically positive margin of excision leaves the patient at very high risk of local recurrence, even if a radical approach to radiation therapy is used.[5] Of 53 sarcomas excised with a negative margin at the NIH, there were no local recurrences. However, eight patients were noted by the pathologist upon final examination of the specimen to have microscopically positive margins of resection. In three of these eight patients local recurrence developed, and two of these three patients later died of systemic disease. Wanebo and colleagues and Rosenberg and colleagues have suggested that there may be a cause-and-effect relationship between local recurrence and systemic disease.[5,6]

PHYSICAL AND RADIOLOGIC EVALUATION FOR DISTANT DISEASE

An essential part of the preoperative workup includes an evaluation seeking distant disease. This includes a search for enlarged local lymph nodes by physical examination and radiologic evaluation. The pulmonary parenchyma should be meticulously examined using computerized tomography taken at 1-cm intervals. If lesions in the lung are found, it may be necessary to perform a thoracotomy or a median sternotomy in order to examine lung tissue before deciding on definitive local therapy. A bone scan is performed to assess spread to the skeleton. Common sites of bony metastases from soft tissue sarcoma include the skull and the ribs.

PHYSICAL AND RADIOLOGIC WORKUP OF THE PRIMARY TUMOR

The preoperative workup of the extremity sarcoma itself includes four different components. First, a careful physical examination must be performed. One tries to determine if the tumor is attached to bony, vascular, or essential nerve structures. The size of the lesion is important in this evaluation, because very large tumors, even when they occur within a muscular compartment, are liable to extend to bone or to an essential artery or nerve and are unlikely to be excised adequately with a negative margin by compartmental excision. It is important to determine whether skin is involved by tumor and to estimate the extent to which skin sacrifice is required around the biopsy site. If hemorrhage into the skin, muscle, or fascia after a previous biopsy was extensive, this hemorrhage may have tumor-contaminated the tissues that blood penetrated. Tumor-contaminated tissues should be included within the wide excision specimen if possible.

Second, the bone scan is used to help determine cortical involvement of bone by tumor. If a bone scan is grossly abnormal in the area of soft tissue sarcoma, one can assume that the tumor involves the bone. This patient then is a better candidate for amputation than for wide excision plus radiation or for compartmental excision. Lesser amounts of increased technetium uptake suggest increased vascularity because of the close proximity of the tumor. If the bone scan is negative, it does not mean that the tumor never involves bone, although usually the periosteum will be clear. It does not mean that a negative margin of excision can be achieved by a wide excision. That assessment can be made definitively only at the time of surgery.

Arteriography and venography are essential, especially with large tumors, to assess the relationship of the sarcoma to major vessels. Also, it is often useful to identify major vessels to the tumor so that these can be ligated early in the wide excision. The association of a tumor blush with major vessels, nerves, and bone may be a great help in estimating resectability.

Finally, a high-quality computerized tomogram is of benefit in assessing the position of the tumor within a muscle group and in assessing its relationship to the major muscle groups of the extremity. However, because tumor and muscle usually cannot be discriminated by differing attenuations on a computerized tomogram, one cannot assume a positive margin on bone or vessels because a tumor mass as seen on the scan is directly adjacent to one of these structures. At surgery, normal muscle may be found compressed between tumor and bone or tumor and vasculature when computerized tomography suggested no adequate margin. Again, one must realize that it is often impossible to determine the adequacy of a local resection before surgical exploration.

IMPORTANCE OF TUMOR BIOLOGY

Adequate margins of resection with a low-grade soft tissue or bony sarcoma may be totally inadequate margins with a high-grade deeply infiltrating tumor. Extension along normal tissue planes, vascular structures, and nerve bundles is to be expected with high-grade cancer, but rarely occurs with the grade I cancers. Penetration of high-grade tumor along lymphatic channels may give rise to daughter metastases that cross muscle bundles so that 1–2-cm margins will leave gross tumor behind. In contrast, dissecting low-grade cancer off bone, major vessels, or major nerve bundles may be acceptable for local recurrence is not inevitable even with inadequate margins with this type of cancer. Even if local recurrence is observed, it may take years to develop and its occurrence is not associated with systemic disease. An amputation or reexcision plus radiation therapy may be the appropriate treatment if local recurrence occurs.

PROCEDURE

For low-grade soft tissue sarcoma wide excision is merely designed to achieve negative margins of resection. In contrast the intent of surgery in a wide local excision for high-grade sarcoma is to optimally prepare the patient for high-dose wide-field irradiation. The surgeon must establish negative margins of resection, but must prevent unnecessary sacrifice of normal tissue so that maximal function is preserved. What follows is an example of the techniques employed in a wide local excision of a high-grade liposarcoma located in the anterior thigh between quadriceps and adductor muscle groups.

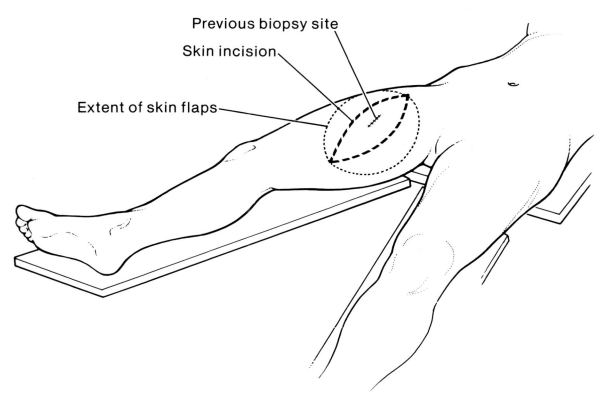

Figure 6–1. INCISION AND SKIN FLAPS. The extremity is prepared and draped from a joint above to a joint below the tumor. If one is working in and around vessels the entire extremity, including the toes, should be excluded from the drapes so that the adequacy of peripheral pulses and perfusion of the extremity distally can be assessed during the procedure. If povidone-iodine is used for skin preparation, it should be washed off with alcohol so that normal skin color can be assessed. The skin incision should be drawn out so that the previous biopsy site and any tumor-contaminated soft tissue are excised. The skin flaps should be marked out to their most distal extent at the margins of palpable tumor. If this is done at the beginning of the procedure, then one is not in danger of dissecting an unnecessarily wide skin flap later in this procedure.

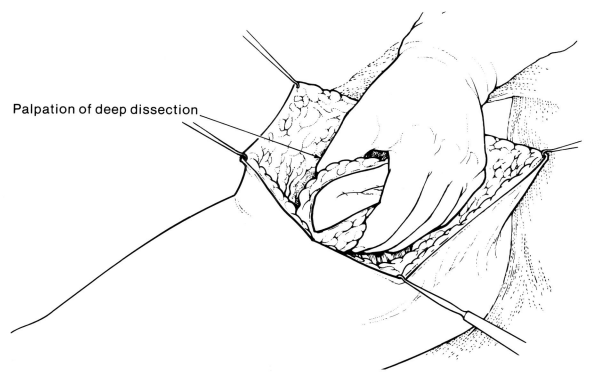

Palpation of deep dissection

Figure 6–2. DETERMINING THE EXTENT OF LATERAL DISSECTION. After the skin flaps are constructed the surgeon can better appreciate the extent of the tumor mass. Muscle and fascia directly over the tumor and for 2 to 3 cm on its sides are sacrificed with the specimen. The adequacy of this excision is grossly monitored by frequent palpation of the mass to assess its extent and its relationship to muscle bundles and other structures.

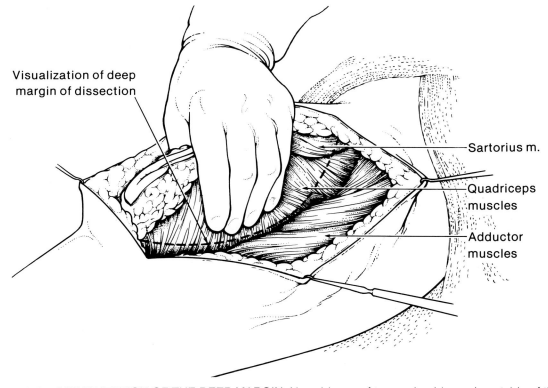

Visualization of deep margin of dissection

Sartorius m.

Quadriceps muscles

Adductor muscles

Figure 6–3. VISUALIZATION OF THE DEEP MARGIN. No evidence of tumor should remain outside of the dissected specimen. In an attempt to eliminate all tumor tissue, the base of the surgical field should be inspected visually. This examination should be repeated frequently during the course of the procedure. Before the incision is closed, the extent of resection is marked with metallic clips and the pathologist is asked to monitor the adequacy of the resection.

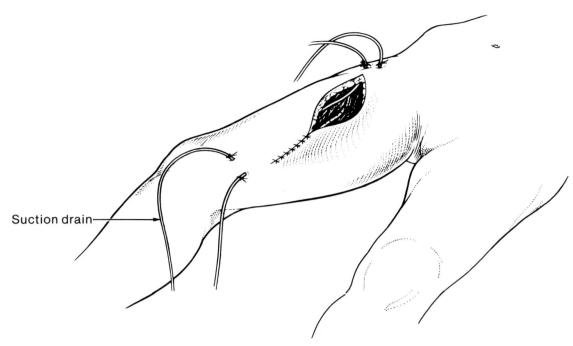

Suction drain

Figure 6–4. CLOSURE OVER GENEROUS SUCTION DRAINAGE. A large surface area of transected muscle tissue may remain after wide excision. Generous suction drainage should be used to hold the skin flaps in direct apposition to the base of the dissection. If the amount of transected muscle and tissue is extensive, prolonged catheter drainage should be expected. To minimize the likelihood of infection ascending along the drain tracts, sterile precautions should be used when the dressing is changed over the suction drains. No circumferential elastic wrap should be used to hold down the skin flaps because this may result in ischemia of the flaps from pressure. Immobilization, elevation of the extremity, and bed rest will help reduce the suction catheter drainage as rapidly as possible.

RADIATION THERAPY FOR SOFT TISSUE SARCOMA

Technical Considerations

In treating patients with truncal or extremity soft tissue sarcoma, one needs to employ optimum techniques for the unique problems of the individual patient to achieve optimal cosmetic and functional results, as well as local tumor control. To maximize the potential benefit of radiation therapy, it is essential that the patient be seen by both the radiation oncologist and the surgeon prior to any surgical procedure. This allows opportunity for discussion of such issues as the tumor extent and location as seen on pre-operative CT and/or MRI scans, the location of the incision site, location of drain sites, the extent of the surgical procedure planned, the anticipated functional result, and the importance of the placement of radio-opaque clips at defined anatomic points in relation to the tumor bed to allow for future planning of radiation portals. The planning for radiation therapy is complex because of the need to treat large sloping anatomic compartments which are not localized to easily identifiable quadrants. For ex-

tremity sarcoma there is the need to spare a contiguous strip of skin and subcutaneous tissue (ie, a sector of the extremity cross section) to allow for lymphatic drainage from the distal extremity. These considerations are critical if the goal of a useful, pain-free, and edema-free limb are to be realized.

Shrinking-Field Technique

The radiation oncologist will typically treat the anatomic compartment with large fields, encompassing the tissues manipulated at surgery to a moderate radiation dose of 5,000 cGy, in hopes of sterilizing microscopic disease. This is best achieved by complex treatment planning, field shaping using customized individual blocks, and the use of wedge filters or tissue compensators to correct for the varied tissue thickness throughout the portals. Additionally, to reduce the risk of radiation osteitis and pathologic fracture in the future, the portals are often angled to avoid the entire circumference of the bone. This may require splints to hold the extremity in an unusual position during the delivery of each treatment. Multiple ports are employed to deliver a uniform dose to the target volume. Each port is treated each day, and a daily tumor dose of 180–200 cGy is delivered, usually five times per week.

The radiation field is then reduced to include only the tumor bed, and an additional 500–1,500 cGy is delivered at the same rate. If the scar is not within the maximally irradiated volume, a bolus is often used to bring the dose given to the surgical scar to 6,000 cGy. Skin sparing seen with the higher megavoltage radiation beams requires this technique. It is at this point in the treatment course that the surgical markers of the tumor bed are critical; they must all be included in the radiation field. The tissue margins extending from the tumor and/or the tumor bed included in the initial volume depend on the grade and size of the mass. For large and/or high-grade tumors the proximal and distal margins are often as wide as 10 cm. Once the fields are reduced, they shrink to 4 to 5 cm.

Radiation Therapy for Patients with Residual Tumor

A final-boost target volume is treated in those patients who were unresectable, and thus treated solely by radiation, or in those patients with gross residual tumor at the time of resection. In this field a 2-cm margin is treated around the detectable tumor or the volume of tissue suspected to contain tumor. The tumor dose is at least 7,000 cGy, depending on the size of the tumor. It should be noted that in certain systemic disease states, such as systemic lupus erythematosis, rheumatoid arthritis, and scleroderma, there is an increased sensitivity to radiation. In those patients only 90% of the normal dose is delivered.

The final tumor dose delivered to an extremity or truncal resection site is governed by normal tissue tolerances. Ideally, one would spare one third or more of the circumference of the limb. Often this is not possible. The minimal width of tissue (as measured from the surface to the center of the extremity) should be 2 cm for the forearm, 3 cm for the lower leg, and 4 cm for the thigh. The preservation of this strip throughout the length of the treated limb helps reduce fibrosis, muscular contractions, pain, and edema. It is also important that while undergoing the course of radiation, which lasts for six to eight weeks, the patient participate in a gentle physical therapy program to help prevent the development of severe muscular contractures and to improve long-term function.

Most soft tissue sarcomas of the extremities today are treated with a combination of surgery and radiation therapy, often with chemotherapy as well. To ensure the optimal integration of these modalities, the surgeon and radiation oncologist should formulate the treatment approach prior to the surgical procedure and conjointly with the medical oncologist. There are many technical hurdles to overcome as one attempts to deliver relatively high doses of radiation to tissues with significant inhomogeneities. At times special needs for extended treatment distances, the need for electron beam capability, the lack of advanced computerized treatment planning systems, and the unavailability of knowledgeable physicists and/or dosimetrists may lead to the referral of difficult patients to more appropriate facilities to offer the best chance for a good result.

DISCUSSION

Unfortunately, anatomic landmarks by which the surgeon can monitor the adequacy of a wide local excision do not exist. The surgeon's task is to reduce the patient's tumor burden to a minimum and yet preserve as much function as possible. The less microscopic residual tumor that remains following surgical excision, the greater the likelihood that radiation therapy will eradicate the disease. This often means that the surgeon attempts to make adequate decisions but has only inadequate information for guidance. To optimize favorable results from surgery, technical requirements for performing a wide excision for sarcoma have evolved. The surgical recommendations for wide excision of an extremity sarcoma are developed here.

The Biopsy Must Not Interfere with Subsequent Definitive Excision.   In performing the initial biopsy, care must be taken that this procedure does not interfere with subsequent definitive therapy. Therefore, all incisions should be made longitudinally, rather than transversely, to the course of the extremity. Also, a majority of tumors should be removed by an incisional rather than excisional biopsy. Only the smallest lesions should be excised in toto. If an excisional biopsy of a large sarcoma is attempted, major bleeding may result and tumor-contaminated hematoma may spread widely along the tissue planes of an extremity. This may make further limb salvage treatment impossible and cause amputation to be the only safe treatment alternative. In general, the minimal procedure to adequately sample the tumor should be recommended. However, a needle biopsy or aspiration cytology is discouraged, because the tumor sample is usually not adequate for satisfactory pathologic examination of a sarcoma.

The Extent of the Margins of Resection May Vary with Tumor Grade. When planning the definitive therapy, the tumor mass and biopsy site with any surrounding tumor-contaminated tissue must be excised with margins negative for tumor; however, the extent of the free margin may vary with tumor type. For example, in a neurofibrosarcoma, tumor may extend many inches above the major tumor mass along a major nerve fascicle. Other tumors may extend several inches along tendon sheaths. This is often true for epithelioid sarcoma and synovial sarcoma. In a low-grade liposarcoma a smaller free margin may be tolerated. No one knows the precise negative margin of excision required for each tumor. Generally, one attempts to leave 2–3 cm of normal tissue on the specimen beyond the tumor. As mentioned previously, the data of Rosenberg and colleagues suggest that a margin microscopically positive for tumor may result in an unusually high local recurrence rate of approximately 40%.[5]

Determine Inoperability Early in the Dissection. The surgeon should plan the procedure to determine if a local resection is feasible as early in the procedure as possible. For instance, if a high-grade sarcoma occurs in and around the superficial and deep femoral arteries and is found to be intimately involved with these structures at the time of surgery, a hemipelvectomy will be required. Determining early in the procedure that these essential vessels are involved may spare a large amount of unnecessary dissection.

Consult the Radiation Therapist Prior to Surgical Intervention. Consultation with the radiation therapist must be obtained before surgery. The radiation therapist must know the extent of the field of radiation and the structures that are within this field. He or she must be aware of the venous and, especially, lymphatic structures that have been sacrificed. If lymphatic damage was extensive with surgery and if the remaining lymphatics are irradiated, then a swollen, painful extremity may result from the combined therapy. Also, with large tumors of the upper thigh and buttock, the radiation field that would be mandated by wide excision may be so enormous that a poor result is expected. In some instances, hemipelvectomy may be a better treatment option than surgery plus wide field radiation.

Mark the Margins of the Dissection with Metal Clips. The extent of surgery must be marked with metal clips after the dissection. These clips allow the radiation therapist to ensure that all potentially tumor-contaminated tissues that were open at the time of tumor resection are included in the radiation field.

The Pathologist Must Monitor the Specimen before Closing the Incision. The surgeon depends heavily on the pathologist to decide on the adequacy of margins and the need for further excision. For some low-grade sarcomas the pathologist's report may suggest no need for postoperative radiation therapy. Before the patient is awakened from anesthesia, the pathologist should report to the surgeon the results of his or her gross observations and cryostat sections. Some small tumors can be removed with a generous margin of muscle and other soft tissues; these tumors are not expected to recur, even without radiation therapy. This is especially true of low-grade malignancies that are unlikely to metastasize distantly and unlikely to be extensively invasive locally. An example of this tumor type is myxoid liposarcoma.

Neither the Surgical Excision nor the Radiation Therapy Should Interfere with Subsequent Amputation. If at all possible, the treatment that is planned, including both surgery and radiation therapy, should not jeopardize subsequent amputation should it be indicated. Radiation therapy should not heavily irradiate buttock skin in treating upper-thigh sarcomas, because this would make hemipelvectomy difficult or impossible.

Use Early and Aggressive Rehabilitation. Physical therapy and psychological counseling may be required as an essential part of this multimodality treatment. Early vigorous physical therapy is indicated. If radiation therapy is used across a joint, physical therapy during the treatment is required for a good functional result. It should be emphasized that the morbidity of this multimodality treatment is not always minimal. Long-term suction catheter drainage may result in wound infection. Extensive sacrifice of soft tissue plus high-dose irradiation may make the quality-of-life advantage of this treatment modality no different than with amputation.[7] The effects of high-dose irradiation around the upper thigh or buttock may result in severe sexual dysfunction. The loss of fertility in young patients that results from radiation therapy may be an overriding consideration and make amputation the preferred treatment.

Systemic Chemotherapy is Indicated for Large High-Grade Soft Tissue Sarcomas. Recent studies have shown that adriamycin and cytoxan chemotherapy improves the survival of patients with extremity soft tissue sarcoma. With the destruction of microscopic foci of tumor that adjuvant chemotherapy is affecting, the role of radiation is less clear. It is possible that chemotherapy alone can eliminate microscopic deposits of tumor in the soft tissue surrounding the wide excision as well as in the lungs. The role of radiation therapy in treating extremity sarcoma, now that chemotherapy seems indicated, is unclear. The problem awaits the results of further clinical trials.

SELECTION OF TREATMENT

Selection of Treatment Alternatives: Amputation versus Limb Salvage

Treatment decisions for patients with soft tissue and bony sarcomas of an extremity depend primarily on the anatomic location of the tumor and the tumor grade. For soft tissue sarcoma, these considerations lead the surgeon to choose amputation, limb salvage surgery plus irradiation, or muscle group excision. In patients with osteosarcoma prosthetic replacement of bone is considered as a reasonable option in selected patients. In other patients amputation is recommended in the local management of the cancer.

Definitely, some soft tissue sarcomas can be treated only by amputation. As discussed in earlier chapters, these tumors are thought to be so extensive that wide excision or muscle group excision would lead to a positive margin of resection. The indications for amputation are shown in Table 6–1.

There are many patients in whom limb salvage surgery is obviously the treatment of choice. With surgery, a negative margin can be obtained, and satisfactory doses of irradiation therapy can be delivered so that local control is expected in almost all of these patients. Systemic chemotherapy may or may not be indicated.

Therapeutic Dilemma

It must be obvious, though, that a spectrum of disease exists with extremity sarcoma. Tumors that are considered in a gray zone where no "obvious treatment plan" can be formulated are frequently encountered. With both soft tissue sarcoma and osteosarcoma, selection of one alternative over another may not always be a straightforward treatment decision. Some clinicians may think that a limb salvage procedure may give reasonable local tumor control; others may only consider amputation. Perhaps a negative margin is possible, but it will be only a few millimeters. Perhaps the tumor involves a major vascular structure or nerve but can be dissected away from those structures with a positive tumor margin. Perhaps the tumor can be excised, but the resulting volume of tissues that will require high-dose wide-field irradiation is so extensive that the adequacy of x-ray therapy is questioned. Not only would the dose of x-ray be suboptimal, but it is entirely possible that the morbidity of such extensive radiation treatment should be expected to be extremely high.

Figure 6–5 illustrates how the treatment alternatives available in the care of extremity soft tissue sarcoma patients may cause a clinical dilemma. Patients shown to be clinically free of disseminated disease are candidates for amputation or limb salvage surgery. A majority of patients (perhaps 60%) are good candidates for wide excision plus irradiation. Another 10% to 20% clearly need amputation because of the great likelihood of a positive margin of resection, or involvement of a major vessel, nerve, or bone. However, in 10% to 20% of patients evaluation of the primary tumor may suggest, but not establish, that limb salvage surgery will result in local treatment failure.

Table 6–1. Indications for Amputation with Extremity Sarcoma

1. *Local recurrence* of a high-grade malignancy.
2. *Major vascular involvement.* The incidence of morbidity and failure associated with resection and reconstruction are significantly higher if a vascular graft is required.
3. *Major nerve involvement.* In general, one nerve may be removed, but a two-nerve deficit results in an extremely poor functional extremity. It does not benefit the patient to preserve a functionless extremity. Nerve grafting has not been effective except in carefully selected anatomic sites.
4. *Involvement of bone* plus surrounding soft tissue so that prosthetic replacement is unlikely to result in local control.
5. *Extensive local soft tissue contamination.* Local contamination often occurs due to prior surgery and/or a poorly planned biopsy. It increases the risk of local recurrence.
6. *Pathologic fracture.* A fracture through a tumor in a weight-bearing bone results in hematoma. Tumor emboli occur within the hemorrhage that dissects along tissue planes. Contamination results beyond the local area, making reliable removal difficult.
7. *Infection.* Infection of the tumor itself or biopsy site will often negate an attempt at local resection and reconstruction. Infection may limit attempts at preoperative and/or postoperative chemotherapy.
8. *Skeletal immaturity.* High doses of radiotherapy result in limb-strength discrepancy and contractures in patients who are not yet fully grown.

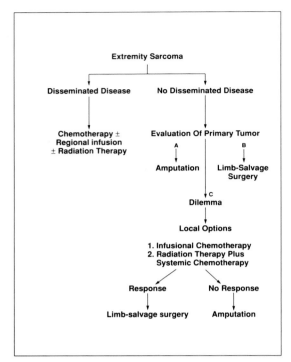

Figure 6–5. Treatment alternatives for extremity soft tissue (A) Amputation is indicated if evaluation of primary tumor shows that proximal margin of resection is positive with limb salvage; major vessel or nerve is involved by primary tumor; or major bone is involved. (B) Limb salvage is indicated if evaluation of primary tumor shows that local treatment failure is unlikely. (C) Problem group of patients exists in whom the examinations of the primary tumor do not give sufficient precise information to choose the optimal treatment alternative.

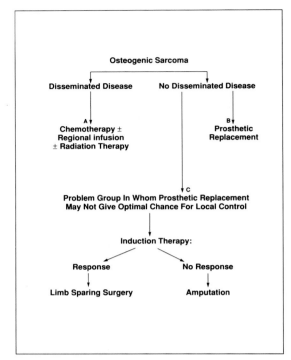

Figure 6–6. Treatment alternatives for osteosarcoma of the femur (A) Amputation is indicated if a high-grade tumor shows extensive soft tissue involvement or positive margin on major nerves and vessels. (B) Prosthetic replacement is indicated with low-grade tumors showing minimal or no soft tissue involvement. (C) Problem group of patients in whom examination of the primary tumor does not give sufficient precise information to choose the optimal treatment alternative.

Although most of this chapter concerns soft tissue sarcoma, it should be pointed out that the treatment alternatives for osteosarcoma of the femur are similar (see Fig. 6–6). Here, a majority of patients need amputation, but, as technology improves, more and more patients may profit from prosthetic replacement of bone. Yet 10% to 20% of patients fall into the "gray area" where examinations of the primary tumor do not give sufficient information to make a clear choice between treatment alternatives.

In recent years the concept of induction therapy has had a definite impact in medical decision making in the Treatment Dilemma Group. As illustrated in Figure 6–5, these patients are considered ideal candidates for preoperative infusional chemotherapy or preoperative radiation therapy plus systemic chemotherapy. Inductive chemotherapy is indicated in the clinical situations listed in Table 6–2. Most simply stated, one should use induction chemotherapy to shrink the primary tumor if a less-than-perfect surgical result is suspected. Above all, if one may enter the tumor mass and disseminate tumor cells within the

operative field with a local resection, inductive treatments are required.

Infusional chemotherapy administered through the relevant arterial supply to the sarcoma can sufficiently shrink a large tumor, allowing one to consider a limb salvage approach (see chapter 7). If a large tumor mass can be reduced in volume, normal tissue planes surrounding the malignancy can be better

---

Table 6–2. Indications for Inductive Chemotherapy

1. When tumor spillage within the operative field is a potential complication of the wide local resection
2. When a large tumor mass is present and is directly adjacent to vital structures (major vessels, major nerves, or major bones)
3. Whenever shrinkage of the primary tumor mass will facilitate surgical resection
4. When the preoperative clinical evaluation suggests disseminated disease
5. When the patient refuses amputation
6. When the primary tumor cannot be removed with a generous margin of excision by an amputation

appreciated by the preoperative radiologic studies. Also, tumor shrinkage may allow the surgeon to work in an operative field that is not so extremely distorted by the presence of a large tumor mass. Working over the top of a large tumor mass can make an otherwise anatomically simple wide excision extremely difficult.

MEDICAL DECISION MAKING AND QUALITY-OF-LIFE ASSESSMENT. IS AN AMPUTATION A REASONABLE TREATMENT ALTERNATIVE?

Quality-of-life issues are usually incorporated into medical decision making in several ways. For example, a patient may refuse to participate in an otherwise medically indicated treatment regimen because of the anticipated adverse effects on life-style. Similarly, a physician may modify or even refuse to follow a treatment protocol because it is assumed that the treatments will have an unacceptable qualitative outcome. For example, the physician may refuse to recommend an amputation when the chance for cure seems remote. In these cases the patient and physician have used quality-of-life issues as the basis for deciding against treatment.

QUALITY-OF-LIFE STUDIES IN EXTREMITY SOFT TISSUE SARCOMA

Attempts to provide quality-of-life data were explored by Sugarbaker, Barofsky, and co-workers.[8-10] In this study all patients had biopsy-confirmed soft tissue sarcoma. The design of the clinical trial in which quality-of-life assessments were performed is shown in Figure 6–7. These sarcoma clinical trials were carried out under the direction of Dr. Steven A. Rosenberg at the Surgery Branch, National Cancer Institute, National Institutes of Health. All histologic

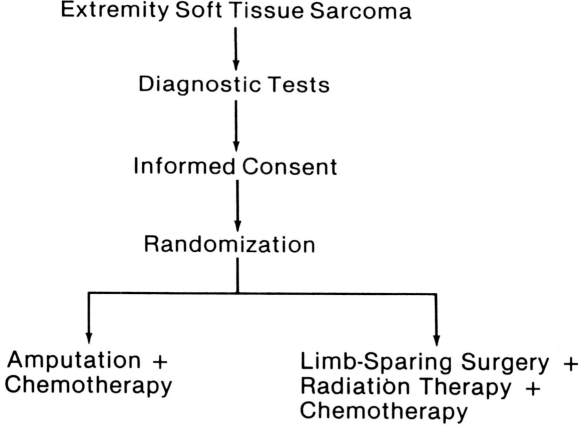

Figure 6–7. Steps to randomization in two arms of an extremity sarcoma protocol. Table 6–3 summarizes the results of the first phase of this study. Statistical analysis of the data failed to reveal substantial differences between the two groups of patients. However, subtest analysis of the various tests did demonstrate some differences. For example, the Sickness Impact Profile revealed that amputees scored better in emotional behavior and in body care and movement (Mann-Whitney statistic).[11] In the Katz Activities of Daily Living Scale, all amputees, but only 7 of 12 limb-sparing procedure patients, reported complete functioning.[12] The Fisher exact probability test indicated that the incidence of reports of less than complete functioning was barely below statistically significant ($P = 0.051$) for the limb-sparing group.[13]

Table 6–3. Assessment Instruments for Patients with Extremity Sarcoma*

ASSESSMENTS	AMPUTATED	LIMB SPARED	P VALUE
Behavioral Assessments			
Sickness Impact Profile (lower scores indicate lesser impairment)			
Total scores	76.3	121.6	NS†
Sleep and rest	8.9	13.8	NS
Emotional behavior	3.6	11.2	<0.05
Body care and movement	2.45	24.5	<0.01
Home management	10.2	12.0	NS
Mobility	9.3	9.0	NS
Social interaction	14.8	12.0	NS
Ambulation	17.9	14.7	NS
Alertness behavior	3.5	5.5	NS
Communication	0.0	2.5	NS
Work	4.4	2.7	NS
Recreation	6.6	11.5	NS
Eating	3.9	2.2	NS
Katz's Activities of Daily Living Scale (lower scores indicate lesser impairment)	1.0	1.5	= 0.051
The Barthel Index (scores indicate % of normal)	100	98.3	NS
Psychosocial Assessment			
Psychosocial Adjustment to Illness Scale (lower scores indicate lesser impairment)			
Total scores	23.9	29.9	NS
Health care orientation	5.6	3.9	<0.10>0.05
Vocational environment	4.5	5.9	NS
Domestic environment	5.3	5.7	NS
Sexual relationships	0.4	3.5	<0.025
Extended family relationships	0.2	0.2	NS
Social environment	1.6	3.7	NS
Psychological distress	6.0	7.0	NS
Economic Assessment			
Number working/number working prior to treatment	3/7 patients	4/11 patients	NS
Change in earning potential	7/9	8/12	NS
Change in home functioning	4/9	6/12	NS
Additional costs (drugs, rehabilitation, etc.)	7/9	8/12	NS
Days in hospital at NIH	51.4	70.9	NS

*From Sugarbaker et al.[10]
†NS = not significant.

types of soft tissue sarcoma except rhabdomyosarcoma and undifferentiated sarcoma in patients under the age of 21 years were included. To rule out distant metastases, patients underwent routine diagnostic tests plus lung tomography, bone scans, and liver scans. If disseminated disease was not apparent, patients were invited to participate in a randomized controlled clinical trial, and written informed consent was obtained. In this trial all patients received chemotherapy with adriamycin and cytoxan followed by methotrexate. Patients were randomized to receive amputation or limb-sparing surgery plus irradiation. The randomization was designed to perform twice as many limb-sparing procedures as amputations. The amputation was at or above the joint proximal to the tumor. Tumors in the leg were treated by above-knee amputation; if the tumors were in the lower thigh, hip disarticulation was performed; and if tumors were in the upper thigh or hip, hemipelvectomy was performed. Patients randomized to receive limb-sparing surgery plus irradiation had the tumor mass removed in toto; if the tumor involved a muscle bundle, that bundle was excised from origin to insertion. However, bone, nerve, and major vascular structures were preserved to maintain limb function even if that resulted in an inadequate margin of tumor resection. Microscopic deposits of tumor were undoubtedly left behind in some extremities. Postoperatively, after the incision was healed, approximately 6,500 rads were administered to the portion of the extremity at risk for local recurrence.

Patients with recurrent cancer were excluded from the quality-of-life assessment. Recurrent disease was considered an overriding variable that would obscure more subtle quality-of-life consequences of treatment. Patients were evaluated one to three years after their initial surgery or surgery plus radiation therapy. This represented a plateau phase of their clinical management and psychosocial status. There was no significant difference in the time between treatment and quality-of-life assessments for patients in the two arms of the protocol. Artificial limbs, if appropriate, had been obtained, and all minor wound-healing problems had been resolved; the chemotherapy with adriamycin and cytoxan was complete.

In the first efforts, a broad range of instruments to assess quality of life was selected; this assessment was extensive because we did not know how these specific cancer treatments would affect psychosocial status.

In the Psychosocial Adjustment to Illness Scale the ratings were ranked and compared with the Mann-Whitney statistic.[14] Ratings of zero on an item indicated no impairment of adjustment. If impairment was seen, its severity was recorded on a $+1$ to $+3$ scale. Total scores ranged from 13 to 35 for the amputees and 8 to 68 for the limb-sparing patients, but were not statistically different. Subtest analysis revealed that the limb-sparing patients were rated as having more often reported disturbed sexual functioning ($P < 0.025$) compared with the amputees. In contrast, the ratings of the patients who underwent amputation approached being statistically significantly different ($P < 0.05$) for health care orientation,

suggesting that their response to the services they received was different from that of the limb-sparing patients.

No significant differences in the economic cost of the two cancer treatments were determined.

At this point a new set of clinical tests included a pain assessment, a mobility scale, an assessment of treatment trauma, and an assessment of sexual functioning. The pain assessment allowed the patient to score severity, frequency, duration, and medicine requirement of pain on a 0 to $+4$ scale. The mobility scale allowed the patient to score his or her posture, walking, gait, sitting, stair climbing, use of hand-held appliances, use of wheelchair, and time usage on a 0 to $+3$ scale. In the treatment trauma questionnaire, patients were asked to rate 34 treatments in the protocol on a 0 to $+10$ scale. The score was computed by adding the numerical value of events of treatments they had experienced. In the assessment of sexual relationships, patients were asked to rate the quality, interest, frequency, and satisfaction of their activity on a 0 to $+3$ scale.

After scoring, results were subjected to statistical analysis using the Fisher exact probability test and the Mann-Whitney statistic. Mean scores for a group and their statistical significance are presented. A value of $P \leq 0.05$ was considered to be statistically significant.

As shown in Figure 6–8, the pain, mobility, and treatment trauma assessments showed no differences between the groups. A trend toward impaired sexual functioning was seen in the limb-sparing group compared with amputees, but statistical analysis failed to confirm the clear defect seen in the first part of this study.

Why was it that the quality-of-life consequences

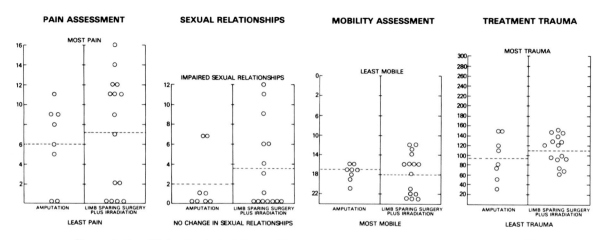

Figure 6–8.   Clinical tests to link specific treatment consequences with quality of life.[10]

for these two treatment alternatives were so similar? During the course of our studies explanations occurred to us. First, the patients who randomized to amputation adjusted to this ablative procedure extremely well with time. After an initial period during which they mourned for the lost limb, they moved on to a seemingly normal existence. Their mood was good, mobility was excellent with the help of prosthetic devices and the automobile, and social interactions often improved. This trend toward better relationships with family members and friends was almost universal. Sexual relationships were not reported impaired; occasionally they were greatly improved. The only complaint regularly elicited was that of phantom limb pain; fortunately, this problem is usually a self-limited one in most patients and was no longer a serious complaint 18 months to 2 years after amputation. Some unfortunate patients continue to have debilitating phantom limb pain even decades after amputation.

The second explanation for the lack of difference between these two groups of patients is seen in the compilation of adverse effects of the multimodality therapy. The combined effects of surgery, radiation, and chemotherapy were devastating to a few patients. In the group of patients undergoing amputation, all recovered from their surgery in a rather predictable fashion and could be discharged from closely supervised medical care within a few weeks. However, five of the patients treated with multimodality therapy had serious long-term medical problems requiring many months of closely supervised medical care. Radiation neuritis was so severe in one patient that subsequent amputation was required. Another needed release of the sciatic nerve from entrapment within radiation fibrosis in the buttock. A third patient had persistent and increasing pain in the irradiated extremity, requiring regular use of narcotics. Two patients had breakdown of their surgical incision within the field of radiation; prolonged healing with its concomitant contractures became long-term problems. This condition was corrected in one patient by a myocutaneous flap, but it persists in the other patient.

One significant difference between the two groups of patients in the standardized tests was sexual functioning. Those patients who underwent limb-sparing surgery, radiation therapy, and chemotherapy reported significant reduction in sexual functioning compared with the amputees. Studies by Shamberger and co-workers[8] have shown persistent decreased spermatogenesis and increased follicle-stimulating hormone (FSH) levels in patients undergoing both thigh irradiation and chemotherapy. Rowley and colleagues[15] showed that as little as 78

rads produced azoospermia in most men receiving testicular irradiation. It is likely that the combined effects of chemotherapy and irradiation scatter caused testicular or ovarian damage and consequent decrease in sexual functioning. However, it is also possible that the decrease mobility associated with radiation fibrosis of the lower leg may interfere with normal sexual activity.

It is possible that a less aggressive plan for sparing an extremity would reduce the morbidity of the protocol treatments, and in so doing show the expected improved quality of life that may result from sparing an extremity. However, lesser local measures to control tumor may result in greater local recurrence rates; an amputation is required in the event of local recurrence, and a high incidence of metastatic disease is associated. Also, more careful case selection may help reduce morbidity; large proximal thigh and hip sarcomas may best be treated by radical amputation so that extremely large-field, high-dose radiation therapy is not required.

QUALITY-OF-LIFE DATA AND THE DECISION TO AMPUTATE

In soft tissue sarcoma trials at the NIH, data have shown that a local recurrence is often associated with an excision in which the margins are several millimeters or less. They also confirmed that local recurrence usually is accompanied by systemic spread of disease. Local control by adequate resection, therefore, must be the primary objective of initial treatment for soft tissue sarcoma. If inadequate margins of resection are a result of wide local excision or muscle group excision, then the surgeon should usually recommend an amputation to the patient. As discussed earlier in this chapter, optimally the surgeon must be able to excise the tumor mass without ever encountering tumor tissue. This philosophy has evolved in part because the quality-of-life data suggest that a very acceptable existence is seen in patients even though they have undergone a major amputation. This reasonable quality of life following amputation becomes even more acceptable when one compares it to the quality of life seen in a group of patients treated by wide excision plus radiation therapy. Our conclusion was that the impact of amputation on a patient's quality of life was not so great that amputation should not be considered as a reasonable treatment alternative. Clinical impressions also confirm that the amputee copes and adapts extremely well, and that although an amputation has the potential to be disabling, it does not necessarily produce a disability. Overzealous selection of the limb salvage approach may result in a less favorable outcome for the population of patients. Of course, this judgment is offered realizing that the unnecessary sacrifice of an extremity can never be recommended by any conscientious oncologist.

REFERENCES

1. Suite HD, Russell WO, Martin RG: Sarcoma of soft tissue: Clinical and histopathologic parameter and response to treatment. *Cancer* 1975;35:1478–1483.
2. Shiu MH, Castro EG, Hjdu SI, et al: Surgical treatment of 297 soft tissue sarcomas of the lower extremity. *Ann Surg* 1975;182:597–602.
3. Lindberg RD, Martin RG, Romsdahl MM, et al: Conservative surgery and postoperative radiotherapy in 300 adults with soft-tissue sarcomas. *Cancer* 1981;47: 2391–2397.
4. Rosenberg SA, Kent H, Costa J, et al: Prospective randomized evaluation of the role of limb-sparing surgery, radiation therapy, and adjuvant chemoimmunotherapy in the treatment of adult soft-tissue sarcomas. *Surgery* 1978;84:62–68.
5. Rosenberg SA, Tepper J, Glatstein E, et al: The treatment of soft tissue sarcomas of the extremities: Prospective randomized evaluations of (1) limb-sparing surgery plus radiation therapy compared to amputation and (2) the role of adjuvant chemotherapy. *Ann Surg* 1982;196:305–315.
6. Wanebo HJ, Shah J, Knapper W, et al: Reappraisal of surgical management of sarcoma of the buttock. *Cancer* 1973;31:97–104.
7. Sugarbaker PH, Barofsky SA, Gianola FJ: Quality of life assessment of patients in extremity sarcoma clinical trials. *Surgery* 1982;91:17–23.
8. Shamberger RC, Sherins RJ, Rosenberg SA: The effects of postoperative adjuvant chemotherapy and radiotherapy on testicular function in men undergoing treatment of soft tissue sarcoma. *Cancer* 1981;47: 2368–2374.
9. Rosenberg SA, Tepper J, Glatstein E, et al: Prospective randomized evaluation of adjuvant chemotherapy in adults with soft tissue sarcomas of the extremities. *Cancer* 1983;52:424–434.
10. Sugarbaker PH, Barofsky I, Rosenberg SA, et al: Quality of life assessment of patients in extremity sarcoma clinical trials. *Surgery* 1982;91:17–23.
11. Bergner M, Bobbit RA, Pollard WE, et al: The sickness impact profile: Validation of a health status measure. *Med Care* 1976;14:57–67.
12. Katz S, Akpom CA: A measure of primary sociobiological function. *Int J Health Serv* 1976;6:493–507.
13. Mahoney FI, Barthel DW: Functional evaluation: The Barthel index. *Md State Med J* 1965;14:61–65.
14. Derogatis LR: Psychosocial adjustment to illness scale (unpublished data 1975).
15. Rowley MJ, Leach DR, Warner GA, et al: Effects of graded doses of ionizing radiation therapy on the human testis. *Radiat Res* 1974;59:665–678.

7

Induction Chemotherapy for Sarcomas of the Extremities

DENNIS A. PRIEBAT, M.D.
RAM S. TREHAN, M.D.
MARTIN M. MALAWER, M.D.
RICHARD S. SCHULOF, M.D., Ph.D.

OVERVIEW

Sarcomas are relatively rare mesenchymal tumors of the soft tissue and bones that exhibit a marked heterogeneity in their clinical presentation, biologic behavior, and histologic features. In 1990, approximately 7,800 new cases will be diagnosed, 5,700 of which arise from the soft tissue and 2,100 from bone.[1] Although the incidence of sarcomas is similar to that of Hodgkin's disease, they are responsible for more than twice as many deaths each year. Major advances in the treatment of these tumors have been limited by problems with accumulating sufficient numbers of similar patients in order to perform significant prospective clinical trials.

Until the 1970s, surgical therapy had been the accepted method for the primary management of most soft tissue and skeletal sarcomas of the extremities. However, surgery alone was associated with frequent treatment failure due to local recurrence after radical wide resection, and less frequently following amputation. Even when local control was achieved, greater than 50% of patients with soft tissue sarcoma and 80% of patients with skeletal sarcoma (osteogenic sarcoma) eventually developed distant metastases and died, usually within two years.[2-6]

Thus, single modality surgical therapy for sarcomas was followed by unacceptably high rates of treatment failure. Conventional treatment modalities, ie, radiation therapy and chemotherapy, were subsequently found to exhibit reproducible antitumor effects against these neoplasms. Over the years, their employment in combined modality therapy has evolved from use solely in the adjuvant (postoperative) setting to preoperative (neoadjuvant, induction) therapy in an attempt to preserve limb function while maintaining or increasing long-term survival.[7-11]

A recent Consensus Development Conference of the National Institutes of Health concluded that limb-sparing surgery for adult soft tissue and osteogenic sarcomas is both a feasible and appropriate approach for a significant proportion of patients, if carefully selected.[12,13] Several investigators have attempted to maximize the number of patients who would be candidates for limb-sparing surgery through the administration of preoperative (induction) chemotherapy. The routes of chemotherapy administration have varied from intravenous bolus, to continuous intravenous infusion, to local (regional) drug delivery directly to the tumor via the feeding artery.[14,15]

REGIONAL CHEMOTHERAPY

Rationale

Any drug that is given intravenously (IV) can be given intra-arterially (IA) if it is titrated to be tolerated by the arterial endothelium. The intra-arterial route has been shown to increase the drug concentration to the tumor by five to nine times (depending on the particular drug).[16] However, the systemic concentration and, thus, systemic toxicity will usually be the same whether the drug is delivered IV or IA.[17,18]

The advantage of an intra-arterial infusion is based on the first-pass effect of the chemotherapy through the tumor bed.[19] Abe et al[20] felt that during the first 3 minutes of infusion, the tumor could be exposed to as much as 250 times the concentration expected from standard intravenous administration (Fig. 7–1). The relative advantage of an intra-arterial infusion is directly proportional to the plasma clearance of the drugs used and inversely proportional to the plasma flow of the tumor.[17]

$$R_1 \text{ (relative advantage)} = \frac{\text{plasma clearance}}{\text{tumor plasma flow}}$$

Thus, the intra-arterial route could be more useful when the tumor blood flow is low and the clearance from the systemic circulation is high.

Most cytotoxic agents have been found to have a steep dose-response curve, ie, the higher the concentration of the drug, the greater the antitumor effect.[22] This has led to the development of techniques that could increase local drug delivery in order to obtain a higher cell kill. Dose dependency has been shown to be important in breast, lung, and ovarian cancer, as well as for the sarcomas.[23] For example, in vitro studies have demonstrated a higher cell kill by prolonged exposure to cisplatin (DDP).[24] It has been felt

Postulated Mechanism of Regional Effect of Neoadjuvant Chemotherapy

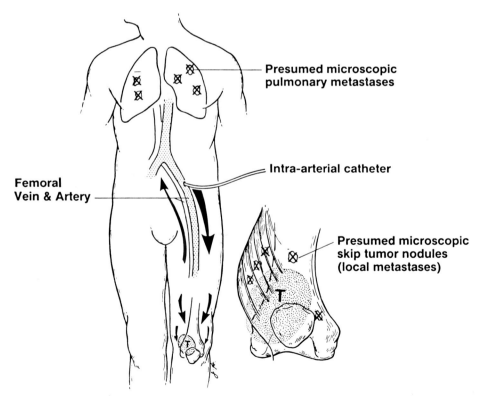

Figure 7–1.   Schematic demonstrating the postulated regional tumor effect of intra-arterial chemotherapy on the presumed local microscopic disease, as well as pulmonary micrometastases. The increased arterial concentration (large arrow) represents increased drug concentration to the local/regional tumor area, which may in turn eradicate local skip lesions as well as the major tumor, thus permitting a safe local procedure to be performed (from Malawer M et al[21]).

that if tumor cell resistance is due to inadequate drug exposure, a higher concentration may help overcome this.[25]

Intra-arterial cisplatin was first used in 1976 in melanoma with the idea that increased local drug concentrations would improve the gradient for penetration across the cell membrane.[26] Jaffe et al[27] showed a higher cisplatin concentration in the vein draining the region of a neoplasm, and also that increased tumor destruction depends on the number of infusions as well as higher drug concentrations.[28] Other chemotherapeutic agents used for intra-arterial use have included adriamycin, 5-FU, FUDR, melphalan (L-PAM), actinomycin-D, nitrogen mustard, and BCNU.

Methods of Administration of Regional Chemotherapy

1. Intra-arterial
2. Intra-arterial with tourniquet infusion
3. Isolation perfusion (IsP) with and without hyperthermia
4. Chemoembolization

Intra-arterial

This technique requires the cannulation of an artery, usually by percutaneous insertion of a catheter, or less often under direct vision by a surgical procedure.[29] The catheter is placed via the femoral artery by using the Seldinger technique. The contralateral femoral artery is used for a lower-extremity tumor. The catheter is then positioned selectively into the feeding artery, as close to the tumor mass as possible, so that the infusion will perfuse the maximum amount of tumor bulk but spare as much normal tissue as possible. It should be left proximal to the first draining vessel, when the tumor mass is bulky and vascular with multiple feeding vessels. Effective intra-arterial therapy depends on appropriate catheter placement.[29] At the time of initial catheter placement and prior to each chemotherapy treatment cycle, a subtraction arteriogram is performed.[30] This better defines the arterial supply serving as a guide to catheter placement. In addition, a nuclear medicine catheter flow study can be done to confirm an adequate distribution of the drug to the tumor. Following treatment, the arteriogram is used as a means to assess tumor response by permitting documentation of tumor neovascularity and stain, and the extent of disease.

Along with the chemotherapeutic agent, aqueous heparin is administered in the IA infusion to mini-mize thrombotic complications.[30] When it is incompatible with the infused drug, ie, adriamycin, then the heparin is given intravenously. If an infusion is given for longer than a 24-hour period, daily radiographs of the area are obtained to check catheter position.

A number of problems can arise with regard to achieving maximal concentrations and the uniform distribution of chemotherapy into the tumor via the intra-arterial approach. Inadequate mixing of chemotherapy can occur due to laminar flow within the infused vessel, which may lead to "streaming" of the infusion for various distances from the catheter tip.[31] A significant proportion of the administered chemotherapy could thus bypass some of the major arterial branches supplying the tumor. The chemotherapy may also unexpectedly flow into a branch draining only part of the tumor or into a distal musculocutaneous branch. With the latter occurrence, necrosis of normal tissues and subsequent scarring may develop. In order to disrupt such infusional streaming, several institutions have utilized a pulsatile infusion pump (Cook, Inc.).[23,30] This releases the infusion in one to three short pulses per second, producing greater turbulence, better drug mixing, and a more homogeneous distribution of drug.

Intra-arterial Tourniquet Infusion (TI)

As described in the previous section, an artery is cannulated and the catheter tip advanced as close as is feasible to maintain good perfusion of the entire tumor area. In addition, this method of drug delivery involves the inflation of a blood pressure cuff to 30 mm above systolic pressure for 10 minutes, proximal to the tumor and the catheter tip. The drug is then delivered over 30 to 60 seconds.[32] Both adriamycin and cisplatin have been employed. It is felt that the drug concentration can be locally increased by up to 30 times.[33] Reversal of the flow in the tumor through collateral circulation may actually end up negating the benefit of occlusion, and has limited the wide use of the tourniquet infusion method.[16,34,35]

Isolation Perfusion

Under surgical guidance, an artery and vein are clamped proximal to the tumor. Catheters are placed in both vessels and connected to an extracorporeal circulation flushed with Ringer's lactate. Perfusion can take from 45 minutes to 2 hours.[25,30,34] Newer methods have utilized a bubble oxygenator and a water-circulated heat exchanger.[24,35] The chemotherapeutic agents most often used have been melphalan (L-PAM), actinomycin-D, and nitrogen mustard.[35,36] Concurrent IsP with hyperthermia has also been tried.[37]

Isolation perfusion is thought to achieve high local blood and tissue levels of chemotherapy with minimal systemic leak.[38] It has been used most often for treating isolated recurrent melanoma of the extremities, as well as extremity sarcomas,[39] but there is no conclusive evidence for its superiority over other regional treatments for sarcoma. The chemotherapeutic agents that have been studied have minimal intravenous activity against sarcomas, and there is little systemic drug delivery in order to treat micrometastatic disease elsewhere. Furthermore, it is a complex, expensive, and labor-intensive technique with significant complications, including tissue necrosis, poor wound healing, persistent extremity edema, and vascular damage.[33,40]

Chemoembolization (CE)

Embolization creates tumor ischemia, which is thought to stop tumor growth and induce regression.[30] When the embolization occurs close to the tumor (in a peripheral vessel), there is less opportunity for collateral circulation. The size and type of particles used will help to determine the site of vascular interruption. Materials such as gel foam powder (40–60 mm), Ivalon polyvinyl alcohol foam particles (150–500 mm), and gel foam cubes (1–3 mm) are most often used for peripheral embolization.[29] Stainless steel coils or gel foam segments (3 × 3 × 20 mm) are used for central occlusion.

The concept of chemoembolization was first introduced by Kato et al.[41] It combines peripheral embolization of the arterial tumor supply with the IA infusion of chemotherapy. In addition to tumor-induced ischemia, the emboli are thought to slow the transit and exposure time of chemotherapy through the vascular bed. Theoretically, this will increase the local drug concentration and enhance the antitumor effect.

The technique involves incorporating a chemotherapeutic agent into microcapsular substances, which are then injected in the artery supplying the tumor, in order to obstruct blood flow and create ischemia. The microcapsule shell then degrades and releases the chemotherapeutic agent into the surrounding tumor in a gradual and sustained manner. Several materials have been used, including ethyl cellulose microencapsulated spheres, biodegradable starch microspheres, and gel foam or polyvinyl foam particles. Vasculitis and extensive tissue damage can occur. Steroids may help in reducing these complications.[16] Again, there appears to be a reduced systemic effect of chemotherapy. Therefore, this technique has been used mostly to treat isolated metastases, ie, hepatic (from colon, breast, etc), rather than high-grade extremity sarcomas.

This review will now focus on the intra-arterial infusion technique via a percutaneous catheter to deliver preoperative (neoadjuvant, induction) chemotherapy. In the examination of the use of regional chemotherapy for the treatment of primary mesenchymal tumors of the extremities, it is important and helpful to separate the clinical studies involving soft tissue from those of bone. Furthermore, the discussion on bone sarcomas will concentrate on osteosarcoma, in which the largest clinical experience has been obtained. The surgical, radiotherapeutic, and chemotherapeutic principles developed in the treatment of osteosarcomas have formed the basis of management strategies for most of the other, rarer, high-grade spindle cell neoplasms of bone.

SOFT TISSUE SARCOMA

Historically, radical surgical excision had been the primary mode of therapy for extremity soft tissue sarcomas. This entailed either amputation (in greater than 35% of cases) or a large compartment resection. Advances in radiologic imaging and orthopedic surgery techniques helped to further reduce the amputation rate to less than 15%–20%.[42,43] Although local tumor control was good, there was still significant functional impairment.[44–46] With the advent of adjunctive radiation therapy, a more limited surgical resection was possible approximately 75% of the time.[44–46] Several investigators have shown this treatment modality to be equally effective in obtaining local tumor control and, for the most part, retaining excellent limb function. However, there still were problems with therapeutic complications and distant metastatic spread. More recently, preoperative regional (IA) chemotherapy with and without radiation therapy has been employed to further improve local tumor control, achieve better limb function with fewer complications, reduce metastatic spread, and increase overall survival (see Table 7–1).[8,25]

Adriamycin is the most active chemotherapeutic agent against soft tissue sarcomas and has been used frequently for IA infusion.[8,25,58,59] Other active agents, ie, methotrexate, DTIC, and ifosfamide, are not satisfactory for IA use.[60,61] Methotrexate has usually been administered intravenously on a weekly basis, and it is thus not logistically feasible to be given intra-arterially. Furthermore, the local venous con-

Table 7-1.   Preoperative Intra-arterial Chemotherapy with Adriamycin (ADR) for Soft Tissue Sarcoma

STUDY	TREATMENT	# PTS	% LIMB SALVAGE	COMPLICATIONS	% LOCAL RECURRENCE	METASTASES	SURVIVAL	MEDIAN FOLLOW-UP (mos)
Azarelli[48] 1983	ADR 100 mg/m² over 8 d	13	85%	8%	8%	38%	DFS 62% OS 92%	15
Mantravadi[49] 1984	ADR 100 mg/m² over 10 d + 2,500 R	32	91%	12%	3%	25%	DFS 57% OS 70%*	36
Denton[50] 1984	ADR 100 mg over 3 d + 3,000 R	15	80%	40%	6%	NM	OS 79%*	36
Eilber[51-55] Protocol 1 (1974-81)	ADR 90 mg over 3 d + 3,500 R	77	96%	43%	5%	NM	OS 62%	96
Protocol 2 (1981-84)	ADR 90 mg over 3 d + 1,750 R	137	95%	25%	12%	NM	OS 77%	48
Protocol 3 (1984-88)	ADR 90 mg over 3 d + 2,800 R	96	99%	14%	8%	NM	DFS 70%	36
		(44-IA)	98%	18%	7%	NM		
		(52-IV)	100%	10%	8%	NM		
Goodnight[56] 1985	ADR 90 mg over 3 d + 3,500 R	17	88%	41%	0%	35%	DFS 59% OS 82%	32
Hoekstra[57] 1989	ADR 60 mg/m² over 3 d + 3,500 R	9	89%	33%	11%	44%	DFS 56% OS 89%	24

ADR = adriamycin; DFS = disease-free survival; OS = overall survival; NM = not mentioned; R = rads; IA = intra-arterial; IV = intravenous.
*Projected survival.

centrations achieved with giving methotrexate via the IA route can probably be attained by giving the drug intravenously at very high doses in conjunction with calcium leucovorin rescue.[62] DTIC and ifosfamide require passage through the hepatic microsomal system for activation.[61]

Clinical Experience

Much of the pioneering work and most extensive experience in utilizing IA adriamycin preoperatively for extremity soft tissue sarcoma has been done by the UCLA group.[51] Several articles have summarized their experience involving four sequential treatment programs over a 15-year period (see Table 7–1).

Serving as an initial basis for comparison, they reported on an historical control group consisting of 63 nonprotocol patients treated from 1972 to 1976.[51,52] These patients received "standard" surgical therapy; 21 patients (33%) had an amputation, 67% had a limb-sparing procedure consisting of a wide excision for 11, and 31 patients had a wide excision followed by 6,000 rads (200 rads/fraction for five days over six weeks). Complications of treatment, namely wound slough, edema, and neuritis, occurred in 22%. A local recurrence developed in 22%, including 16% of patients who had an amputation.

In 1974, a prospective study group received preoperative treatment consisting of continuous-infusion IA adriamycin 30 mg per day for three days, followed by radiation therapy 3,500 rads (350 rads per day for 10 days).[51,53] Of these patients, 96% were able to undergo a limb-sparing procedure, and only 5% had a local tumor recurrence. With a median follow-up of more than eight years, overall survival was 62%. Unfortunately, complications occurred in 43% of the patients, requiring reoperation in 23%. Wound slough was the most common complication. Additionally, in 10%, fracture of adjacent long bones occurred, which necessitated an open intramedullary fixation procedure. Pathologic evaluation in all these cases revealed no evidence of recurrent tumor.

In order to reduce the high complication rate, the treatment program was changed in 1981 with a decrease in the radiation dose from 3,500 rads to 1,750 rads (350 rads/day × 5).[51,54] Of 137 total patients, 95% were able to have a limb-sparing procedure. Complications occurred in 25% of patients, with 5% requiring reoperation, but only 1% developed fractures of the adjacent bone. Overall survival was 77% at a median follow-up of 48 months. Nevertheless, the local recurrence rate of 12% was significantly inferior when compared with the previously higher radiation dose regimen.

Therefore, the protocol was again modified in 1984, incorporating an intermediate radiation dose of 2,800 rads (350 rads/day × 8).[51] In addition, the preoperative adriamycin treatment was randomized to be given at the same dose either as an IA or as an IV infusion.[51,55] Now, 99% of patients were able to receive a limb-sparing procedure, with only an 8% local recurrence rate. Complications occurred in 14%, with a slightly higher rate in the IA group. Median tumor necrosis was 65%.[55] At a median follow-up of 36 months, there was no significant difference in the limb salvage rate, local recurrence rate, complication rate, percent histologic necrosis, and disease-free survival between the IA and IV groups.[55]

Huth et al evaluated the histological effects of treatment outcomes observed with the UCLA protocols.[63] The degree of necrosis did not seem to be related to pathologic grade or radiation dose. As in other studies, tumor grade and size were shown to be important factors for influencing overall patient survival. Patients were also randomized to receive or not to receive postoperative (adjuvant) chemotherapy. There was no benefit of adjuvant chemotherapy found on patient survival. This was in agreement with the majority of other adjuvant chemotherapy studies reported in the literature.[64]

All three UCLA studies, utilizing preoperative IA adriamycin and radiation therapy, allowed for a very high percentage of patients to receive nonamputative surgery compared with the historical control group of no preoperative therapy. The local control rate was improved and the complication rate reduced with the intermediate radiation dose. In this specific combined modality neoadjuvant scheme, there was no significant advantage found for IA *v* IV route of adriamycin administration. However, at the time of initial randomization, the two treatment groups were not stratified for tumor size and grade, and the IA group contained a greater percentage of patients with large (>10 cm) high-grade (III) tumors.[55]

Several investigators have attempted to reproduce the UCLA results by using similar or slightly modified treatment programs of IA adriamycin and radiation (see Table 7–1).[25,48–50,56,57] Unfortunately, all these studies contain small patient numbers and have a short duration of follow-up. Goodnight et al,[56] using a higher preoperative radiation dose of 3,500 to 4,000 rads, also noted the development of pathologic fractures of the long bones, but this was not noted by Hoekstra et al,[57] using the same radiation dose. Mantravadi et al[49] and Denton et al,[50] using a lower radiation dose, noted no pathologic fractures, but Denton et al's overall complication rate was still high. Azzarelli et al[48] obtained excellent results utilizing an extended IA adriamycin infusion alone without concomitant preoperative radiation therapy.

The results of these multiple studies are equally impressive, yet it is hard to compare them with each other or with other types of treatment. Most of the data have been compared to historical controls from the investigators' own institution or published reports in the literature, both of which can obviously be flawed. When compared with contemporary results achieved with preoperative and/or postoperative radiation therapy alone,[7,47,65–67] preoperative IA adriamycin appears to have a slightly lower local recurrence rate and greater overall survival.[8,25] But there is still a lack of prospective randomized studies comparing these different treatment modalities, performed in similar patient populations, with equal distributions for patient age, performance status, histologic heterogeneity, and tumor size, grade, and site.

Although local tumor control and limb salvage rates appear much improved from the past, metastatic spread remains a significant problem and a continuing challenge, occurring in more than 30% of patients. In addition, the problem of musculocutaneous necrosis from the IA adriamycin regimen is still of concern. New innovative approaches are needed to reduce the complication rate and to better control systemic disease.

Drawing from the experience in osteosarcoma, our group and others are evaluating the use of IA cisplatin.[68–74] This drug has previously been tested in soft tissue sarcoma via the intravenous route and has only minor activity (having a response rate of approximately 0%–15% in refractory disease and 4%–21% in untreated patients).[75–77] However, its use as an intra-arterial agent and its synergistic activity with adriamycin[78] have not been rigorously tested in soft tissue sarcoma. Along with intra-arterial cisplatin, adriamycin has been given either as an IV bolus,[69] as a two-day to three-day continuous IV infusion through a central venous catheter,[72,74] or as an IA infusion.[70,71] Preliminary results appear promising. Rosen and Eilber at UCLA are also evaluating this two-drug regimen, but given with concomitant preoperative radiation therapy (280–350 cGy × 8 doses).[72,73,171]

Osteosarcoma

Osteosarcoma is a rare tumor, yet it is the most frequently occurring malignant tumor of bone in adolescence and young adults. It is more common in males and has a strong predilection for the distal femur, proximal tibia, and proximal humerus. Approximately 80% of patients have localized disease at the time of initial diagnosis.[6]

Prior to 1970, the primary treatment of nonmetastatic osteosarcoma of the extremities consisted of surgical obliteration alone (usually amputation) and/or high-dose radiation therapy of the primary tumor. The five-year disease-free survival was no more than 20%, with lung metastases being the most common reason for treatment failures. Early investigations of chemotherapy for osteosarcoma were unrewarding, and it was considered a chemoresistant tumor.[5,6,79–83]

It was not until the early 1970s, and continuing through the 1980s, that reports emerged of effective drugs to treat patients with osteosarcoma, ie, adriamycin,[84] high-dose methotrexate with calcium leucovorin rescue[85–87,] cisplatin,[88] and, most recently, ifosfamide.[89] It was demonstrated that these chemotherapeutic agents could eradicate overt and micrometastatic disease and improve survival.[90] To a large extent the major advances made over the past two decades in the treatment of osteosarcoma are a consequence of the development of effective chemotherapy. The introduction of these chemotherapeutic agents has helped generate multidisciplinary treatment strategies in order to perform more conservative limb-sparing procedures and to help improve overall patient survival.

With the demonstration of effective chemotherapy for metastatic disease, therapeutic investigations were initiated to determine the efficacy of these agents to destroy micrometastases thought to be present in the majority of patients at the time of initial primary surgery (ie, adjuvant chemotherapy).[90] There have been conflicting reports from different institutions concerning the value of adjuvant chemotherapy *v* historical surgery alone controls.[91–96] The exact contribution of adjuvant chemotherapy was heatedly debated. Some felt that an increased survival for osteosarcoma patients had occurred over time. They believed that this was solely related to new diagnostic advancements for staging and the earlier detection of metastases, and to improvements in surgical techniques and supportive care. This finally prompted the initiation of definitive prospectively randomized control studies. The results of two recent randomized trials have now demonstrated that intensive multidrug adjuvant chemotherapy exerts a significant impact on prolonging the disease-free, and probably overall, survival of patients with osteosarcoma of the extremities.[97,98] Adjuvant chemotherapy has also been shown to alter the pattern of development of pulmonary metastases, with a reduction in number and delay in appearance, thus possibly facilitating their surgical removal.[99–102] It has changed the natural history of this neoplasm, with more patients developing extrapulmonary metastases (ie, skin, brain, heart, etc).[103,104]

Currently, one standard form of therapy for patients with osteosarcoma of the extremities and no evidence of metastases is amputation followed by adjuvant systemic chemotherapy for approximately one year. This type of multimodality therapy has yielded an approximately 40%–65% long-term (five-year) disease-free survival.[10,90,93–98] However, amputation leads to loss of a limb. In addition, there can be a delay in the early administration of chemotherapy to treat possible micrometastases because of the recovery time needed for adequate healing following surgery.

At the same time that chemotherapy was developing, advanced and improved techniques in primary surgical resection were attempted with a search for alternative methods short of amputation, ie, limb-sparing surgery. With these new procedures there was a presurgical delay of two to three months necessary for the production of a custom-made endoprosthesis. From the increasing enthusiasm of orthopedic surgeons to do limb-sparing surgery, there evolved a strategy to use preoperative (neoadjuvant, induction) chemotherapy which was introduced as a maneuver to treat patients early while awaiting manufacture of the prosthesis.[9,10,12,105]

Preoperative chemotherapy was felt to be an early defense against the possible presence of pulmonary micrometastases, with the theoretical advantage of a reduction in the emergence of drug-resistant tumor cells.[9,10,12,105] It was also thought to be helpful in downstaging a tumor by decreasing the size of an accompanying soft tissue mass and forming a surrounding reactive rim (confining it within a calcified periosteum), thereby leading to better tumor demarcation and permitting successful tumor removal with a limb-sparing resection[106,107] (Fig. 7–2). In addition, the response of the tumor to preoperative chemotherapy could possible provide an in vivo drug sensitivity test for selecting the best postoperative (adjuvant chemotherapy), ie, "customizing" or "tailoring" postoperative chemotherapy.[9,10,12,108]

The responses of osteosarcoma to preoperative chemotherapy may be assessed by clinical, laboratory, radiologic, and pathologic parameters. Clinical responses are seen with a reduction in pain, swelling, and heat.[109] A laboratory response can occur with a reduction of an elevated alkaline phosphatase.[110,111] On plain radiography and CT scan, there can be a reduction and/or complete disappearance of any associated soft tissue mass, revisualization of the fat planes between muscle bundles, healing of pathologic fractures and organized deposition of calcium within the neoplastic bone (calcified periosteum)[112–116] (Fig. 7–3). With angiography, responses are manifest by a diminution and/or disappearance of tumor vascularity and stain (Fig. 7–4). An arteriogram offers a less subjective means of assessing tumor response.[113,117,118] Other techniques undergoing further evaluation as to their benefit include technetium-99 methylene diphosphonate functional imaging,[119] gallium,[9] thallium-201,[9,120] and NMR scans.[121,122]

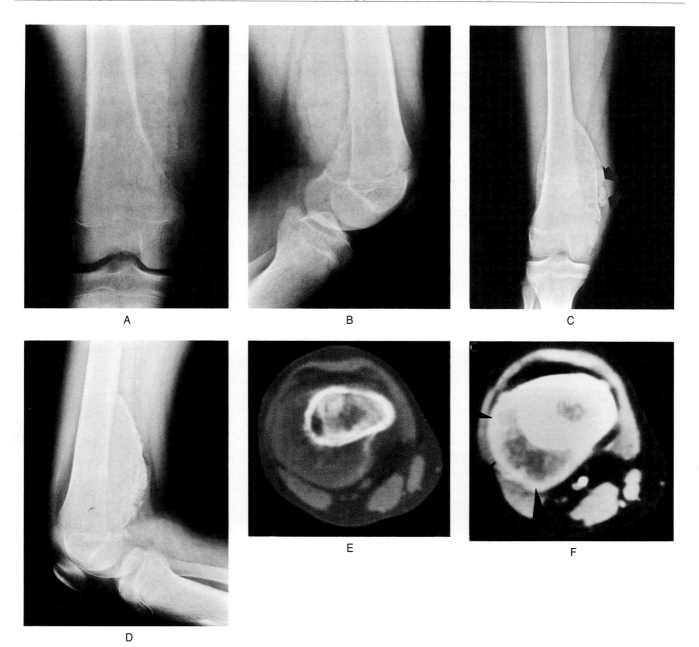

Figure 7–2. Osteosarcoma of the distal femur treated with regional intra-arterial chemotherapy. Plain radiographs (anterior and lateral views) of a 16-year-old patient with a distal femoral osteosarcoma prior to (**A and B**) and following (**C and D**) two cycles of intra-arterial cisplatin and intravenous adriamycin. There is a marked reossification of both the intraosseous and extraosseous components. Note the smooth margins of the new bone and reossification (arrows) of several small tumor nodules along the medial aspect. A CAT scan prior to and following chemotherapy. (**E and F**). There is a large posterior soft tissue mass in close proximity to the popliteal vessels. Following intra-arterial chemotherapy there is marked "rimming" (arrows) of the extraosseous component, which indicates a good tumor response, even though the size did not significantly decrease. This patient initially was considered for amputation and was converted to a limb-sparing procedure. The gross specimen showed >90% tumor necrosis (from Malawer M et al[21]).

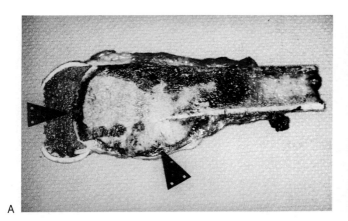

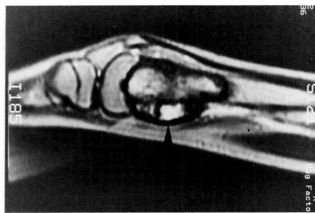

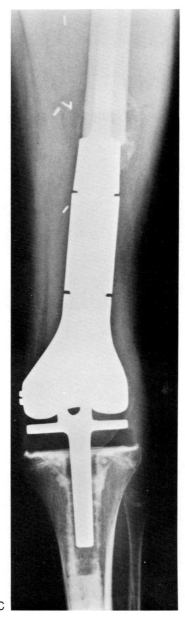

Figure 7–3.   The gross specimen, corresponding MRI, and postoperative radiograph of the patient in Figure 7–2. The patient underwent a limb-sparing procedure with a segmental modular prosthesis. (**A**) The gross specimen demonstrates almost complete necrosis. The arrows correspond to the rim of new bone formation seen on the MRI (**B**). The thick black rim on the MRI represents new bone formation as seen on the CT (Fig 7–2E, F) and indicates the formation of new (nonneoplastic) bone around the necrotic tumor. This is a reliable sign of the tumor response to preoperative therapy. (**C**) Postoperative radiograph showing a modular segmental replacement prosthesis (from Malawer et al[21]).

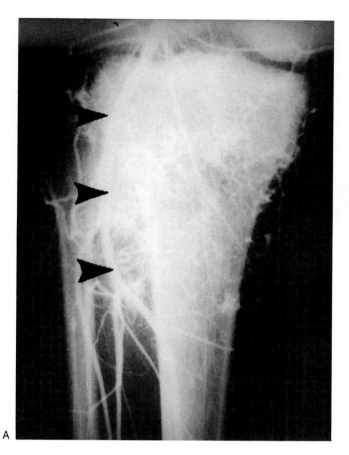

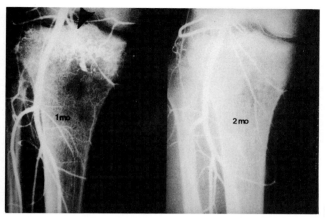

Figure 7–4. Typical angiographic response of an osteosarcoma to intra-arterial chemotherapy. (**A**) Angiogram of an osteosarcoma of the proximal tibia prior to intra-arterial chemotherapy. Note the marked vascularity and displacement of the popliteal as well as the anterior tibial artery (solid arrows). (**B**) Angiograms following the first (1 mo) and second (2 mo) cycles of intra-arterial cisplatin and adriamycin. Note the marked decrease in tumor vascularity. This is considered one of the most reliable radiographic criteria for a good tumor response (necrosis). The popliteal vessels are still displaced. This indicates the tumor matrix is still present, although the tumor cells are necrotic (common finding). The gross specimen had >95% tumor necrosis.

Nevertheless, the histologic appearance of the resected primary tumor specimen after preoperative chemotherapy has emerged as the gold standard for evaluating and measuring a therapeutic response[108] (Fig. 7–5). A number of pathologic grading systems have been devised for this assessment, all of which are based on the degree of tumor cellularity and necrosis within the resected specimen (see chapter 3).[123–125] Unfortunately, the percentage of tumor necrosis is difficult to evaluate, and most investigators have not graded tumor necrosis in a similar fashion as first proposed by Huvos and Rosen,[108,123] This ambiguity in the definition of a complete (good) pathologic response prevents a fully adequate and direct comparison between different preoperative chemotherapy regimens.

The initial concept of preoperative chemotherapy for osteosarcoma of the extremities was introduced and pioneered by Rosen and Marcove at the Memorial Hospital, starting in 1973.[105,126] Rosen's strategy evolved over a ten-year period and used systemic intravenous chemotherapy in four successive nonrandomized treatment protocols (T-4, T-7, T-10, T-12).[127] Refinements were made based on the che-

motherapy available at the time and by direct observation of responses on the primary tumor.[9,120]

With the second-generation T-7 protocol,[105] the introduction of the combination of BCD[128] (bleomycin, cytoxan, and dactinomycin being substituted for cytoxan alone) plus high-dose methotrexate 8–12 g/m² (increased from 200 mg/kg) resulted in an increase in the reported disease-free survival from approximately 50% to over 70% at a follow-up time between six and eight years. Surgery was performed at approximately week 10, and chemotherapy was resumed postoperatively for about ten months. Of 37 patients receiving preoperative chemotherapy, 62% underwent a limb-sparing procedure.

It became apparent from this protocol that those patients having a complete (good) response had almost a 100% disease-free survival (if they did not develop a local recurrence). A good response was defined as a clinical complete response (CR), with the additional histologic finding of only a few microscopic foci of viable tumor or no viable tumor (Huvos grade III or IV). Therefore, the responsiveness of the primary tumor to preoperative chemotherapy (as assessed by histologic examination) was found to be

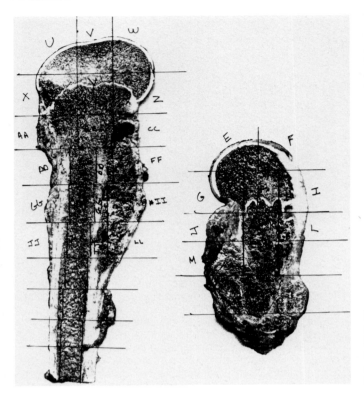

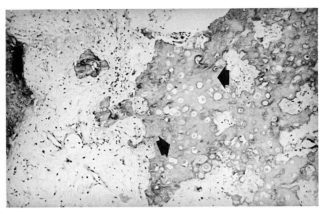

Figure 7–5. Technique of examination of the gross specimen following resection in order to determine the percent tumor necrosis. Square sections of 1 cm are drawn on an actual photocopy of the specimen, and each box is sampled. A map and percentage of the actual tumor necrosis can easily be determined and recorded.

a powerful predictor of tumor recurrence. Those patients at high risk for relapse could then be identified early, based on a poor response to preoperative chemotherapy.[108]

In 1978, Rosen initiated the T-10 protocol, which has yielded one of the best reported outcomes to date (see Table 7–2).[108] This was based on the emergence of cisplatin as an effective agent in osteosarcoma and the need for better therapy for the subset of patients

who had a poor histologic response (Huvos grades I and II) on the T-7 regimen. All patients received the same intensive pre-op T-7 regimen. After surgery, good responders continued to receive the same regimen (T-10B), in order to spare the toxic effects of cisplatin and adriamycin, whereas those patients having a partial or lesser response (fair and poor) received cisplatin, adriamycin, and BCD (T-10A).

Of 87 patients treated, 62% had a limb-sparing

Table 7–2. Preoperative Intravenous Chemotherapy with T-10 Like Regimens for Osteosarcoma

STUDY	# PTS	% GOOD RESPONDERS	% LIMB SALVAGE	% LOCAL RECURRENCE	SURVIVAL	MEDIAN FOLLOW-UP (mos)
Rosen T-10[108,127] MSKCC	87	48% (H-III,IV)	62%	2%	DFS 77% OS 82%	58
Rosen T-12[9,108,127] MSKCC	51	49% (H-III,IV)	84%	12%	DFS 75% OS 76%	25
Kalifa[129] Gustave Roussy	60	55% (>95% N)	82%	0	DFS 58% OS 85%	48
Provisor[130] CCSG, #782	192	30% (>95% N)	NM	NM	DFS 61%	24
Winkler[131,132] GPO, COSS-80	113	67% (>50% N)	55%	4%	DFS 68%	54
Winkler[132,133] GPO, COSS-82	125	43% (>90% N)	26%	2%	DFS 58%	34
Weiner[134] Mount Sinai	25	88% (H-III,IV)	64%	12%	DFS 72%	36

H = Huvos grade III, IV pathologic response; N = necrosis; DFS = disease-free survival; OS = overall survival, NM = not mentioned.

procedure; there was only a 2% local recurrence rate, and 48% had a good or complete histologic response. At a median follow-up of 58 months, 77% of patients were disease-free, with an 82% overall survival.[9,127] There was no difference in survival between those who underwent amputation and those who underwent en bloc resection. The disease-free survival of the poor-responding group was significantly better than the comparable T-7 regimen cohort ($P < .001$) and was almost the same as the good-responding group. The poor responders appeared to be "salvaged" by the selection of alternative postoperative chemotherapy. Thus, Rosen found that using the response to preoperative chemotherapy as the basis for the selection of a postoperative regimen (ie, "tailoring") was a helpful strategy.

The T-10 regimen became the prototype for several studies utilizing presurgical chemotherapy in the United States and around the world. However, recent trials attempting to confirm Rosen's T-10 single institution observations have yielded variable results.

Kalifa, at The Gustave Roussy (Villejuif, France), applied the T-10 regimen in 60 patients treated preoperatively over 12 weeks.[129] Eighty-two percent of patients underwent limb-sparing surgery, and 55% achieved a good histologic response. At a median follow-up of 48 months, 58% of all patients were continuously disease-free. Poor responders were switched to postoperative cisplatin/adriamycin chemotherapy. Yet, the disease-free survival rates for good and poor responders were 75% and 32%, respectively.

The Children's Cancer Study Group (CCSG) conducted a large multi-institutional trial of 192 patients with a modified T-10 regimen (preoperative adriamycin omitted).[130] The results were not as favorable as those reported by Rosen, with only 30% having a good histologic response (again defined as greater than 95% tumor necrosis) and 29% a fair response (50%–95% necrosis). The disease-free survival for these good responders was 91%; however, the disease-free survival for fair and poor responders was 83% and 40%. The disease-free survival for all patients was 61% at a median of two years follow-up. This larger cooperative trial further defined a subset of patients who appeared not to respond to salvage chemotherapy.

Rosen next developed the T-12 protocol in an attempt to improve the results of the T-10 regimen by intensifying preoperative chemotherapy with six courses of high-dose methotrexate and two of BCD. In addition, the postoperative treatment for good histologic responders was shortened to only five weeks of BCD and high-dose methotrexate (excluding adriamycin).[9,127] Of 51 patients treated, 84%

had a limb-sparing procedure. Unfortunately, the good histologic response rate was similar to the T-10 regimen at 49%, and the local recurrence rate was increased to 12%. At a median follow-up of 25 months, the disease-free survival for the entire group was 75%.

In the COSS-82 trial performed by the German Pediatric Oncology Group (GPO), switching postoperative chemotherapy for histologic nonresponders produced no better results than a previous trial (COSS-80) in which patients received identical preoperative and postoperative chemotherapy.[131–133] Similar to the other studies, the results suggest that patients demonstrating a poor response of the primary tumor will have a poor prognosis, and that poor responders will not be salvaged by alternative chemotherapy regimens. The GPO concluded that the active agents, ie, cisplatin and adriamycin, should not be withheld from the initial therapy of newly diagnosed patients (despite their toxicity).[133]

Weiner et al, from Mount Sinai, initiated a small nonrandomized study utilizing cisplatin and adriamycin.[134] Twenty-five patients received high-dose methotrexate ($8–12$ g/m^2) given for two consecutive weeks followed a week later by intravenous push cisplatin 75 mg/m^2 and adriamycin 75 mg/m^2 (25 mg/m^2/day $\times$ 3 days). After a two-week rest, this was repeated for two to four cycles. The same chemotherapy was continued postoperatively, regardless of the histologic response outcome. Sixty-four percent of patients had a successful limb salvage procedure, and the local recurrence rate for all patients was 12%. At surgery, 88% of patients had a good histologic response (Huvos grade III or IV). There was no difference between the number of cycles of preoperative chemotherapy received and the histologic tumor response. At a median follow-up of 36 months, there was a 72% disease-free survival. Interestingly, the high percentage of good responding patients has not translated into a dramatically better disease-free survival.

The results of these multiple preoperative intravenous chemotherapy studies represented a marked improvement compared with the investigators' previous experiences from their own institutions. However, the outcomes were not as good as Rosen had previously reported (T-10). Also, the strategy of salvaging poor histologic responders with alternative drug regimens failed to be duplicated. This problem has been further accentuated by the report of disparate histologic responses in primary and metastatic osteosarcoma treated simultaneously with preoperataive chemotherapy (some patients having a poor local response to chemotherapy showed an excellent response in pulmonary metastases that were excised

Table 7-3. Preoperative Intra-arterial Chemotherapy without Cisplatin for Osteosarcoma

STUDY	TREATMENT	# PTS	% LIMB SALVAGE	% LOCAL RECURRENCE	SURVIVAL	MEDIAN FOLLOW-UP (mos)
Akahoshi[136] 1976	MMC 8-12 mg/biw 5-FU 1-1.5 g/wk MTX 100-150 mg/wk (over 8-48 d)	56	NM	NM	OS 31% (44% with >3 wk infusion)	60
Eilber[137] 1987	ADR 90 mg over 3 d + 1,750 R	27 (control)	74%	33%	DFS 11% OS 25%	40
		32 (T-10B adjuvant)	75%	6%	DFS 38% OS 52%	40
Denton[50] 1984	ADR 100 mg over 3 d + 3,000 R	10	90%	0%	OS 89%*	12
Goodnight[56] 1985	ADR 90 mg over 3 d + 3,500-4000 R	8	75%	0%	DFS 63% OS 75%	34

ADR = adriamycin; 5-FU = 5-fluorouracil; MMC = mitomycin-C; MTX = methotrexate; NM = not mentioned; DFS = disease-free survival; OS = overall survival; R = rads.
*Projected survival. % necrosis not mentioned in all of the above studies.

simultaneously).[135] Nevertheless, Rosen has attributed the poor results of other investigators to (1) improper administration of methotrexate, with use of lower doses (ie, <8–12 g/m^2) and excessive, instead of restricted, hydration within the first 24 hours of administration, and to (2) misinterpretation of the Huvos histologic response criteria with less stringent definitions for a good response.[9,120]

In order to improve the results of preoperative intravenous systemic chemotherapy, to further downstage tumors, and to increase the limb-sparing procedure rate, other investigators (see Tables 7–3 to 7–5) began utilizing preoperative chemotherapy via the *intra-arterial route.* This allows for a higher cytotoxic concentration of chemotherapy to be directed to the primary tumor (increase the local drug concentration) and possible improved penetration of drug across the cell membrane. Several pharmacologic studies have confirmed an increased regional drug concentration, drug uptake, and tumor destruction.[18,117,155,156] Furthermore, the concentration of chemotherapy reaching the systemic circulation after initial intra-arterial passage is similar to that attained via the intravenous route and therefore should be enough to possibly destroy microscopic pulmonary metastases.[18]

Table 7-4. Single-Agent Preoperative Intra-arterial Cisplatin (DDP) alone for Osteosarcoma

STUDY	TREATMENT	# PTS	>60% NECROSIS	% LIMB SALVAGE	% LOCAL RECURRENCE	SURVIVAL	MEDIAN FOLLOW-UP (mos)
Jaffe[138] 1985	DDP 150 mg/m^2 over 2 h Q 2-3 wk (for 6-12 wk)	15	60% (47% GR)	NM	NM	NM	NM
	MTX 12.5 g/m^2 over 6 h (IA initially, then IV) QWK (for 6-12 wk)	15 (pediatric)	27%	NM	NM	NM	NM
Jaffe[139] 1987	DDP 150 mg/m^2 over 2 h Q 2 wk (1-7 courses)	35 (pediatric)	69% (40% GR)	40%	9%	DFS 56%	36
Jaffe[28] 1989	DDP 150 mg/m^2 over 2 h Q 2 wk	42					
	(1-3 courses)	9	11%	NM	NM	NM	NM
	(4-7 courses)	33 (pediatric)	79% (52% GR)	NM	NM	NM	NM
Epelman[140,141] & Petrelli 1987	DDP 100 mg/m^2 over 2 h Q 2 wk (for 3-5 courses)	58	NM	33%	2%	DFS 61% OS 89%	24

DDP = cisplatin; MTX = methotrexate; NM = not mentioned; DFS = disease-free survival; OS = overall survival; GR = good response (>90% necrosis); Pediatric = <16 years old.

Table 7-5. Multiagent Preoperative Chemotherapy with Intra-arterial Cisplatin (DDP) for Osteosarcoma

STUDY	TREATMENT	# PTS	% GOOD RESPONDERS	% LIMB SALVAGE	% LOCAL RECURRENCE	SURVIVAL	MEDIAN FOLLOW-UP (mos)
Benjamin[142,143] 1987	ADR 90 mg/m^2 IV over 4 d DDP 120 mg/m^2 IA over 2 h (for 3-7 courses)	37 (adult)	59%	60%	6%	DFS 53% OS 62%	60
Benjamin[144] 1989	ADR 90 mg/m^2 IV over 4 d DDP 160 mg/m^2 IA over 24 h (given till max response)	50 (adult)	71%	86%	NM	DFS 72%	48
Picci[145-149] 1988	MTX *750 mg/m^2 IV over 30 min* DDP 120-150 mg/m^2 IA over 3 d *or*	54	(42%)			(DFS 43%)	48
	MTX 7.5 g/m^2 IV over 6 h DDP 120-150 mg/m^2 IA over 3 d (for 2 courses)	*58* 112	*(61%)* 52%	72%	5%	*(DFS 64%)* DFS 54%	48 48
Picci[150] 1989	MTX 8 g/m^2 IV over 6 h DDP 120 mg/m^2 IA over 3 d ADR 60 mg/m^2 IV over 8 h (for 2 courses)	116	76%	87%	1%	DFS 89%	24 (mean)
Stine[151] 1989	ADR 90 mg/m^2 IV over 4 d DDP 150 mg/m^2 IA over 2 h (for 3-4 courses)	8 (pediatric)	75% (>80%N)	75%	13%	DFS 63% OS 100%	18 23
Malawer[152,153] 1989	DDP 120 mg/m^2 IA ADR 60 mg/m^2 IV over 3 d (for 2 courses)	31	60%	87%	3%	DFS 68%	30
Weiss[154] 1989	ADR 8 mg/m^2/d FUDR 0.5 mg/kg/d (until systemic toxicity) DDP 120 mg/m^2 IA over 6 h (for 2 courses)	18	90% (>85%N)	86%	0%	DFS 89%	24 (mean)

ADR = adriamycin; DDP = cisplatin; FUDR = floxuridine; MTX = methotrexate; NM = not mentioned; DFS = disease-free survival; OS = overall survival; Adults = ≥16 years old; Pediatric = <16 years old; N = necrosis; Good Response = ≥90% necrosis.

For most studies involving IA chemotherapy, the pathologic evaluations of a response have consisted of less strict criteria than Rosen and Huvos, ie, good response being greater than 90% tumor necrosis, fair response being 60%–90% tumor necrosis, and poor response being less than 60% tumor necrosis.

An early study by Akahoshi used a combination of minimally active drugs (ie, mitomycin-C, 5-FU, and low-dose methotrexate) all given IA over an 8- to 48-day period.[136] Those patients receiving a greater than three-week infusion had a 44% survival at five years. However, 60% of patients developed metastases within one year. Eilber et al utilized adriamycin given as a three-day infusion, followed by radiation therapy of 1,750 rads (350 rads/day for five days) to the involved bone (similar to that for soft tissue sarcoma).[137,157] A high proportion of patients received limb salvage surgery. Overall survival was 68% at 30 months, with only a 2% local recurrence rate. A fairly high degree of tumor destruction was described, but no specific detailed histologic response was reported. Both Denton and Goodnight in much smaller patient series have obtained similar results to Eilber (see Table 7–3) but their follow-up was much shorter.[50,56] Unfortunately, the intra-arterial adriamycin treatment was complicated by erythema and ulceration of the underlying skin and subcutaneous tissue, with extensive necrosis of nor-

mal tissues. Furthermore, a complete histologic response in the primary tumor was rarely noted. Because of the potential for normal tissue destruction, preoperative intra-arterial adriamycin has not been universally endorsed or accepted.

An alternative drug for preoperative intra-arterial use was cisplatin. Jaffe et al has made numerous contributions utilizing intra-arterial cisplatin as a single agent for the treatment of osteosarcoma in the pediatric population (patients ≤ 16 years old). A preoperative dose of 150 mg/m^2 given every two to three weeks was found to be safe and effective for producing a clinical response.[117] In another study (see Table 7–4), Jaffe compared intra-arterial cisplatin with high-dose methotrexate given either IA and/ or IV (pharmacologic studies showed no significant differences in terms of response if methotrexate was given by the IA or IV route).[62,138] A greater proportion of patients were found to respond to intra-arterial cisplatin, and the number of pathologic good responses (≥90% tumor necrosis) was significantly higher. In addition, two patients failing to respond to methotrexate achieved a complete response with intra-arterial cisplatin, whereas no patient failing to respond to cisplatin subsequently responded to high-dose methotrexate. Unfortunately, there was still a high rate of metastases (almost 50%) with this therapy.

Recently, Jaffe has shown that the primary tumor response to intra-arterial cisplatin depends on the number of courses of cisplatin administered.[28] When used as a single agent, at least four courses were required to achieve an optimum effect. Only 11% of patients receiving one to three courses of therapy achieved a pathologic response (≥60% necrosis), compared to 79% of patients receiving four to seven courses. There was no further significant difference in histologic degree of tumor destruction among patients receiving four to five *v* six to seven courses of cisplatin. However, clinical and radiologic differences were felt to be more impressive with the extra courses.

The complete (good) response rate for intra-arterial cisplatin alone in the Jaffe studies was 40%–50%. One study reported a 40% limb salvage procedure rate, with 9% local recurrences.[139] Postoperatively, patients received 12 months of rotating cycles of intravenous high-dose methotrexate, adriamycin, and cisplatin. In patients with <60% tumor necrosis, the intravenous cisplatin was omitted. Disease-free survival in this study was 56% at 36 months (see Table 7–4). Life table analysis as a function of good *v* poor responders was 72% and 36%, respectively. These data are difficult to evaluate since they include patients receiving variable courses of preoperative cisplatin.

Epelman and Petrelli utilized a lower dose of intra-arterial cisplatin 100 mg/m² over three to five courses and achieved almost similar results.[140,141] Postoperatively, cisplatin and adriamycin were given to all patients with no alteration for the tumor histologic response. The limb salvage rate was 33% with only a 2% local recurrence. At a median of 24 months, disease-free survival was 61% with an overall survival of 89%.

There have also been several multiagent preoperative chemotherapy studies incorporating concomitant intra-arterial cisplatin (see Table 7–5). In the adult osteosarcoma population (≥16 years old) Benjamin et al developed a combination preoperative regimen consisting of adriamycin 90 mg/m² given on an outpatient basis as a 96-hour continuous intravenous infusion through a central venous catheter, followed by intra-arterial cisplatin 120 mg/m².[142,143] Adriamycin was given as a four-day intravenous infusion to avoid dose-limiting local toxicity, to reduce the acute toxicity of nausea and vomiting, and to decrease cumulative cardiac toxicity.[158] On the fifth day, the infusion was discontinued; the patient was then admitted to the hospital for hydration, prior to an arteriogram and the intra-arterial infusion of cisplatin on day 6. Postoperatively, the same drugs were given IV. DTIC was substituted for cisplatin if there was evidence of significant neurotoxicity and/or ototoxicity.

Between 1979 and 1982, 37 patients were treated and 59% had a good histologic response (≥90% tumor necrosis).[142,143] At a median of five years follow-up, the disease-free survival was 53% and the overall survival 62%. Limb salvage procedures were performed in 60% of patients, and the local recurrence rate was 6%. As part of a prognostic factor analysis evaluating independent variables, Benjamin found (similar to Rosen) that a good histologic response was over 1000 times more important than the combination of four previously identified pretreatment prognostic variables (ie, primary site in the lower extremity; differentiated, small-cell, or high-grade surface-tumor histology; soft tissue mass >1 cm; and male sex). This single prognostic factor essentially displaced all other pretreatment prognostic factors from the equation. Patients with a good histologic response had a five-year survival of 84% compared to 14% for those with a partial or no response.

Since 1983, Benjamin et al increased the intra-arterial dose of cisplatin to 160 mg/m² for patients with three or more poor pretreatment prognostic factors.[143,144] Also, any patient not having a good angiographic response to lower-dose cisplatin received the intensified regimen. Most patients received four or more courses of chemotherapy prior to surgery, it being continued until maximum response was judged by subtraction arteriography. Patients with a complete response received only three postoperative cycles of intravenous cisplatin and adriamycin, and patients with <90% necrosis were switched to a 9- to 12-month alternating postoperative chemotherapy regimen of high-dose methotrexate, adriamycin with DTIC, and BCD. With 71% achieving a complete histologic response, limb salvage procedures were performed in 86% of patients.[144] At a median follow-up of four years, the disease-free survival was a respectable 72% (81% for good responders).[144] This compares favorably with a three-year disease-free survival (DFS) rate of 20% in an historical untreated control series, 50% DFS in an adriamycin-based adjuvant chemotherapy series, and to a 60% DFS in the previous lower-dose intra-arterial cisplatin study. Although patients received a prolonged and intensified preoperative regimen, the excellent DFS for good responders was achieved with only three courses of postoperative chemotherapy. Patients with <90% tumor necrosis had a 51% DFS at four years compared with 14% (at three years) in the previous series treated before 1983. This could be related to the change in postoperative adjuvant chemotherapy (salvage therapy), but could also be contributed by the more prolonged intense primary treatment (since most of these patients achieved a partial response).

In these two intra-arterial series from Benjamin, only 8% of patients were felt to be candidates for limb salvage prior to preoperative intra-arterial chemotherapy. But as a direct result of this chemotherapy, 60% of patients in the first group and 86% in the second group were able to undergo a limb salvage procedure.[143] The incidence of local relapse was low and almost identical for patients having a limb salvage procedure *v* an amputation. Survival was more closely related to the response to chemotherapy than to the type of surgery performed. Furthermore, the local complication rate was lower and more acceptable than that found in the studies that used local radiation and intra-arterial adriamycin.

Stine et al, in a few pediatric patients, utilized a preoperative regimen similar to Benjamin's given for two to five courses.[151] Seventy-five percent of patients were able to undergo a limb salvage procedure. The postoperative chemotherapy was different, consisting of rotating cycles of BCD, cisplatin with adriamycin, and cisplatin with etoposide. Study comparisons of the histologic response are difficult to make since a less strict definition for a good response was used; 75% of patients had *>80% tumor necrosis*. The DFS was less than the Benjamin series, being 63% at 18 months.

Investigators at the Rizzoli Institute (Bologna, Italy) have reported on the largest series of localized osteosarcoma patients (including both pediatric and adult) treated with preoperative intra-arterial cisplatin.[145–149] From 1983 to 1986, 127 patients were given two cycles (six weeks) of preoperative methotrexate and cisplatin; adriamycin was not used because of its cardiac toxicity. Patients were randomized to receive either intravenous high dose (7.5 g/m^2 in a 6-hour infusion) or moderate dose (750 mg/m^2 over 30 minutes) methotrexate. Six days later, cisplatin 120–150 mg/m^2 was administered as a 72-hour *continuous intra-arterial* infusion in order to reduce the potential renal toxicity of the methotrexate/cisplatin combination and to possibly obtain greater cell killing.[159,160] This regimen had first been tried in a pilot study in which seven patients received preoperative intra-arterial cisplatin and six received intravenous cisplatin. Pathologic review of the surgical specimens revealed that the percentage of patients with good histologic necrosis was higher in the intra-arterial group (five of seven—71%) than in the intravenous group (zero of six). Based on the results from this small series, *intra-arterial* cisplatin was then used in the definitive protocol.

Surgery was performed seven weeks after the start of the preoperative chemotherapy. Seventy-two percent of patients were able to undergo a limb salvage procedure. The local recurrence rate was only 5%, which was not significantly different from the rate observed in a previous study with amputation and adjuvant chemotherapy alone.[149] There was no significant difference for methotrexate dose (high *v* moderate) or type of surgery performed (amputation *v* limb-sparing procedure). Two factors seemed to influence the rate of local recurrence: the extent of surgical margins, and the percent of histologic necrosis induced by the preoperative regimen.[149,161] Limb salvage surgery appeared to be as safe as ablative surgery if adequate margins were achieved. For good responders, a wide margin of resection was sufficient, whereas for fair and poor responders a radical margin was the minimum required.[149,161]

The histologic response induced by this preoperative regimen was respectable, with 52% of patients having a good response (≥90% necrosis) and 35% a fair response (60%–89% necrosis). The rate of good responders was significantly higher in the high-dose methotrexate group compared with the moderate dose (62% *v* 42%, $P < 0.04$).[149]

Postoperative (adjuvant) intravenous chemotherapy was begun one week after surgery in amputated patients and three weeks later in patients having a limb salvage procedure, and it was based on the histologic response to preoperative chemotherapy ("salvage" treatment). Initially, good responders received a short post-op course with only two cycles of the same preoperative regimen (without adriamycin). Fair responders received 24 weeks of adriamycin 45 mg/m^2 × 2 days, methotrexate, and cisplatin. Poor responders were treated with a 45-week regimen of adriamycin and BCD. However, when four early relapses (lung metastases) occurred among the first 15 good-responding patients treated with the short post-op regimen, this study arm was closed. Thereafter, all other good responders were treated with the same postoperative schedule as fair responders (ie, including adriamycin).[145–149]

Excluding the above 15 patients, the DFS for the remaining 112 patients was 54% at a median follow-up of four years (Table 7–5). There was a statistically significant DFS for the high-dose methotrexate group (64% *v* 43%, $P < 0.05$).[149] There was no significant difference in survival based on patient age, or type of surgery (amputation *v* limb-sparing procedure). A multivariate analysis of several other prognostic factors revealed that only the preoperative alkaline phosphatase level and percent histologic necrosis correlated with patient survival.[149]

The DFS rate for good-responding patients receiving post-op adriamycin was 78%, compared with

27% for the 15 patients treated with the short post-op, no-adriamycin regimen, and the DFS for fair and poor responders was 42% and 10%, respectively. This study again showed that changing the post-op chemotherapy regimen based on the tumor response to pre-op chemotherapy ("salvage therapy") did not significantly increase patient survival for poor responders.

When the results in DFS for the 112 patients in this trial were compared with the DFS for 106 patients treated at the Rizzoli Institute between 1980 and 1982 with surgery and adjuvant chemotherapy alone (regimen including adriamycin and methotrexate), there was a slight advantage for preoperative chemotherapy (54% *v* 43%).[94,149] Furthermore, 78% of patients in the adjuvant chemotherapy alone group required an amputation *v* only 27% in the present study. Preoperative chemotherapy did, however, increase the overall complication rate; five infectious complications led to later amputation.[149,162]

Investigators at the Rizzoli Institute began a second study in September 1986 with the aim of increasing the number of histologic good responders by modifying the previous regimen with more intensive chemotherapy.[150] Methotrexate was increased to 8 g/m^2, and on the third day of the intra-arterial cisplatin infusion, adriamycin 60 mg/m^2 was added as an eight-hour intravenous infusion. Patients again received two cycles of preoperative chemotherapy (each cycle lasting 28 days), and surgery was performed during the eighth week. Thus far, the preliminary results reported are extremely encouraging. The good-response rate ($\geq$90% necrosis) was 76%. Of 116 patients, limb salvage procedures were able to be performed in 87%, with only a 1% local recurrence rate.[150]

Postoperatively, good-responding patients received three cycles (12 weeks) of the same preoperative chemotherapy, and patients with <90% tumor necrosis had a longer duration of treatment with adriamycin and methotrexate, plus ifosfamide (2 g/m^2 $\times$ 5 days) and etoposide (120 mg/m^2 $\times$ 3 days). Follow-up was still short, but at a *mean duration* of 24 months 89% of patients are continuously disease-free (for 51 patients with a $\geq$24-month follow-up, the DFS is 84%). Compared with their first intra-arterial neoadjuvant study, there was a significant increase in limb salvage procedures performed (87% *v* 77%), good response rate (76% *v* 52%), and two-year continuous DFS (84% *v* 59%), without there being significant differences found in chemotherapy toxicity.[149,150]

The role of drug dose intensity (DDI) was also examined by calculating the average percentage of the originally planned drug doses per week for each patient.[163] The DFS in patients with a DDI $\geq$ 75% was 91% compared with 79% with a DDI < 75% (*P* = .04). Furthermore, within the good-responding group the relapse rates with a $\geq$75% DDI and <75% DDI were 8% and 16%, respectively (*P* = .05). Therefore, DDI, in addition to percent tumor necrosis, appears to be an important determinant for prognosis.

Recently, we have studied the combined use of IA cisplatin and IV adriamycin (without methotrexate), limited to two preoperative courses.[152,153] The regimen differed from Benjamin et al in that slightly lower doses of the same drugs were given in reverse sequence for fewer cycles (six total cycles—two preoperative and four postoperative). Cisplatin was administered IA 120 mg/m^2 over 2 hours followed by adriamycin 60 mg/m^2 given as a continuous intravenous infusion over three days through a central venous catheter. After surgery, postoperative therapy continued for all patients with the same two drugs given IV for four cycles. Following preoperative chemotherapy, a limb-sparing procedure was possible in 87% of patients, and only 3% had a local recurrence. Of interest, 82% of patients initially deemed unresectable were able to be converted to a limb-sparing procedure (Fig. 7–6). Sixty percent of patients had a good histologic response ($\geq$90% necrosis), and the local recurrence rate was 3% (Fig. 7–7). At a median follow-up of 30 months, DFS was 68%. Although this is a small study and requires confirmation, it appears that a short course of active drugs (cisplatin and

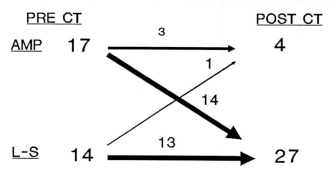

SURGICAL PROCEDURES
AMPUTATION V. LIMB-SPARING SURGERY

Figure 7–6. The impact of regional (intra-arterial) chemotherapy for high-grade bone sarcomas as recently reported by the authors. The schematic shows the relationship of the initial surgical decision (prechemotherapy, Pre CT) *v* the actual procedure performed following 2 cycles of intra-arterial chemotherapy (Post CT) with respect to amputation (Amp) and limb-sparing (L-S) surgery. The initial limb-sparing rate was 45% (if no chemotherapy was to be given) *v* 87%, the actual limb-sparing rate. Fourteen of 17 patients (82%) requiring an amputation converted to a limb-sparing procedure (from Malawer et al[21]).

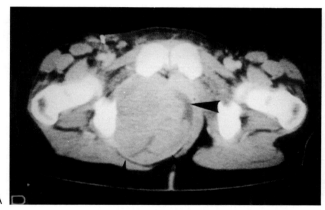
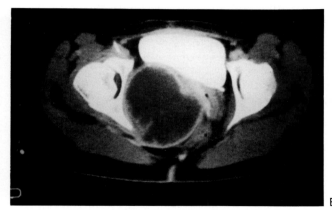

A   B

Figure 7–7. Computerized tomography (CT) scan of a large sarcoma arising from the pelvic floor (**A**) demonstrating a good response to intra-arterial chemotherapy. This tumor (solid arrow) was considered inoperable even by a hemipelvectomy. The patient underwent two courses of intra-arterial chemotherapy. CT prior to treatment and (**B**) following intra-arterial chemotherapy. Note the complete necrosis as represented by the "liquefaction" (decreased density) of the tumor. This patient underwent a limb-sparing (pelvic floor, type III) resection and remains alive without recurrence at five years. Examination of the gross specimen showed 100% necrosis.

adriamycin) can provide almost comparative response rates to more-intensive and longer-duration chemotherapeutic regimens.

Weiss et al, in another small study, also used two courses of preoperative intra-arterial chemotherapy.[154] FUDR and adriamycin were administered as a continuous intravenous infusion until systemic toxicity was reached. On the fourth and last day of this infusion, cisplatin 120 mg/m^2 was administered IA over 6 hours. Among 18 patients, limb salvage was performed in 86% with no local recurrences. The pathologic response reported was excellent, but it was based on a less stringent histologic standard—90% of patients having *greater than 85% tumor necrosis*. All patients received two years of postoperative treatment consisting of adriamycin, actinomycin-D, methotrexate, and cyclophosphamide. Although follow-up is short, overall survival was 89% at a *mean* follow-up of two years.

Whether preoperative *intra-arterial* chemotherapy is superior or equivalent to the *intravenous* route is still questionable, and this was not fully answered by the very small comparative pilot trial performed by the Rizzoli Institute. Two other studies have tried to address this important issue (see Table 7–6). Graham-Pole et al gave two courses of high-dose methotrexate followed by two courses of cisplatin and adriamycin preoperatively.[164] Intra-arterial cisplatin 100 mg/m^2 administered over one hour was compared with the identical intravenous dose over 6 hours. Postoperatively, all patients were given the same three drugs intravenously for five cycles. These were in reality two sequential trials without a prospective randomization; the patients receiving pre-

operative intravenous cisplatin were those diagnosed in the first year of the study (before the use of intra-arterial cisplatin was adopted), all those between 10 and 30 years old, and those who chose not to receive intra-arterial cisplatin. The histologic tumor response (>80% necrosis) was found to be equivalent between the intra-arterial and intravenous cisplatin groups (57% v 54%). The responses in both groups were inferior to other studies, possibly related to the lower doses of cisplatin and adriamycin used. The limb salvage rate was found to be higher in the intra-arterial group (63% v 47%), although this was not statistically significant (both being higher than a historical control group rate of 30%). At a median follow-up of only 18 months, disease-free and overall survival were slightly better in the intra-arterial group, but again this was not statistically significant. Unfortunately, this study lacked a prospective randomization, utilized suboptimum doses of cisplatin and adriamycin, had a short duration of intra-arterial administration (most studies using 2 hours or more), and had a short duration of follow-up.

In a second study investigating the use of more intensive preoperative chemotherapy (COSS-86), Winkler et al compared the effects of cisplatin given by either intra-arterial tourniquet infusion or by intravenous infusion.[165] Following cycles of intravenous adriamycin and high-dose methotrexate, the cisplatin was administered over one hour with concomitant intravenous ifosfamide (Table 7–6). As in other studies, the authors showed that the amount of drug available to act against micrometastatic disease was not compromised by regional therapy. They

Table 7–6. Comparison of Preoperative Intravenous versus Intra-arterial Cisplatin for Osteosarcoma

STUDY	TREATMENT	# PTS	% NECROSIS (N)	% LIMB SALVAGE	PROJECTED 2-YEAR SURVIVAL
Graham-Pole, 1988[164]	MTX 7.5 g/m² IV over 6 h (2 courses) plus 2 courses DDP 100 mg/m² *IV* over 6 h ADR 40 mg/m² IV push	17	(>80%N) 54%	47%	DFS 65% OS 69%
	or DDP 100 mg/m² *IA* over 1 h ADR 40 mg/m² IV push	19	57%	63%	DFS 77% OS 81%
Winkler, 1989[165] (COSS-86)	ADR 90 mg/m² IV over 2 d MTX 12 g/m² IV (2 courses) IFOS 3 g/m² IV × 2d (2 courses) plus 2 courses DDP 150 mg/m² *IV* over 1 h	15	(>90%N) 47%		
	or DDP 120 mg/m² *IV* over 5 h	26	77%		
	or DDP 150 mg/m² *IA* over 1 h	36	75%		

ADR = adriamycin; DDP = cisplatin; IFOS = ifosfamide; MTX = methotrexate; DFS = disease-free survival; OS = overall survival.

found an identical systemic availability for cisplatin (with similar plasma, ultrafiltrate, and urinary concentrations) regardless of the route used.[18] There was also no correlation between the deposition of cisplatin in tumor tissue and the mode of cisplatin administration or histologic response of the sarcoma to preoperative chemotherapy.[18] When the pharmacokinetic data showed equal systemic drug availability for either cisplatin route, the dose was reduced from 150 to 120 mg/m². Additionally, the intravenous cisplatin infusion was extended from 1 to 5 hours in order to decrease ototoxicity. The 1-hour intra-arterial tourniquet infusion had a good response rate (≥90% necrosis), 28% higher than the 1-hour intravenous infusion (75% v 47%, P = .04), but was found to be similar to the 5-hour intravenous infusion (77%).[165] The authors assumed that a regional advantage for a more prolonged intra-arterial infusion without a tourniquet would be markedly less and probably not worthwhile (but this may not be true). Patient accrual for each treatment was not fully prospectively randomized, and the doses of cisplatin were variable and changed in mid-study. The intensive doses of the concomitant intravenous chemotherapy may have negated or obscured any effect of regional chemotherapy. Of consequence, comparisons of the limb salvage rate, disease-free, and overall survival were not reported.

Winkler's COSS-86 data has been further updated and continues to show no advantage for IA cisplatin over IV cisplatin in terms of good histologic tumor response (34/50—68% vs. 41/59—69%). Even though this was a large study involving 53 institutions, 46% (94/203) of the patients were excluded from the analysis because of changes in the timing of surgery (early, late, or none), major protocol violations and missing data.[172] Also, as mentioned, this was not a strict randomized trial but a sequential study, and modifications of cisplatin infusion time and dosage were made in mid-study.

In summary, over the past two decades the prognosis for patients with osteosarcoma of the extremities has markedly improved, with more than two thirds of patients who present with nonmetastatic disease being cured. The impact of postoperative adjuvant chemotherapy now appears indisputable. Newer approaches of preoperative (neoadjuvant) chemotherapy and limb-sparing surgery have in nonrandomized studies shown durable local control with further improved disease-free survival. However, some investigators have felt that these superior results may reflect the use of more intensive multiagent chemotherapy (ie, incorporating cisplatin) and are unrelated to the timing (pre-op v post-op) or route of administration (IV v IA) of chemotherapy. They have argued that equally intensive adjuvant chemotherapy regimens need to be tested against preoperative chemotherapy in a prospectively randomized fashion.[10,166] The Pediatric Oncology Group trial (POG-8651) has been designed to examine the benefit of standard adjuvant chemotherapy alone v preoperative chemotherapy. Unfortunately, this trial may not accrue a sufficient number of patients because of the reluctance of orthopedic surgeons to operate without preoperative chemotherapy.

Preoperative intra-arterial chemotherapy appears to allow for more limb-sparing procedures to be performed without substantially increasing the risk of local recurrence and still controlling micrometastatic disease. It converts a marginal resection to a wide resection, allowing for a safer surgical procedure. Despite variations in the definition of a good response by various research groups, there appears to be a consistently improved DFS for good-responding patients. The benefit of "tailoring" adjuvant chemotherapy based on the response of the primary tumor to preoperative chemotherapy has not been substantiated. Most current preoperative protocols include a multidrug regimen given for 6 to 24 weeks, followed by resection of the primary tumor and 4 to 12 months of adjuvant intravenous chemotherapy. The essential drugs in the preoperative regimens include cisplatin, adriamycin, and/or high-dose methotrexate. Benjamin and Jaffe's strategy has been to treat preoperatively with multiple cycles of chemotherapy until the patient has achieved a maximal clinical/angiographic response, whereas other investigators administer only two preoperative chemotherapy cycles.

Whether preoperative intra-arterial chemotherapy when compared with intravenous chemotherapy will further increase the limb-sparing rate with an equivalent or increased long-term survival is not yet known. To date, the technique has been limited to centers with excellent angiographic support and facilities. There is a need to determine whether the cost, complexity, time commitment, and morbidity are justifiable. Furthermore, it is essential to note that patients receiving this treatment need to be followed closely, since a small number may be completely insensitive to the prescribed drugs. In this case, the tumor may continue to progress, and these patients need to be identified early so that they can be switched either to another chemotherapy regimen and/or have an immediate operation.

CONCLUSIONS

For the future, we will need to build upon this foundation of recent preoperative regional chemotherapy studies. With current treatment regimens, it appears that limb salvage will be possible for the majority of patients with sarcomas of the extremities. Although these clinical trials appear to be encouraging, several are, for the most part, preliminary, have limited patient accrual, and/or are not well controlled. Larger prospectively randomized multi-

institution studies will be needed. Further refinement of the use of existing chemotherapeutic agents as to dose intensity, duration, and site of administration will be required. Innovative trials incorporating new drugs into the best-known treatment regimens will have to be further developed (ie, ifosfamide and new platinum analogues having reduced toxicity).[167–170]

Further dose escalation of active chemotherapy with concomitant utilization of hematopoietic growth factors (ie. G-CSF—granulocyte colony stimulating factor, GM-CSF—granulocyte/macrophage colony stimulating factor) should also be examined.

Clearly, only time will tell whether the new regional (neoadjuvant) treatment regimens are more beneficial. Nevertheless, one important outgrowth of these studies has been the development of a meaningful dialogue and cooperation between a variety of different health professionals involved in the care of these patients. A continued multidisciplinary team approach will be absolutely necessary in order to further advance the goals of local tumor control, limb salvage with optimum extremity function, minimal morbidity from treatment, and improved long-term survival.

REFERENCES

1. Silverberg E, Boring CC, Squires TS: Cancer statistics 1990. *CA* 1990;40:18–19.
2. Fine G, Chorodnik JM, Horn RC, et al: Soft tissue tumors: Their clinical behavior and course and influencing factors, in *Seventh National Cancer Center Conference Proceedings*. Philadelphia, JB Lippincott, 1973; pp 873–882.
3. Shiu MH, Castro EB, Hajdu SI, et al: Surgical treatment of 297 soft tissue sarcomas of the lower extremity. *Ann Surg* 1975;182:597–602.
4. Sim FH, Pritchard DJ, Reiman HM, et al: Soft tissue sarcoma: Mayo Clinic experience. *Sem Surg Oncol* 1988;4:38–44.
5. Friedman MA, Carter SK: The therapy of osteogenic sarcoma: current status and thoughts for the future. *J Surg Oncol* 1972;4:482–510.
6. Goorin AM, Abelson HT, Frei E III: Osteosarcoma: Fifteen years later. *N Engl J Med* 1985;313:1637–1643.
7. Kalnicki S: Radiation therapy in the tratment of bone and soft tissue sarcomas. *Orthop Clin N Am* 1989; 20:505–512.
8. Bramwell VHC: Current perspectives in the management of soft tissue sarcomas: The role of chemotherapy in multimodality therapy. *Can J Surg* 1988; 31:390–396.
9. Rosen G: The current management of malignant bone tumors: Where do we go from here? *Med J Austral* 1988;148:373–377.
10. Nachman JB: Controversies in the treatment of osteosarcoma. *Med J Austral* 1988;148:405–410.
11. Jaffe N: Chemotherapy for malignant bone tumors. *Orthop Clin N Am* 1989;20:487–503.

12. Consensus Conference: Limb-sparing treatment of adult soft-tissue sarcomas and osteosarcomas. *JAMA* 1985;254:1791–1794.

13. National Institutes of Health Consensus Development Panel: Limb-sparing treatment of adult soft tissue sarcomas and osteosarcomas: Introduction and conclusions. *Cancer Treat Symp* 1985;3:1–5.

14. Simon MA, Nachman J: Current concepts review: The clinical utility of preoperative therapy for sarcomas. *J Bone Joint Surg* 1986;68:1458–1463.

15. Klopp CT, Alford TC, Bateman J, et al: Fractionated intra arterial cancer chemotherapy with methyl bisamine hydrochloride. *Ann Surg* 1950;132:811–832.

16. Wallace S, Charnsangavej JC, Carrasco CH, et al: Infusion embolization. *Cancer* 1984;54:2751–2765.

17. Chen HSG, Gross JF: Intraarterial infusion of anticancer drugs: Theoretic aspects of drug delivery and review of responses. *Cancer Treat Rep* 1980;64:31–40.

18. Bielack SS, Erttmann R, Looft G, et al: Platinum disposition after intraarterial and intravenous infusion of cisplatin for osteosarcoma. *Cancer Chemother Pharmacol* 1989;24:376–380.

19. Howell SB: Improving the therapeutic index of intraarterial cisplatinum chemotherapy. *Eur J Cancer Clin Oncol* 1989;25:775–776.

20. Abe R, Akiyoski T, Koba F, et al: "Two route chemotherapy", using intraarterial cis-platinum & intravenous sodium thiosulfate; its neutralizing agent, for hepatic malignancies. *Eur J Cancer Clin Oncol* 1988;24:1671–1674.

21. Malawer M, Priebat D, Buch R, et al: The impact of a short course (2 cycles) of neoadjuvant chemotherapy with *cis*-platinum and adriamycin on the choice of surgical procedure for high grade bone sarcomas of the extremities. *Clin Orthop Rel Res*, to be published.

22. Holland JF, Frei E III: Effect of dose and schedule on response, in Holland JF, Frei E III (eds): *Cancer Medicine*. Philadelphia, Lea & Febiger, 1973.

23. Carrasco CH, Charnsangavej JC, Richli WJ, et al: Intraarterial cisplatinum in osteosarcoma. *Haematol Blut Transfus* 1987;31:52–56.

24. Drewinko B, Gottlieb JA: Action of cis-dichlorodiammine-platinum II on cultured human lymphoma cells and its therapeutic implications. *Cancer Chemother Rep* 1973;33:3091–3095.

25. Bramwell VHC: Intraarterial chemotherapy of soft tissue sarcomas. *Sem Surg Oncol* 1988;4:66–72.

26. Pritchard D, Mavligit GM, Benjamin RS, et al: Regression of regionally confined melanoma with intraarterial cis-dichlorodiammine platinum. *Cancer Treat Rep* 1979;63:555–558.

27. Jaffe N, Robertson R, Takaue Y, et al: Control of primary osteosarcoma with chemotherapy. *Cancer* 1985;56:461–466.

28. Jaffe N, Raymond AK, Ayala A, et al: Effect of cumulative courses of intraarterial cis-diamminedichloroplatinum II on the primary tumor in pediatric osteosarcoma. *Cancer* 1989;63:63–67.

29. Chuang VP, Wallace S: Arterial infusion and occlusion in cancer patients. *Sem Roent* 1981;16:13–25.

30. Wallace S: Interventional radiology—intraarterial chemotherapy. *J Radiol* 1984;65:499–508.

31. Stewart DJ: Pros and cons of intra-arterial chemotherapy. *Oncology* 1989;3:20–26.

32. Karakousis CP, Kanter PM, Park HC, et al: Tourniquet infusion versus hyperthermic perfusion. *Cancer* 1982;49:850–858.

33. Anderson JH, Gianturco C, Wallace S: Experimental transcatheter intraarterial infusion—occlusion chemotherapy. *Invest Radiol* 1981;16:496–500.

34. Krementz ET, Carter RD, Sutherland CM, et al: Chemotherapy of sarcomas of limbs by regional perfusion. *Ann Surg* 1977;185:555–564.

35. Krementz ET: Regional perfusion: Current sophistication, what next? *Cancer* 1986;57:416–432.

36. Hoekstra HJ, Schraffordt Koops H, Molenaar WM, et al: Results of isolated regional perfusion in the treatment of malignant soft tissue tumors of the extremities. *Cancer* 1987;60:1703–1707.

37. Lehti PM, Stephens MH, Janoff K, et al: Improved survival for soft tissue sarcoma of the extremities by regional hyperthermic perfusion, local excision and radiation therapy. *Surg Gynecol Obstet* 1986;162:149–152.

38. McBride CM: Sarcoma of the limbs: Results of adjuvant chemotherapy using isolation perfusion. *Arch Surg* 1974;109:304–308.

39. Muchmore JH, Carter RD, Krementz ET: Regional perfusion for malignant melanoma and soft tissue sarcoma: A review. *Cancer Invest* 1985;3:129–143.

40. Klaase JM, Kroon BBR, Benckhuijsen C, et al: Results of regional isolation perfusion with cytostatics in patients with soft tissue tumors of the extremities. *Cancer* 1989;64:616–621.

41. Kato T, Nemoto R, Mori H, et al: Arterial embolization with microencapsulated anticancer drugs. *JAMA* 1981;245:1123–1127.

42. Lawrence W, Donegan W, Natarjan N, et al: Adult soft tissue sarcomas: A pattern of care survey of the American College of Surgeons. *Ann Surg* 1987;205:349–359.

43. Lawrence W: Concepts in limb sparing treatment of adult soft tissue sarcomas. *Sem Surg Oncol* 1988;4:73–77.

44. Brennan MF, Shiu MH: Multimodality therapy for soft tissue sarcoma, in Shiu MH, Brennan MF (eds): *Surgical Management of Soft Tissue Sarcoma*. Philadelphia, Lea and Febiger, 1989, pp 277–290.

45. Antman KH, Eilber F, Shiu MH: Multidisciplinary approaches to soft tissue sarcoma. *Am Soc Clin Oncol Education Booklet* 1988, pp 14–27.

46. Yang JC, Rosenberg SA: Surgery for adult patients with soft tissue sarcomas. *Sem Oncol* 1989;16:289–296.

47. Tepper JE: Role of radiation therapy in the management of patients with bone and soft tissue sarcomas. *Sem Oncol* 1989;16:281–288.

48. Azzarelli A, Quagliuolo V, Audisio RA, et al: Intraarterial adriamycin followed by surgery for limb sarcomas. Preliminary report. *Eur J Cancer Clin Oncol* 1983;19:885–890.

49. Mantravadi RVP, Trippon MJ, Patel MK, et al: Limb salvage in extremity soft tissue sarcoma: Combined modality therapy. *Radiology* 1984;152:523–526.

50. Denton JW, Dunham WK, Salter M, et al. Preoperative regional chemotherapy and rapid fraction irradiation for sarcomas of the soft tissue and bone. *Surg Gynecol Obstet* 1984;158:545–551.

51. Eilber FR, Giuliano A, Huth J, et al: Neoadjuvant chemotherapy, radiation and limited surgery for high grade soft tissue sarcoma of the extremity, in Ryan

JR, Baker LO (eds): *Recent Concepts In Sarcoma Treatment.* Boston, Kluwer Academic Publishers 1988, pp 115–122.

52. Morton DL, Eilber FR, Townsend CN Jr, et al: Limb salvage from a multidisciplinary treatment approach for skeletal and soft tissue sarcomas of the extremity. *Ann Surg* 1976;184:268–278.

53. Eilber FR, Morton DL, Grant TT, et al: Is amputation necessary for sarcoma? A seven year experience with limb salvage. *Ann Surg* 1980;192:431–437.

54. Eilber FR, Morton DL, Eckhardt J, et al: Limb salvage for skeletal and soft tissue sarcomas: Multidisciplinary preoperative chemotherapy. *Cancer* 1984; 53:2579–2584.

55. Eilber FR, Giuliano AE, Huth JF, et al: Intravenous vs. intraarterial adriamycin, 2800 R radiation and surgical excision for extremity soft tissue sarcomas: A randomized prospective trial. *Proc Am Soc Clin Oncol* 1990;9:309. (data from abstract and presentation at meeting)

56. Goodnight JE, Bargar WL, Voegeli T, et al: Limb sparing surgery for extremity sarcomas after preoperative intra-arterial doxorubicin and radiation therapy. *Am J Surg* 1985;150:109–113.

57. Hoekstra HJ, Koops HS, Molenaar WM, et al: A combination of intraarterial chemotherapy, preoperative & postoperative radiotherapy, and surgery as limb-saving treatment of primary unresectable high grade soft tissue sarcomas of the extremities. *Cancer* 1989;63:59–62.

58. Eilber FR, Eckhardt J, Morton DL: Advances in the treatment of sarcomas of the extremity. *Cancer* 1984;54:2695–2701.

59. Lokich JJ, Lochman R, Weiss AJ: Soft tissue and osteogenic sarcomas, in Lokich J (ed): *Cancer Chemotherapy by Infusion* 1987, pp 380–387.

60. Chang AE, Rosenberg SA, Glatstein EJ, et al: Treatment of soft tissue sarcomas, in De Vita VT, Helman SH, Rosenberg SA (eds): *Cancer: Principles and Practice of Oncology.* Philadelphia, JB Lippincott, 1989, pp 1379–1390.

61. Chabner BA, Myers CE: Clinical pharmacology of cancer chemotherapy, in De Vita VT, Rosenberg SA, Helman S (eds): *Cancer: Principles and Practice of Oncology.* Philadelphia, JB Lippincott, 1989, pp 367–385.

62. Jaffe N, Prudich J, Knapp J, et al: Treatment of primary osteosarcoma with intraarterial and intravenous high-dose methotrexate. *J Clin Oncol* 1983; 1:428–431.

63. Huth JF, Mirra JJ, Eilber FR: Assessment of in vivo response to preoperative chemotherapy and radiation therapy as a predictor of survival in patients with soft tissue sarcoma. *Am J Clin Oncol* 1985;8:497–503.

64. Elias AD, Antman KH: Adjuvant chemotherapy for soft tissue sarcoma: An approach in search of an effective regimen. *Sem Oncol* 1989;16:305–311.

65. Tepper JE, Suit HD: Radiation therapy of soft tissue sarcomas. *Cancer* 1985;55:2273–2277.

66. Suit H, Mankin HJ, Wood WC: Preoperative, intraoperative, and postoperative radiation in the treatment of primary soft tissue sarcoma. *Cancer* 1985;55:2659–2667.

67. Barkley HT, Martin RG, Romsdahl MM, et al: Treatment of soft tissue sarcomas by preoperative irradiation and conservative surgical resection. *Intl J Radiat Oncol Bio Phys* 1988;14:693–699.

68. Kempf RA, Irwin LE, Menendez LR, et al: Intraarterial cisplatin for extremity soft tissue and bone sarcoma in adults and teenagers—A limb salvage protocol. *Proc Am Soc Clin Oncol* 1988;7:276.

69. Benedetto P, Mnaymneh W, Ghandur-Mnaymneh L, et al: Neoadjuvant chemotherapy for extremity soft tissue sarcomas. *Proc Am Soc Clin Oncol* 1989;8:323.

70. Lachman R, Bennan J, Gunn W, et al: Therapy of sarcoma of the extremities with intraarterial FUDR, doxorubicin and platinol. *Proc Am Soc Clin Oncol* 1987;6:128.

71. Lachman RD, Weiss AJ, Sullivan K, et al: Therapeutic approach to unresectable extremity soft tissue sarcomas. *Proc Am Soc Clin Oncol* 1990;9:315.

72. Rosen G: Spindle cell sarcomas of soft tissue, in Schein PS (ed): *Decision Making in Oncology.* Marcel Dekker Inc, 1989, pp 174–179.

73. Antman KH, Eilber FR, Shiu MH: Soft tissue sarcomas: Current trends in diagnosis and management. *Curr Probl Cancer* 1989;13:340–367.

74. Malawer M, Schulof R, Priebat D, et al: Unpublished data.

75. Antman KH, Elias AD: Chemotherapy of advanced soft tissue sarcomas. *Sem Surg Onc* 1988;4:53–58.

76. Budd GT, Metch B, Balcerzak SP, et al: High dose cisplatin for metastatic soft tissue sarcoma. *Cancer* 1990;65:866–869.

77. Sordillo PP, Magill GB, Brenner J, et al: Cisplatin: A phase II evaluation in previously untreated patients with soft tissue sarcomas. *Cancer* 1987;59:884–886.

78. Pratt CB, Champion JE, Senzer N, et al: Treatment of unresectable or metastatic osteosarcoma with cisplatin or cisplatin/doxorubicin. *Cancer* 1985;56:1930–1933.

79. Cade S: Osteogenic sarcoma. A study based on 133 patients. *J R Coll Surg Edin* 1955;1:79–111.

80. Dahlin DC, Coventry MB: Osteogenic sarcoma. A study of 600 cases. *J Bone Joint Surg* 1967;49A:101–110.

81. Marcove RC, Mike V, Hajeh J, et al: Osteogenic sarcoma under the age of twenty-one. A review of 145 operative cases. *J Bone Joint Surg* 1970;52:411–423.

82. Uribe-Botero G, Russel WO, Sutow W, et al: Primary osteosarcoma of bone: A clinicopathological investigation of 243 cases with necropsy study in 54. *Am J Clin Pathol* 1977;67:427–435.

83. Companacci M, Bacci G, Bertoni F, et al: The treatment of osteosarcoma of the extremities. Twenty years experience at the Instituto Orthopedico Rizzoli. *Cancer* 1981;48:1569–1581.

84. Cortes E, Holland J, Wang J: Doxorubicin in disseminated osteosarcoma. *JAMA* 1972;221:1132–1138.

85. Jaffe N, Paed D: Recent advances in the chemotherapy of metastatic osteogenic sarcoma. *Cancer* 1972;1622–1631.

86. Pratt C, Howarth C, Ransom J, et al: High dose methotrexate used alone and in combination for measurable primary and metastatic osteosarcoma. *Cancer Treat Rep* 1980;64:11–20.

87. Grem JL, King SA, Wittes RE, et al: Review: The role of methotrexate in osteosarcoma. *J Natl Cancer Inst* 1988;80:626–656.

88. Ochs J, Freeman A, Douglas H, et al: Cis-dichlorodi-

ammine platinum in advanced osteogenic sarcoma. *Cancer Treat Rep* 1978;62:239–245.

89. Marti C, Kroner T, Remagen W, et al: High dose ifosfamide in advanced osteogenic sarcoma. *Cancer Treat Rep* 1985;69:115–117.

90. Eilber FR, Rosen G: Adjuvant chemotherapy for osteosarcoma. *Sem Oncol* 1989;16:312–323.

91. Carter SK: Adjuvant chemotherapy in osteogenic sarcoma: The triumph that isn't? *J Clin Oncol* 1984;2:147–148.

92. Taylor WF, Ivins JC, Pritchard DI, et al: Trends and variability in survival among patients with osteosarcoma. A 7-year update. *Mayo Clin Proc* 1985;60:91–104.

93. Goorin AM, Delorey M, Gelber RE, et al: Dana Farber Institute/The Children's Hospital adjuvant chemotherapy trials for osteosarcoma: Three sequential studies. *Cancer Treat Symp* 1985;3:155–159.

94. Bacci G, Gherlinzoni F, Picci P, et al: Adriamycin methotrexate high dose versus adriamycin methotrexate moderate dose as adjuvant chemotherapy for osteosarcoma of the extremities. A randomized study. *Eur J Cancer Clin Oncol* 1986;22:1337–1345.

95. Ettinger LJ, Douglas HO, Mindell ER, et al: Adjuvant adriamycin and cisplatin in newly diagnosed nonmetastatic osteosarcoma of the extremity. *J Clin Oncol* 1986;4:352–362.

96. Pratt CB, Champion JE, Fleming ID, et al: Adjuvant chemotherapy for osteosarcoma of the extremity: Long term results of two consecutive prospective protocol studies. *Cancer* 1990;65:439–445.

97. Link MP, Goorin AM, Miser AW, et al: The effect of adjuvant chemotherapy on relapse free survival in patients with osteosarcoma of the extremity. *N Engl J Med* 1986;314:1600–1606.

98. Eilber F, Giuliano A, Eckhardt J, et al: Adjuvant chemotherapy for osteosarcoma. A randomized prospective trial. *J Clin Oncol* 1987;5:21–26.

99. Jaffe N, Smith E, Abelson HT, et al: Osteogenic sarcoma: alterations in the pattern of pulmonary metastases with adjuvant chemotherapy. *J Clin Oncol* 1983;1:251–254.

100. Goorin AM, Delorey MJ, Lack EE, et al: Prognostic significance of complete surgical resection of pulmonary metastases in patients with osteogenic sarcoma. Analysis of 32 patients. *J Clin Oncol* 1984;2:425–431.

101. Meyer WH, Schell MJ, Kumar APM, et al: Thoracotomy for pulmonary metastases in osteosarcoma: An analysis of prognostic indicators of survival. *Cancer* 1987;59:376–379.

102. Huth JF, Eilber FR: Patterns of recurrence after resection of osteosarcoma of the extremity. Strategies for treatment of metastases. *Arch Surg* 1989;124:122–126.

103. Giuliano AE, Feig S, Eilber F: Changing metastatic patterns of osteosarcoma. *Cancer* 1984;54:2160–2164.

104. Goorin AM, Shuster JJ, Miser A, et al: Osteosarcoma: Pattern of relapse for patients receiving immediate adjuvant chemotherapy compared to patients receiving delayed chemotherapy following relapse. Results of the Multi-Institutional Osteosarcoma Study. *Proc Am Soc Clin Oncol* 1988;7:258.

105. Rosen G, Marcove RC, Caparros B: Primary osteosarcoma. The rationale for preoperative chemotherapy and delayed surgery. *Cancer* 1979;43:2163–2177.

106. Bacci G, Springfield D, Capanna R, et al: Neoadjuvant chemotherapy for osteosarcoma of the extremity. *Clin Orthop* 1987;224:268–276.

107. Gherlinzoni M, Mercuri M, Avella M, et al: Surgical implications of neoadjuvant chemotherapy: The experience at the Instituto Orthopedico Rizzoli in osteosarcoma and malignant fibrous histiocytoma, in Jacquillat C, Weil M, Khayat D (eds): *Neoadjuvant Chemotherapy*. John Libbey Eurotext Ltd., 1988, vol 169, pp 541–544.

108. Rosen G, Caparros B, Huvos AG, et al: Preoperative chemotherapy for osteosarcoma. Selection of postoperative adjuvant chemotherapy based on response of primary tumor to preoperative chemotherapy. *Cancer* 1982;49:1221–1239.

109. Chuang VP, Wallace S, Benjamin RS, et al: The therapy of osteosarcoma by intraarterial cisplatinum and limb preservation. *Cardiovasc Intervent Radiol* 1981;4:229–235.

110. Bacci G, Picci P, Orlandi M, et al: Prognostic value of serum alkaline phosphatase in osteosarcoma. *Tumori* 1987;73:331–336.

111. Saleh RA, Graham-Pole J, Cassano W, et al: Response of osteogenic sarcoma to the combination of etoposide and cyclophosphamide as neoadjuvant chemotherapy. *Cancer* 1990;65:861–865.

112. Smith J, Heela RT, Huvos AG, et al: Radiographic changes in primary osteogenic sarcoma following intensive chemotherapy. *Radiology* 1982;145:355–360.

113. Chuang VP, Benjamin R, Jaffe N, et al: Radiographic and angiographic changes in osteosarcoma after intraarterial chemotherapy. *Am J Roentg* 1982;139:1065–1069.

114. Jaffe N, Spears R, Eftekhari F, et al: Pathologic fracture in osteosarcoma. Impact of chemotherapy on primary tumor and survival. *Cancer* 1987;59:701–709.

115. Mail JT, Cohen MD, Mirkin LD, et al: Response of osteosarcoma to preoperative intravenous high dose methotrexate chemotherapy: CT evaluation. *AJR* 1985;144:89–94.

116. Shirkoda A, Jaffe N, Wallace S, et al: Computed tomography of osteosarcoma after intraarterial chemotherapy. *AJR* 1985;144:95–99.

117. Jaffe N, Knapp J, Chuang VP, et al: Osteosarcoma: Intraarterial treatment of the primary tumor with cisdiammine dichloroplatinum II (CDP). Angiographic, pathologic and pharmacologic studies. *Cancer* 1983;51:402–407.

118. Carrasco CH, Charnsangavej C, Raymond KA, et al: Osteosarcoma: Angiographic assessment of response to preoperative chemotherapy. *Radiology* 1989;170:839–842.

119. Sommer HJ, Joachim K, Ulricht H, et al: Histophotometric changes of osteosarcoma after chemotherapy: Correlation with 99mTc methylene diphosphonate functional imaging. *Cancer* 1987;59:252–257.

120. Rosen G: The medical management of osteogenic sarcoma. *Am Soc Clin Oncol Education Booklet*, 1990, pp 90–93.

121. Nathanson SD, Haggar A, Froelich J, et al: Preoperative magnetic resonance imaging of sarcomas: Assessment of in vivo response to neoadjuvant chemo and radiotherapy. *Proc Am Soc Clin Oncol* 1988;7:274.

122. Hoekstra HJ, Hogeboom WR, Mooyart WR, et al: Evaluation of neoadjuvant chemotherapy for extremity osteosarcomas with magnetic resonance imaging and bone biopsies. *Proc Am Soc Clin Oncol* 1988; 7:275.

123. Huvos AG, Rosen G, Marcove R: Primary osteogenic sarcoma: Pathologic aspects in 20 patients after treatment with chemotherapy, en bloc resection and prosthetic bone replacement. *Arch Pathol Lab Med* 1977;101:14–18.

124. Picci P, Bacci G, Campanacci M, et al: Histologic evaluation of necrosis in osteosarcoma induced by chemotherapy. Regional mapping of viable and nonviable tumor. *Cancer* 1985;56:1515–1521.

125. Raymond AK, Chawla SP, Carrasco CH, et al: Osteosarcoma chemotherapy effect: A prognostic factor. *Sem Diagnos Pathol* 1987;4:212–236.

126. Rosen G, Murphy ML, Huvos AG, et al: Chemotherapy, en bloc resection, and prosthetic bone replacement in the treatment of osteogenic sarcoma. *Cancer* 1976;37:1–11.

127. Rosen G: Preoperative (neoadjuvant) chemotherapy for osteogenic sarcoma. A ten year experience. *Orthopedics* 1985;8:659–664.

128. Mosende C, Guttierez M, Caparros B, et al: Combination chemotherapy with bleomycin, cyclophosphamide and dactinomycin for the treatment of osteogenic sarcoma. *Cancer* 1977;40:2779–2786.

129. Kalifa C, Mlika N, Dubousset J, et al: The experience of T10 protocol in the pediatric department of the Gustave Roussy Institute, in Ryan JR, Baker LO (eds): *Recent Concepts in Sarcoma Treatment*. Boston, Kluwer Academic Publishers 1988, pp 301–305.

130. Provisor A, Nachman J, Krailo M, et al: Treatment of nonmetastatic osteogenic sarcoma of the extremities with pre- and postoperative chemotherapy. *Proc Am Soc Clin Oncol* 1987;6:217.

131. Winkler K, Beron G, Kotz R, et al: Neoadjuvant chemotherapy for osteosarcoma: Results of a cooperative German/Austrian study. *J Clin Oncol* 1984; 2:617–624.

132. Winkler K, Juergens H: The German Pediatric Oncology (GPO) cooperative study on osteosarcoma, in Ryan JR, Baker LO (eds): *Recent Concepts in Sarcoma Treatment*. Boston, Kluwer Academic Publishers 1988, pp 269–300.

133. Winkler K, Beron G, Delling G, et al: Neoadjuvant chemotherapy of osteosarcoma: Results of a randomized cooperative trial (COSS-82) with salvage chemotherapy based on histological tumor response. *J Clin Oncol* 1988;6:329–337.

134. Weiner MA, Harris MB, Lewis M, et al: Neoadjuvant high dose methotrexate, cisplatin, and doxorubicin for the management of patients with nonmetastatic osteosarcoma. *Cancer Treat Rep* 1986;70:1431–1432.

135. Nachman J, Simon MA, Dean L, et al: Disparate histologic responses in simultaneously resected primary and metastatic osteosarcoma following intravenous neoadjuvant chemotherapy. *J Clin Oncol* 1987;5:1185–1190.

136. Akahoshi Y, Takeuchi S, Chen SH, et al: The results of surgical treatment combined with intraarterial infusion of anticancer agents in osteosarcoma. *J Clin Orthop* 1976;120:103–109.

137. Eilber FR, Giuliano AE, Eckhardt J, et al: A randomized prospective trial of adjuvant chemotherapy for osteosarcoma, in Salmon S (ed): *Adjuvant Therapy of Cancer V*. Grune and Stratton, 1987, pp 691–699.

138. Jaffe N, Robertson R, Ayala A, et al: Comparison of intraarterial cis-diamminedichloroplatinum II with high dose methotrexate and citrovonum factor in the treatment of primary osteosarcoma. *J Clin Oncol* 1985;3:1101–1104.

139. Jaffe N, Raymond AK, Ayala A, et al: Intraarterial cis-diamminedichloroplatinum II in pediatric osteosarcoma. Relationship of effect on primary tumor to survival, in Ryan JR, Baker LO (eds): *Recent Concepts in Sarcoma Treatment*. Boston, Kluwer Academic Publishers 1988, pp 275–282.

140. Petrilli S, Gentil F, Quadros J: Preoperative treatment with intraarterial cis-diamminedichloroplatinum II (CDP) and postoperative adjuvant treatment with CDP and adriamycin for osteosarcoma of the extremities. *Proc Am Soc Clin Oncol* 1986;5:202.

141. Epelman S, Petrilli AS, Franco EL: Factors influencing survival of patients with non-metastatic osteosarcoma treated with intraarterial cisplatinum. *Proc Am Soc Clin Oncol* 1987;6:223.

142. Benjamin RS, Chawla SP, Carrasco C, et al: Arterial infusion in the treatment of osteosarcoma in Ryan JR, Baker LO (eds): *Recent Concepts in Sarcoma Treatment*. Boston, Kluwer Academic Publishers 1988, pp 269–274.

143. Benjamin RS: Regional chemotherapy for osteosarcoma. *Sem Oncol* 1989;16:323–327.

144. Benjamin RS, Raymond AK, Carrasco CH, et al: Primary chemotherapy of osteosarcoma of the extremities with systemic adriamycin and intraarterial cisplatinum. *Proc Am Soc Clin Oncol* 1989;8:322.

145. Bacci G, Springfield D, Capanna R, et al: Neoadjuvant chemotherapy for osteosarcoma of the extremity. *Clin Orthop* 1987;224:268–276.

146. Picci P, Bacci G, Caparros R, et al: Neoadjuvant chemotherapy for localized osteosarcoma of the extremities. Experience related to 112 cases treated between March 1983 and June 1986, in Salmon S (ed): *Adjuvant Therapy of Cancer V*. Grune and Stratton, 1987, pp 711–717.

147. Picci P, Bacci G, Capanna R, et al: Neoadjuvant chemotherapy for osteosarcoma—Results of a prospective study, in Ryan JR, Baker LO (eds): *Recent Concepts in Sarcoma Treatment*. Boston, Kluwer Academic Publishers, 1988, pp 291–295.

148. Picci P, Bacci G, Campanacci M, et al: Neoadjuvant chemotherapy in osteosarcoma: Results of a multicentric study in Italy, in Jacquillat C, Weil M, Khayat D (eds): *Neoadjuvant Chemotherapy*. John Libbey Eurotext Ltd, 1988, vol 169, pp 509–513.

149. Bacci G, Picci P, Ruggieri P, et al: Primary chemotherapy and delayed surgery (neoadjuvant chemotherapy) for osteosarcoma of the extremities. *Cancer* 1990;65:2539–2553.

150. Ruggieri P, Picci P, Marangolo M, et al: Neoadjuvant chemotherapy for osteosarcoma of the extremities. Preliminary results in 116 patients treated preoperatively with methotrexate (IV), cisplatinum (IA) and adriamycin. *Proc Am Soc Clin Oncol* 1990;9:310.

151. Stine KC, Hockenberry MJ, Harrelson J, et al: Systemic doxorubicin and intraarterial cisplatin preoperative chemotherapy plus postoperative adjuvant chemotherapy in patients with osteosarcoma. *Cancer* 1989;63:848–853.

152. Malawer M, Reaman G, Priebat D, et al: Impact of a short course (2 cycles) of neoadjuvant chemotherapy with cisplatinum (DDP) and adriamycin (ADR) on the choice of surgical procedure for high grade bone sarcomas of the extremities. *Proc Am Soc Clin Oncol* 1989;8:320.

153. Malawer M, Priebat D, Schulof R, et al: Additional unpublished data.

154. Weiss A, Lackman R, Bennan J: Intraarterial preoperative chemotherapy for osteosarcoma. *Proc Am Soc Clin Oncol* 1989;8:321.

155. Stewart DJ, Benjamin RS, Siefert W, et al: Clinical pharmacology of intraarterial cis-diamminedichloroplatinum II. *Proc Am Assoc Cancer Res, Am Soc Clin Oncol* 1980;21:237.

156. Stewart DJ, Benjamin RS, Zimmerman S, et al: Clinical pharmacology of intraarterial cis-diamminedichloroplatinum (II). *Cancer Res* 1983;43:917–920.

157. Eilber FR, Grant T, Morton DL: Adjuvant therapy for osteosarcoma. Preoperative treatment. *Cancer Treat Rep* 1978;62:213–216.

158. Legha SS, Benjamin RS, Mackay B: Reduction of doxorubicin cardiotoxicity by prolonged continuous intravenous infusion. *Ann Int Med* 1982;96:133–139.

159. Goren MP, Wright RK, Horowitz ME, et al: Enhancement of methotrexate nephrotoxicity after cisplatin therapy. *Cancer* 1986;58:2617–2621.

160. Jaffe N, Keifer R III, Robertson R, et al: Renal toxicity with cumulative doses of cis-diamminedichloroplatinum in pediatric patients with osteosarcoma. *Cancer* 1987;59:1577–1581.

161. Picci P, Bacci G, Neff JR, et al: The influence of preoperative chemotherapy in the surgical planning in patients with osteosarcoma. A histopathological study on 205 patients. *Proc Am Soc Clin Oncol* 1990;9:310.

162. McDonald DJ, Capanna R, Gherlinzoni F, et al: Influence of chemotherapy on perioperative complications in limb salvage surgery for bone tumors. *Cancer* 1990;65:1509–1516.

163. Prasad R, Bacci G, Campanacci M, et al: Does drug dose intensity (DDI) of chemotherapy determine the prognosis of primary high grade osteosarcoma. *Proc Am Soc Clin Oncol* 1990;9:311.

164. Graham-Pole J, Saleh R, Springfield D, et al: Neoadjuvant chemotherapy for limb osteosarcoma, in Jacquillat C, Weil M, Khayat D (eds): *Neoadjuvant Chemotherapy. Proceedings of the Second International Congress on Neoadjuvant Chemotherapy.* John Libbey Eurotext Ltd, 1988, vol 169, pp 515–520.

165. Winkler K, Bielack S, Delling G, et al: Influence of intraarterial tourniquet infusion versus intravenous infusion of cisplatinum in osteosarcoma on histological response rate. *Proc Am Soc Clin Oncol* 1989; 8:296.

166. Link MP, Eilber F: Osteosarcoma, in Pizzo PA, Poplack DG (eds): *Principles and Practice of Pediatric Oncology.* Philadelphia, JB Lippincott Co., 1989, pp 703–706.

167. Reddel RR, Kefford RF, Grant JM, et al: Ototoxity in patients receiving cisplatin. Importance of dose and method of administration. *Cancer Treat Rep* 1982; 66:19–23.

168. Chawla SP, Rosen G, Lowenbraun S, et al: Role of high dose ifosfamide in recurrent osteosarcoma. *Proc Am Soc Clin Oncol* 1990;9:310.

169. Meyer WH, Schell MJ, McHaney VA, et al: Increased hearing loss in patients with osteosarcoma receiving both cisplatin and ifosfamide. *Proc Am Soc Clin Oncol* 1990;9:291.

170. Miser J, Pritchard D, Sim F, et al: Treatment of osteosarcoma with a new chemotherapy regimen of ifosfamide, adriamycin and high dose methotrexate. *Proc Am Soc Clin Oncol* 1990;9:295.

171. Chawla SP, Rosen G, Eilber F, et al: Cisplatin and adriamycin as neoadjuvant chemotherapy and adjuvant chemotherapy in the management of soft tissue sarcomas in Salmon SE (ed) Adjuvant Therapy of Cancer VI. W.B. Saunders Co., 1990, p 567–573.

172. Winkler K, Bielack S, Delling G, et al: Effect of intraarterial versus intravenous cisplatin in addition to systemic doxorubicin, high-dose methotrexate, and ifosfamide on histologic tumor response in osteosarcoma (Study COSS-86) *Cancer* 1990;66:1703–1710.

8

Posterior Flap Hemi-pelvectomy

PAUL H. SUGARBAKER, M.D.
PAUL B. CHRETIEN, M.D.

OVERVIEW

Hemipelvectomy is most frequently indicated for sarcoma of the upper thigh, hip, or pelvis. With the patient in the lateral position the incision is made through the anterior abdominal wall, and the iliac vessels are dissected free and divided just distal to the aortic bifurcation. The multiple visceral branches of the internal iliac vessels are divided and ligated to expose the sacral nerve roots deep within the pelvis. The posterior skin flap is dissected free, and the gluteus maximus muscle severed from its origin on the sacrum. Back muscles are detached from the wing of the ilium, and the psoas muscle with accompanying obturator and femoral nerves is divided. The pelvis begins to open as the symphysis pubis is divided. Next the sacral nerve roots are divided, and the anterior capsule of the sacroiliac joint is transected. The muscles and ligaments of the pelvic floor are severed, including the urogenital diaphragm, levator ani muscle, sacrotuberous ligament, and sacrospinalis ligament. The specimen is released by severing the sacroiliac joint posteriorly. The operative defect is closed by suturing gluteal fascia to the inguinal ligament over suction drains.

INTRODUCTION

Early descriptions of the surgical technique of hemipelvectomy emphasized the need for careful selection of patients and the importance of immediate replacement of blood loss.[1-15] Other, later technical descriptions of this procedure have been published.[16-22] Recent reports of series of hemipelvectomy patients have shown this procedure to have a low mortality rate and to offer an acceptable survival in carefully selected patients.[20-22] Quality-of-life studies would suggest that the long-term morbidity that accompanies this radical amputation is not greater than that experienced with other cancer treatments.[23] Possible alternatives to hemipelvectomy in selected patients are limb-sparing procedures combined with radiation therapy.[24,25] Surgical techniques for excision of the hemipelvis with limb preservation have also been described and offer new possibilities for improved function.[26-29] The consideration of an anterior myocutaneous flap for closure of the operative defect should always be considered because of an improved cosmetic and functional result.[30,31]

We describe a surgical technique of hemipelvectomy in detail with an attempt to develop an orderly sequence of steps in the procedure. The patient is placed in the lateral and modified Trendelenburg position; this position facilitates performance of the operation for several reasons: (1) Intraperitoneal structures, bladder, and rectum fall by gravity out of the surgeon's field, thus minimizing the amount of retraction required and improving exposure. (2) The posterior skin flap is constructed under optimal visualization. (3) Flexing the operating room table allows the angle between the ilium and lumbar vertebrae to open, thus facilitating the release of back muscles from the iliac crest and division of the iliolumbar ligament under direct vision.

Two surgical principles will be emphasized: (1) Movement of the extremity maintains the tissues to be divided under tension. (2) Muscles are divided as close to their origin or insertion on bone as possible to minimize blood loss and maximize the margin of resection.

GENERAL INDICATIONS FOR POSTERIOR FLAP HEMIPELVECTOMY

Hemipelvectomy is often required for *recurrent sarcoma* of the thigh treated by local excision plus radiation therapy. In this clinical situation care must be taken to develop skin flaps that have not been irradiated. Occasionally a large soft tissue tumor occurring high in the anterior thigh must be removed by posterior flap hemipelvectomy. The preferred approach is a wide local excision plus postoperative radiation therapy (Fig. 8–1). Small lesions superficially located toward the lateral aspect of the thigh are optimal for the limb salvage approach (chapter 6). The closer the primary tumor mass is to the femoral vessels, the greater the likelihood of a local recurrence after wide excision plus radiation therapy. Osteosarcoma of the proximal femur of the pelvis almost always requires a hemipelvectomy for its complete removal (Fig. 8–2). Soft tissue sarcomas of the upper thigh or groin area may involve the superficial femoral artery and vein and thereby require hemipelvectomy. Occasionally patients with soft tissue sarcomas arising within the true pelvis may be curatively resected using the hemipelvectomy procedure. The abdominal-inguinal incision may be utilized to remove a portion of the hemipelvis and spare the extremity (chapter 11). Other patients occasionally benefiting are those with recurrent carcinoma of the rectum, anus, or penis that extends to the side wall of the pelvis. *Pathologic fractures* through a bony sarcoma of the upper femur or pelvis require hemipelvectomy in that the hematoma that develops causes wide dissemination of tumor cells into the surrounding soft tissue. Also hematoma may develop from spontaneous rupture of a tumor mass or hemorrhage following an open biopsy procedure.

Skeletal immaturity may result in marked leg-length discrepancy if wide excision plus radiation therapy is used to treat cancer in the proximal femur. Approximately 80% of the growth of the femur is from the proximal epiphysis. Marked leg-length discrepancy may result in a young patient and cause hemipelvectomy to be used rather than wide local excision plus radiation therapy for soft tissue sarcomas of the proximal thigh.

CLINICAL CONSIDERATIONS

The timing for this major surgical procedure is important. Both physiologic and psychological factors must be optimized. If the patient has received preoperative chemotherapy, it is essential that both leukocytes and platelets be permitted to return toward normal. Significant deficits in red blood cell mass should be corrected by preoperative transfusion. Although vascular insufficiency is rarely a complicating factor in these patients, suboptimal wound healing may be a problem in patients who have received high-dose regional or systemic chemotherapy preoperatively. Also poor nutrition from nausea

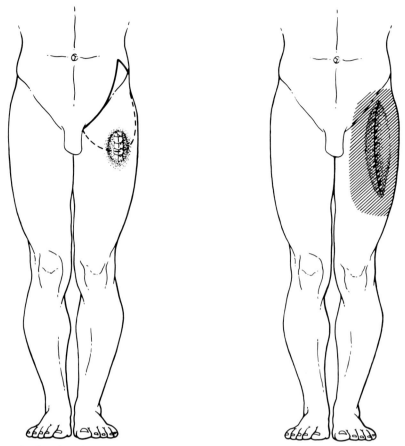

Figure 8–1. Posterior flap hemipelvectomy may be required for high-grade large soft tissue sarcomas of the proximal thigh, especially if they are adjacent to or *invade the neurovascular bundle* (**left**). Wide local excision plus radiation therapy is the preferred approach if negative margins can be obtained by limb salvage surgery (**right**).

and vomiting induced by preoperative chemotherapy may further complicate wound-healing problems. Because of potential wound-healing difficulties, fascia and skin closure must be securely and meticulously performed. Hematoma and seroma must be avoided by the use of adequate closed suction drainage. One should defer removal of skin sutures for three to four weeks. Often unusual skin flaps will be used, and this may require a considerable time period to mold the amputation site.

REHABILITATION AND EMOTIONAL SUPPORT

The cancer patient faces unique psychological problems with hemipelvectomy. Not only is there a threat to the loss of a lower limb and hemipelvis, but also there is a threat to life itself. Rehabilitation of the

patient undergoing this major amputation begins at the time of the staging studies. The entire health care team must develop an honest relationship with the patient and include him or her in the early stages of decision making. Building upon trust and understanding, the patient will be better able to accept the amputation and set realistic goals.

All patients undergoing hemipelvectomy will experience considerable phantom limb sensation. This may be a major problem with the hemipelvectomy. As a matter of fact, it may end up being a more disruptive long-term problem to the patient than the loss of the limb itself. The patient should understand that phantom limb sensations are to be expected and that they can be treated with analgesics. It should be emphasized that the discomfort will lessen over time. The patients who report severe disabling pain are often those who find it most difficult to adapt to surgery and to the malignant process.

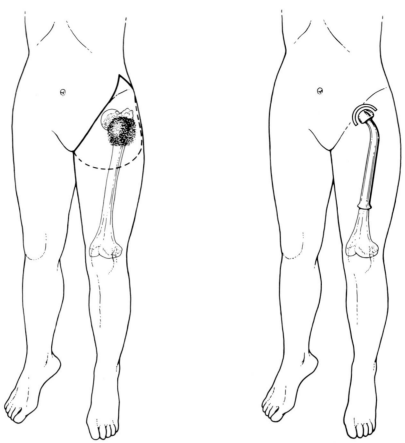

Figure 8–2.   Posterior flap hemipelvectomy is the procedure required for most osteosarcomas of the proximal femur. Only occasionally is a prosthetic replacement of the femur an option. Prosthetic replacement of the upper femur or pelvis is infrequent. If *infection* has resulted from tumor invading through the skin or is introduced at the time of biopsy, prosthetic materials are contraindicated.

Although successful rehabilitation depends to a great extent on the patient's attitude, the physiatrist can help tremendously in these efforts. A *positive attitude* toward functional recovery augmented by early postoperative ambulation may move the patient rapidly to his or her goals. A positive approach is amplified by contact with other patients who have successfully met some of the rehabilitation challenges. This can provide an immeasurable psychological boost to the patient. The oncologist, rehabilitation therapist, and others involved in the postoperative care must coordinate their efforts carefully. There may be conflicting demands on the patient's time. There may be a different interpretation by the patient and family of the same clinical information presented by several different caregivers. The entire team must not only be coordinated but must be positive about the complete rehabilitation that can be achieved following hemipelvectomy.

LEVEL OF AMPUTATION

The standard procedure for a hemipelvectomy involves a disarticulation through the symphysis pubis and lumbosacral joint. However, a modified hemipelvectomy with the bony incision through the ilium (rather than the lumbosacral joint) at the level of the sciatic notch may be elected for lesions of the medial thigh region, especially those in the adductor muscle group. The segment of ilium preserved with a modified hemipelvectomy may be used to support a belt or help stabilize a prosthesis postoperatively. Posterior lesions that involve the buttocks should be treated by buttockectomy or anterior flap hemipelvectomy (chapters 9 and 12).

In an extended hemipelvectomy the sacroiliac joint itself is included in the operative specimen. The bony incision through the pelvis passes through the sacral neural foramina. Papaioannou and co-workers have described long-term disease-free survival following compound hemipelvectomy.[32] In these operations contiguous structures infiltrated by or adherent to the tumor were also excised. The resections may include en block resection of bladder, rectum, or female internal genitalia. An occasional patient may profit greatly. Other modifications of the hemipelvectomy procedures indicated for selected tumors include an intraperitoneal approach with possible cross utero-ureterostomy if a portion of ureter needs to be sacrificed (chapter 13).

The internal hemipelvectomy should be considered in patients with small lesions of the hemipelvis or soft tissue tumors that closely approximate the hemipelvis. Internal hemipelvectomy is discussed in chapter 10.

RADIOLOGIC STUDIES

The patient should be carefully studied with computerized tomograms of the lungs, abdomen, and pelvis. The computerized tomogram is the most effective means for ruling out lung metastases. Retroperitoneal and iliac lymphadenopathy should also be ruled out.

CT, MRI, and bone scan should be used to determine that a free margin of excision can be achieved with the hemipelvectomy procedure. Barium enema may be required in order to rule out involvement of the rectal ampulla. Cystogram and cystoscopy are frequently indicated along with retrograde pyelogram if there is a pelvic extension of the malignancy.

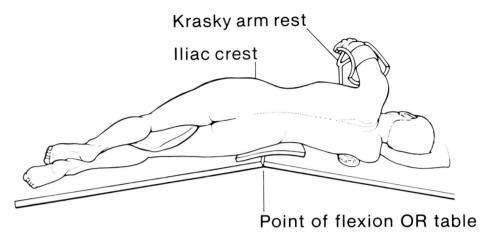

Krasky arm rest

Iliac crest

Point of flexion OR table

Figure 8–3. POSITION. The patient is placed on the operating table with the iliac crest over the point for table flexion. Indwelling venous cannula and arterial lines are secured, and a Foley catheter is placed in the bladder. A cushion is placed beneath the iliac crest and greater trochanter. Then the patient is rolled into a fully lateral position. Padding is placed beneath the axilla to allow full excursion of the chest wall. The upper arm is positioned on a Krasky arm rest, and the anus is sutured shut. The nonoperative lower extremity is wrapped to prevent venous pooling. The operating table is flexed to open the angle between the iliac crest and the vertebral column. A single piece of wide tape across the upper chest secures the patient to the table. As the skin is prepared, the lower extremity to be amputated is covered and wrapped so that it is draped free. One member of the operating team is assigned the primary responsibility of moving the leg during dissection so that all tissues are severed under tension.

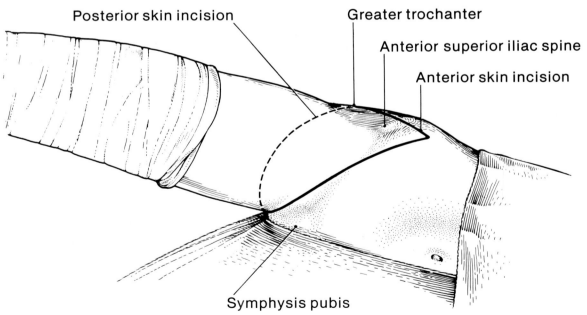

Posterior skin incision

Greater trochanter

Anterior superior iliac spine

Anterior skin incision

Symphysis pubis

Figure 8–4. INCISION. Anteriorly, the incision extends from approximately 2 in above the anterior superior iliac spine to the pubic tubercle. Laterally, the incision courses over the anterior portion of the greater trochanter and then parallels the gluteal crease posteriorly around the thigh. The incision should be made progressively more distal to the gluteal crease when the pelvis has a large anteroposterior diameter. Previous biopsy sites must be widely excised by the incision and included in the operative specimen.

The surgeon is positioned anterior to the patient. The incision is made through Scarpa's fascia, external oblique aponeurosis, and internal oblique and transversus muscles. The spermatic cord is swept medially and the inguinal lymph nodes laterally with the specimen. By means of blunt dissection, the iliac fossa is exposed.

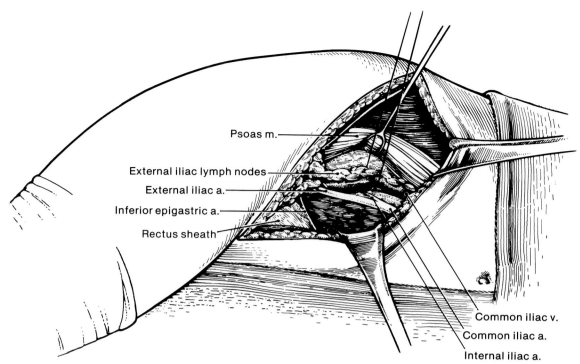

Figure 8–5. DISSECTION OF THE ILIAC VESSELS. The parietal peritoneum is elevated off the iliac vessels and falls inferiorly with the viscera. The inferior epigastric vessels are identified at the lower aspect of the incision and clamped, divided, and ligated. The right rectus muscle and its sheath are freed from their insertion on the pubis to the midline. The common and external iliac arteries and veins are dissected free; the external and common iliac lymph nodes are removed and submitted as a separate specimen for histopathologic examination. The common iliac vessels are traced superiorly to their origin at the aorta and vena cava where they are ligated and divided. Care is taken to exclude the ureter by moving it medially.

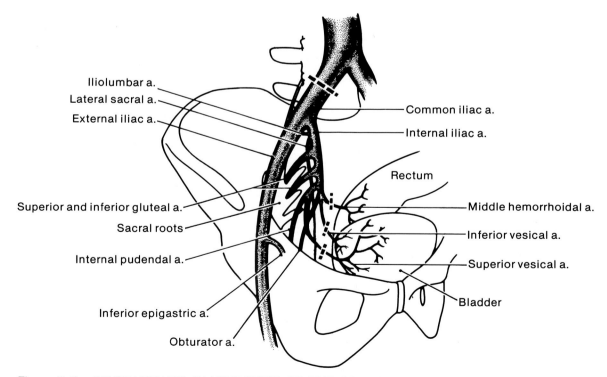

Figure 8–6. DIAGRAMMATIC ILLUSTRATION OF THE POINTS OF TRANSECTION OF THE ILIAC ARTERIES. This drawing emphasizes that the internal iliac artery in the pelvis is removed with the specimen, and all its branches are transected in their course to the side wall of the pelvis, the rectum, and the bladder. Vessels to be divided to expose the sacroiliac joint and pelvic diaphragm include the iliolumbar and lateral sacral arteries to the neural foramina, the superior and inferior gluteal arteries, the internal pudendal artery to the perineum, the middle hemorrhoidal artery to the rectum, and the inferior and superior vesicular arteries to the bladder.

127

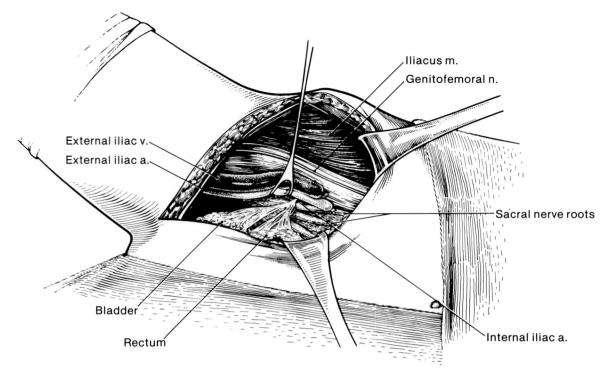

Figure 8–7. DIVISION OF BRANCHES OF THE INTERNAL ILIAC VESSELS. With lateral traction on the internal iliac artery and vein, vessels coursing toward the sacrum and into the viscera are isolated, clamped, divided, and ligated. The fibroareolar tissues over bladder and rectum are retracted medially so that vascular branches to these structures are identified. To visualize the sacral nerve roots for their later transection, branches of the internal iliac artery coursing to the pelvic side wall should also be divided. When this dissection is completed, the rectum and bladder should be completely separable from the pelvic side wall, and sacral nerve roots should be skeletonized, but with all nerve trunks remaining intact. Nerves coursing through the pelvis to the rectum, prostate, and bladder from the area of the sacral promontory and from the sacral nerve roots should be preserved if possible. Transection of these nerves may increase the severity of sexual and bladder dysfunction associated with this procedure.

If a tumor mass in the pelvis obscures access to the branches of the internal iliac artery, the surgeon may consider opening the pelvis by division of the sacroiliac joint and pubic symphysis prior to division of the vessels. This allows more adequate visualization behind the tumor and greatly increases the safety of transection of these vessels.

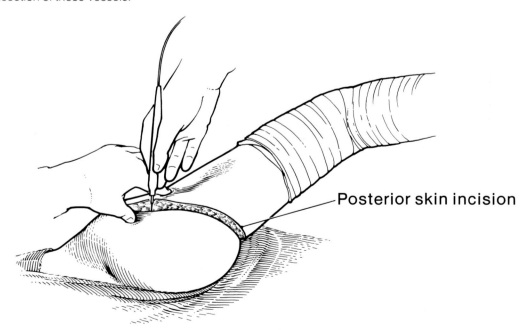

Posterior skin incision

Figure 8–8. POSTERIOR SKIN INCISION. The anterior dissection is now packed with warm, moist gauze. The extremity is rotated anteriorly to obtain tension on the buttock skin and fascia. The posterior skin incision is made and continues down through the gluteal fascia; inferiorly, the incision should be extended to the medial aspect of the thigh where it connects with the anterior incision.

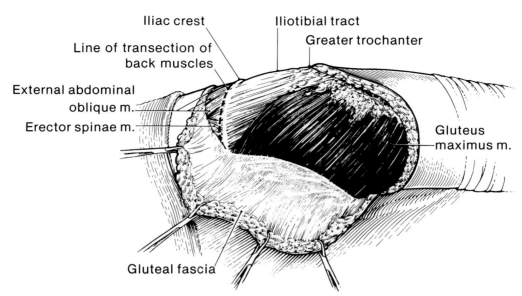

Iliac crest

Iliotibial tract

Line of transection of
back muscles

Greater trochanter

External abdominal
oblique m.

Erector spinae m.

Gluteus
maximus m.

Gluteal fascia

Figure 8–9. CONSTRUCTION OF THE POSTERIOR SKIN FLAP. Adair clamps are secured to the full thickness of the skin and gluteal fascia for traction. The posterior skin flap is fashioned by dissecting the gluteal fascia directly off the muscle, after dividing its attachments to the iliotibial tract and the tensor fascia lata. In constructing the posterior skin flap, extreme care must be taken to preserve the gluteal fascia with the subcutaneous tissue and skin that compose the flap. If this is done, the blood supply to the flap is protected and undue stretching of the subcutaneous tissue is avoided. The flap is dissected from the anterolateral to the posteromedial position until one is free of tumor with a wide (>5 cm) margin. Then the gluteus maximus is incised to include it with the flap. One can preserve a portion of the gluteus muscle, and the viability of the long portion of the posterior skin flap will be ensured. According to Karakousis and coworkers at the Roswell Park Memorial Institute, flap necrosis does not occur if a generous portion of gluteus maximus muscle is left attached to the posterior skin flap (33). Superiorly, the flap must be elevated over the iliac crest.

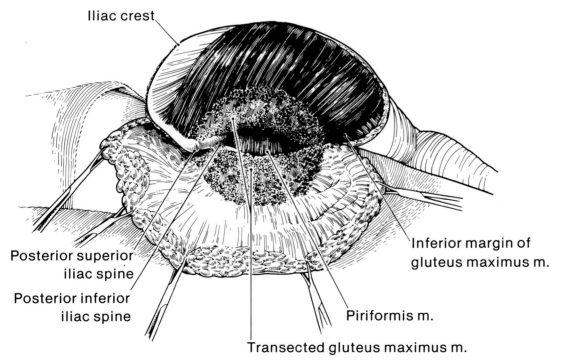

Iliac crest

Inferior margin of
gluteus maximus m.

Posterior superior
iliac spine

Posterior inferior
iliac spine

Piriformis m.

Transected gluteus maximus m.

Figure 8–10. RELEASE OF THE MUSCLES OF THE BACK FROM THE ILIAC CREST AND GLUTEUS MAXIMUS MUSCLE FROM THE SACRUM. The muscles and fascia of the back that insert into the right iliac crest are transected as close to the bone as possible. These structures include the external oblique aponeurosis, the rector spinae, the latissimus dorsi, and the quadratus lumborum muscles. The gluteus maximus muscle is detached from the sacrotuberous ligament, coccyx, and sacrum. This is accomplished by first locating the inferior margin of the gluteus maximus muscle, which presents as a rolled edge; then while the surgeon bluntly dissects beneath the muscle, it is released from the sacrum by means of electrocautery.

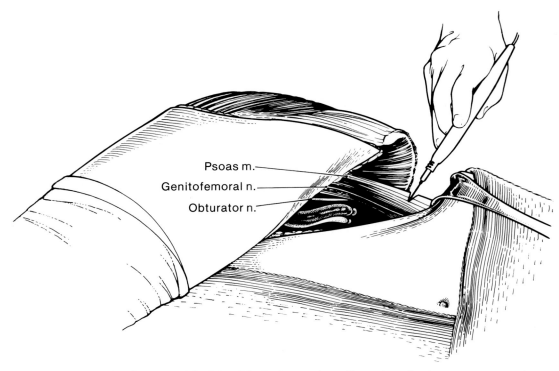

Figure 8–11. DIVISION OF THE PSOAS MUSCLE. The previous dissection affords easy access to the psoas muscle, which is divided with electrocautery at the level of the iliac crest. Multiple bleeding points in this muscle may produce serious postoperative hemorrhage if not properly controlled at this time. The genitofemoral nerve, which lies on the superficial surface of the psoas muscle, and the obturator and femoral nerves, which lie deep to it, are transected. Transection of the lumbosacral nerve trunk may be done at this time.

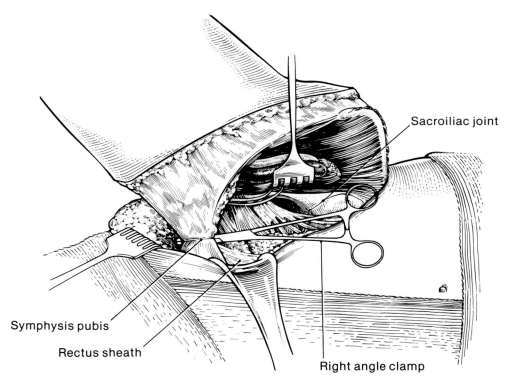

Figure 8–12. TRANSECTION OF SYMPHYSIS PUBIS. The hip is abducted to place tension on the ligaments of the symphysis pubis. A long right-angle clamp is passed beneath the symphysis so as not to disrupt venous channels that are beneath it and surround the prostate and bladder. If injured, these veins may bleed profusely and are difficult to control before removal of the specimen. With the bladder, prostate, and urethra protected by the right-angle clamp, a scalpel is used to probe for the joint space and divide its capsule. The arcuate ligament on the inferior aspect of the symphysis pubis should also be transected. After the symphysis is divided, the bleeding points in the corpora cavernosa are packed to minimize blood loss.

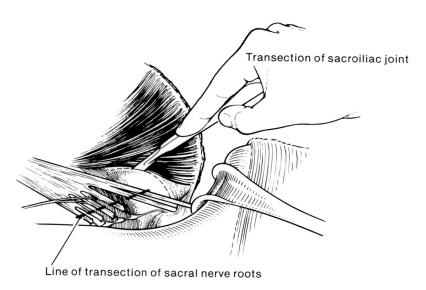

Transection of sacroiliac joint

Line of transection of sacral nerve roots

Figure 8–13. LINE OF TRANSECTION OF THE SACRAL NERVE ROOTS AND DIVISION OF THE ANTERIOR CAPSULE OF THE SACROILIAC JOINT. The sacral nerve roots should be ligated and then transected 1 to 2 cm from the neural foramina. If possible, the nervi erigentes that course from the sacral nerve roots to the pelvic plexus should be identified and preserved.

The anterior surface of the sacroiliac joint is exposed by retracting overlying iliacus muscle. The joint space courses parallel to the anterior surface of the ilium; it is located by probing through the thick fascial capsule with a knife blade at the brim of the pelvis. When the joint space is entered, the capsule is transected on the anterior and inferior aspects of the joint. Occasionally in elderly patients a bony union of sacrum and ilium has formed, which requires an osteotome for release. If there is the possibility of extension of tumor to the sacroiliac joint, an extended hemipelvectomy should be performed.

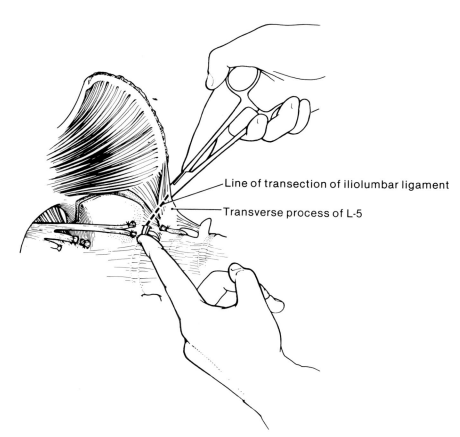

Line of transection of iliolumbar ligament

Transverse process of L-5

Figure 8–14. DIVISION OF THE ILIOLUMBAR LIGAMENT. A space between the transverse process of the fifth lumbar vertebra and the sacrum is localized anteriorly. Before transection the L-4 and L-5 sacral nerve roots were just medial to this point. The tip of a large Kelly clamp is passed behind the transverse process of the fifth lumbar vertebra and guided up into the space previously defined. The clamp is forced through this space; transection of the dense fibrous tissue above the clamp with electrocautery results in division of the iliolumbar ligament.

131

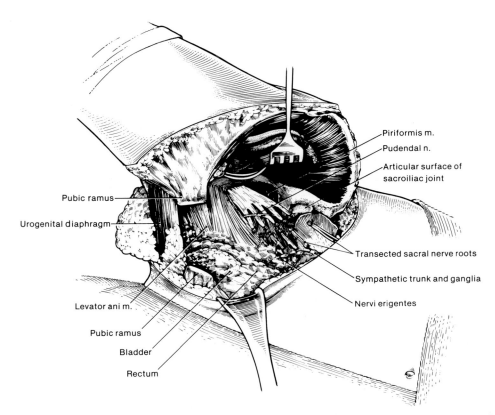

Figure 8–15. THE OPEN HEMIPELVIS. At this point division of the vascular structures anteriorly and completion of the skin flap posteriorly have been accomplished. The remaining structures to be transected are those that constitute the pelvic diaphragm.

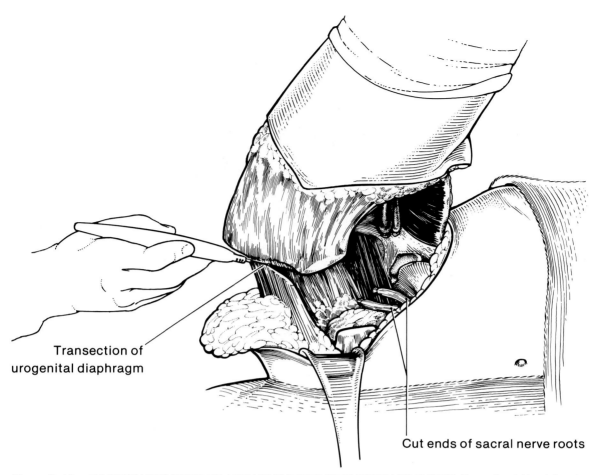

Transection of
urogenital diaphragm

Cut ends of sacral nerve roots

Figure 8–16.   DIVISION OF MUSCLES AND LIGAMENTS OF THE PELVIC FLOOR. Care should be taken to protect the bladder, urethra, and rectum for they may be easily damaged at this point in the dissection. The essential requirement for safe transection of the pelvic diaphragm is maximal upward traction on the leg. If the flexed knee is draped over the second assistant's shoulder, traction elongates the structures of the pelvic diaphragm and separates pubis and ischium from urethra, bladder, and rectum. A thorough irrigation of the operative field for complete visualization of these structures is often helpful at this time. The dissection commences at the right symphysis pubis and proceeds toward the ischial tuberosity with division of the muscles of the urogenital diaphragm and pubococcygeus at their point of attachment on the inferior pubic ramus; if the muscles are transected on the lower pubic ramus, minimal bleeding from ischiocavernosus muscle will be encountered. The dissection proceeds from ischial tuberosity to coccyx, further dividing ischiococcygeus, iliococcygeus, and piriformis muscles followed by the sacrotuberous and sacrospinalis ligaments. As these structures are transected, the leg is moved progressively more medially and superiorly; this is done to keep muscles and ligaments to be transected under tension.

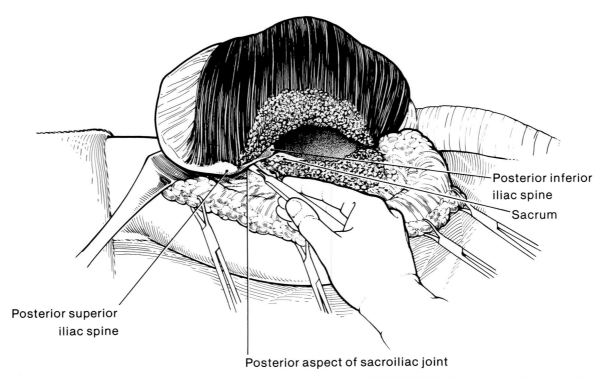

Posterior inferior
iliac spine

Sacrum

Posterior superior
iliac spine

Posterior aspect of sacroiliac joint

Figure 8–17. DIVISION OF SACROILIAC JOINT CAPSULE POSTERIORLY. Now the leg is moved far anteriorly to facilitate release of the specimen by dividing the posterior aspect of the sacroiliac joint capsule. After the specimen is removed, the operative site is copiously irrigated and any bleeding points are secured.

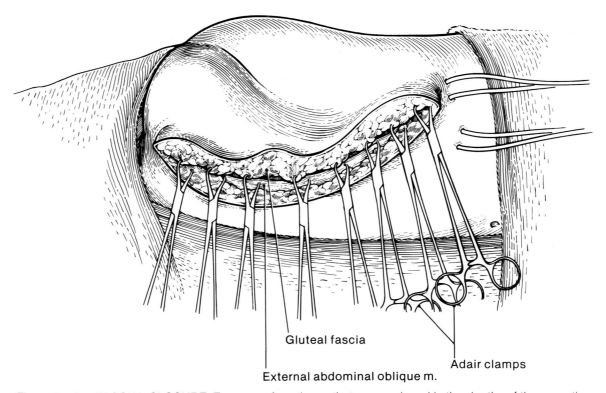

Gluteal fascia

External abdominal oblique m.

Adair clamps

Figure 8–18. FASCIAL CLOSURE. Two sets of suction catheters are placed in the depths of the operative defect; one set is secured in the hollow of the sacrum, another set beneath the abdominal wall. Adair clamps are used to adjust the longer skin flap posteriorly to the less lengthy fascia anteriorly. The gluteal fascia is sutured to the fascial structures of the abdominal wall and pubic symphysis.

134

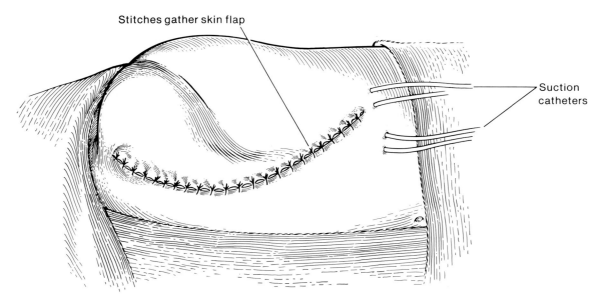

Stitches gather skin flap

Suction catheters

Figure 8–19.   SKIN CLOSURE AND POSTOPERATIVE CARE. The skin is closed with monofilament sutures. Postoperatively pressure is kept off the sacral region and off the operative side to maximize blood flow to the skin flap. Bed rest is maintained for seven to ten days, but the patient is encouraged to exercise the remaining leg and the arms in bed. A trapeze is often well utilized. The Foley catheter should remain in place until the patient begins ambulation. Family and sex counseling begun preoperatively should continue postoperatively. Because much bone marrow is lost in the specimen, blood transfusion in the postoperative period is often required.

DISCUSSION

Hemipelvectomy performed as indicated here is rarely accompanied by postoperative or intraoperative mortality. Blood loss of 500 to 2000 mL is customary. Only if the tumor is located anteriorly within the pelvis and covering the major vessels is extensive blood loss to be expected.

In the first postoperative week the patient is usually more comfortable in bed. Increased pressure on the incision from the abdominal wall and viscera while standing is usually quite painful. Using a tilt table (chapter 4) to first ambulate the patient has proven to be of value. Prolonged sitting may cause ischemia of the posterior skin flap. Prone lying and turning onto the nonoperative side should be encouraged. The suction drains usually put out serous material for one to two weeks. As long as these skin exit sites are dressed in a sterile and occlusive fashion, there is no hurry to remove them (Fig. 8–20).

The morbidity of this amputation is often extensive. Approximately 10% of patients will have ischemia of the posterior skin flap. If this does occur, prompt revision in the operating room is almost always in the patient's best interest; this should be done on the fourth to tenth postoperative day before the flap heals to underlying tissue and after the ischemic process has fully declared itself. Miller has described the excision of a wedge-shaped section of the posterior flap.[21] This is indicated at the time of amputation if the flap is noted to be ischemic. However, in our experience, prediction of the exact area that will eventually become necrotic is not possible. Also, only a lesser percentage of patients will require it, and occasionally the wedge excision seems to extend the area of ischemia at the edges of the posterior skin flap. Preservation of gluteus maximus muscle over the medial portion of the posterior skin flap will prevent ischemic necrosis in nearly all patients.[33,34]

Infection is a second postoperative problem seen in approximately 15% of patients; it may retard wound healing for many months if it occurs. Several procedures have been followed to help reduce the incidence of this serious complication.

1. Preoperative scrub of the perineal area with a surgical soap.
2. Complete mechanical and antibiotic bowel preparation prior to surgery.
3. Perioperative broad spectrum antibiotics.
4. Suture the anus shut in a watertight fashion prior to skin preparation.
5. Antibiotic-moistened gauze pads placed over all exposed tissue surfaces intraoperatively.
6. Generous suction drainage. When caring for the skin exit sites of these drains, wear surgical masks and sterile gloves.

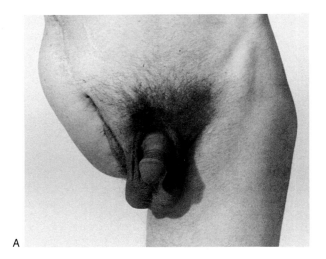

A

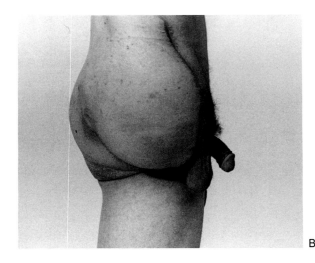

B

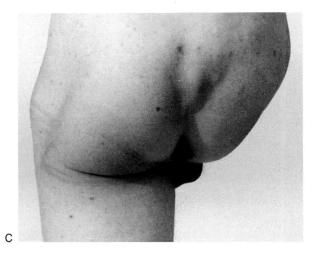

C

Figure 8–20. (**A**) Anterior, (**B**) lateral, and (**C**) posterior views of the operative site following hemipelvectomy. The skin is the only coverage of the sacrum and opposite pubic symphysis. For this reason, weight bearing on the resection site is poorly tolerated.

Phantom limb pain is experienced by virtually all patients in the early postoperative period. It is most severe in the second and third postoperative weeks. It will remain as a serious and debilitating problem in approximately 10% of patients. In our experience, phantom limb pain is the most serious long-term problem that impairs quality of life in hemipelvectomy patients. Fortunately, in most patients the pain gradually diminishes to a tolerable level over the first postamputation year. No definite solution of this problem is currently known. Transcutaneous nerve stimulation is occasionally helpful; anticonvulsive drugs, such as diphenylhydantoin, also work well in some patients. Injection of severed nerve ends has been advocated by some but is not of proven merit. Others have suggested that unusually deep anesthesia at the time the nerves are divided will prevent late persistence of the problem. A complete discussion of the problem and an explanation of the dorsal root entry zone operation are in chapter 5.

Bladder atony and impotence are occasionally observed. If care is taken to preserve the nervi erigentes, as shown in Figure 8–13, this should rarely occur.

The greatest obstacle to recovery of mobility is obesity. This occurs all too frequently and may progress rapidly to a morbid extent. Patients need to be warned.

Herniation of bowel into the amputation site occasionally occurs. It often is associated with the development of obesity. Preservation of a portion of the gluteus muscle and the gluteus fascia on the posterior skin flap, as shown in Figure 8–9, will minimize this late complication. Postoperatively, if the patient is kept recumbent for seven days, the hernia problem may also be lessened.

REFERENCES

1. Pringle JH: The interpelvic-abdominal amputation; notes on two cases. *Br J Surg* 1916;4:283–295.
2. Speed K: Hemipelvectomy. *Ann Surg* 1932;95:167–173.
3. Gordon-Taylor G, Wiles P: Interinnomino-abdominal (hindquarter) amputation. *Br J Surg* 1935;22:671–681.
4. Morton JJ: Interinnomino-abdominal (hindquarter) amputation. *Ann Surg* 1942;115:628–646.
5. Leighton WE: Interpelviabdominal amputation. Report of three cases. *Arch Surg* 1942;45:913–923.
6. King D, Steelquist J: Transiliac amputation. *J Bone Surg* 1943;25A:351–367.
7. Sugarbaker, ED, Ackerman LV: Disarticulation of the innominate bone for malignant tumors of the pelvic parietes and upper thigh. *Surg Gynecol Obstet* 1945;81:36–52.
8. Pack GT, Ehrlich HE: Exarticulation of the lower extremity for malignant tumors: Hip joint disarticulation (with and without deep iliac dissection) and sacroiliac disarticulation (hemipelvectomy). *Ann Surg* 1946;124:1–27.
9. Pack GT, Ehrlich HE, Gentile F deC: Radical amputations of the extremities in the treatment of cancer. *Surg Gynecol Obstet* 1947;84:1105–1116.
10. Wise RA: Hemipelvectomy for malignant tumors of the bony pelvis and upper part of the thigh. *Arch Surg* 1949;58:867–874.
11. Beck NR, Bickel WH: Interinnomino-abdominal amputations. Report of twelve cases. *J Bone Joint Surg* 1948;30A:201–209.
12. Slocum DB: *An Atlas of Amputations.* St. Louis, CV Mosby, 1949, pp 244–249.
13. Ravitch MM: Hemipelvectomy. *Surgery* 1949;26:199–207.
14. Saint JH: The hindquarter (interinnomino-abdominal) amputation. *Am J Surg* 1950;80:142–160.
15. Gordon-Taylor G: The technique and management of the "hindquarter" amputation. *Br J Surg* 1952;39:536–541.
16. Banks SW, Coleman S: Hemipelvectomy: Surgical techniques. *J Bone Joint Surg* 1956;384:1147–1155.
17. Phelan JT, Nadler SH: A technique of hemipelvectomy. *Surg Gynecol Obstet* 1964;119:311–318.
18. Higinbotham NL, Macrov RC, Casson P: Hemipelvectomy: A clinical study of 100 cases with 5 year follow up on 60 patients. *Surgery* 1966;59:706–708.
19. Francis KC: Radical amputations, in Nora PF (ed): *Operative Surgery.* Philadelphia, Lea & Febiger, 1974.
20. Douglas HO, Rajack M, Holyoke D: Hemipelvectomy. *Arch Surg* 1975;110:82–85.
21. Miller TR: Hemipelvectomy in lower extremity tumors. *Orthop Clin N Am* 1977;8:903–919.
22. Sugarbaker PH, Chretien PB: Hemipelvectomy in the lateral position. *Surgery* 1981;90:900–909.
23. Sugarbaker PH, Barofsky I, Rosenberg SA, et al: Quality of life assessment of patients in extremity sarcoma clinical trials. *Surgery* 1982;91:17–23.
24. Sugarbaker PH, Chretien PB: The surgical technique of buttockectomy. *Surgery* 1982;91:104–107.
25. Rosenberg SA, Kent H, Costa J, et al: Prospective randomized evaluation of the role of limb-sparing surgery, radiation therapy, and adjuvant chemoimmunotherapy in the treatment of adult soft-tissue sarcomas. *Surgery* 1978;84:62–69.
26. Ariel IM, Shah JP: The conservative hemipelvectomy. *Surg Gynecol Obstet* 1977;144:407–413.
27. Enneking WF, Dunham WK: Resection and reconstruction for primary neoplasms involving the innominate bone. *J Bone Joint Surg* 1978;60A:731–746.
28. Eilber FR, Grant TT, Skai D, et al: Internal hemipelvectomy-excision of the hemipelvis with limb preservation. An alternative to hemipelvectomy. *Cancer* 1979; 43:806–809.
29. Johnson JTH: Reconstruction of the pelvic ring following tumor resection. *J Bone Joint Surg* 1978;60A:747–751.
30. Steel HH: Partial or complete resection of the hemipelvis. An alternative to hindquarter amputation for periacitabular, chondrosarcoma of the pelvis. *J Bone Joint Surg* 1978;60A:719–730.
31. Frey C, Mathew LS, Benjamin H, et al: A new technique for hemipelvectomy. *Surg Gynecol Obstet* 1976;143:753–756.
32. Papaioannou AN, Critselis AN, Volk H: Long term survival after compound hemipelvectomy. *Surg Gynecol Obstet* 1977;144:175–178.
33. Sugarbaker PH, Chretien PB: Hemipelvectomy for buttock tumors utilizing an anterior myocutaneous flap of quadriceps femoris muscle. *Ann Surg* 1983; 197:106–115.
34. Karakousis CP, Enrich L, Driscoll D: Variants of hemipelvectomy and their complications. *Am J Surg* 1989;158:404–408.

9

Anterior Flap Hemi-pelvectomy

PAUL H. SUGARBAKER, M.D.
PAUL B. CHRETIEN, M.D.

OVERVIEW

Hemipelvectomy utilizing an anterior myocutaneous flap is indicated for aggressive tumors of the buttock and proximal portion of the posterior thigh. A large operative defect created posteriorly by amputation of the lower extremity, hemipelvis, and buttock is covered by a myocutaneous flap of quadriceps femoris muscle and overlying skin and subcutaneous tissue. The superficial femoral artery is preserved to sustain the myocutaneous flap.

INTRODUCTION

Bowden and Booher,[1] in reporting their treatment of sarcoma of the buttock, described a hemipelvectomy procedure in which the buttock skin flap could be partially sacrificed with the specimen. To cover the operative defect posteriorly, the external iliac vessels and a small portion of the superficial femoral vessels were preserved to nourish an anterior skin flap. Frey and co-workers[2] reported the use of an anterior myocutaneous flap of the quadriceps femoris muscle. We describe in detail a hemipelvectomy procedure in which a large operative defect posteriorly is closed with a myocutaneous flap that is composed of the quadriceps femoris muscle and nourished by the superficial femoral vessels. The results of treatment are excellent except for phantom limb pain and sensations experienced in some patients.

INDICATIONS

The anterior flap hemipelvectomy is indicated for buttock tumors that cannot be adequately excised by buttockectomy.[3] If at the time of excision of the gluteus maximus muscle, involvement of the pelvic bones, upper femur, or sciatic nerve is observed, the anterior flap hemipelvectomy should be recommended. Tumors of the ilium or ischium that do not extend into the pelvic cavity may be curatively resected by this operation, but the medial bony margin should be carefully radiologically assessed preoperatively. For a curative resection the tumor must not have anterior extension with involvement of the common or external iliac vessels; these must be preserved to supply the myocutaneous flap of quadriceps femoris muscle (Fig. 9–1).

A great advantage of this procedure is that the medial margin of resection, usually the closest margin, can be determined prior to operative events that make amputation mandatory. By exposing the sacrum and removing the outer table of the sacrum, the medial margins of resection and the sacral nerve roots may be examined grossly and histologically.

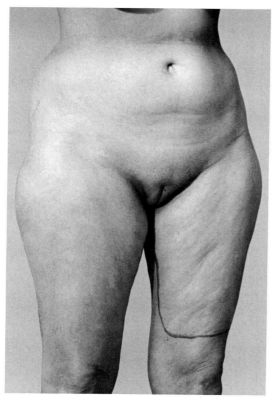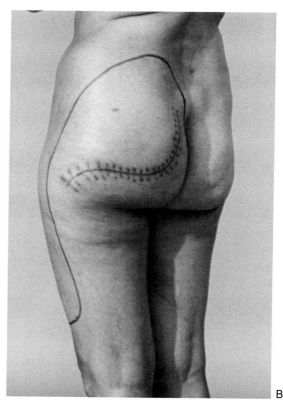

Figure 9–1. Anterior (**A**) and lateral (**B**) view of patient showing skin incision used for anterior flap hemipelvectomy in a patient with a large buttock sarcoma.

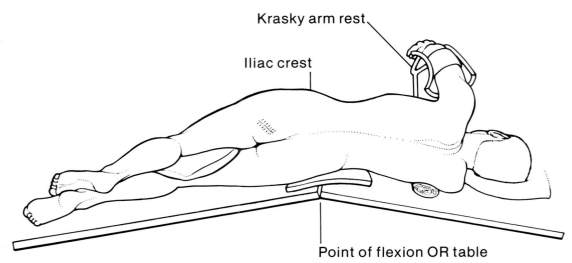

Krasky arm rest

Iliac crest

Point of flexion OR table

Figure 9–2. POSITION. Preoperative preparations include correction of blood deficits and a complete bowel preparation. In females, the vagina is also prepared. Venous and arterial lines are secured, and a drainage catheter is placed in the bladder. After being placed supine on the operating table, the patient is rolled into the lateral position with the iliac crest at the flexion point of the table. As the patient is positioned, a cushion is placed beneath the right iliac crest and greater trochanter to prevent pressure necrosis of the skin. Padding beneath the right axilla is used to allow full excursion of the chest wall and as prophylaxis against injury to the brachial plexus. The left arm is placed on a Krasky arm rest. An elastic wrapping or a support stocking is used to prevent blood pooling in the right lower extremity. The operating room table is flexed to open the angle between the crest of the ilium and the lumbar vertebra. The anus is sutured shut. The left lower extremity is prepared and draped free with the skin exposed circumferentially from the knee to the iliac crest.

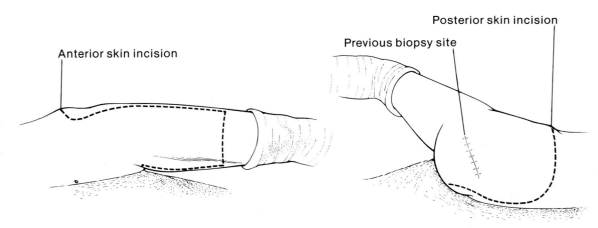

Anterior skin incision

Posterior skin incision

Previous biopsy site

Figure 9–3. INCISION. It is critical to determine before the operation that the myocutaneous flap created from the tissue overlying the quadriceps muscle will cover the operative defect created in the buttock. The location of the proposed incision is mapped out with a marking pen and the width and length of the flap compared with the anticipated defect in the buttock. Once it is ascertained that the flap is adequate to cover the defect, the remainder of the incision is determined. First, draw the location of the incision medial to the tumor at or near the midline posteriorly above the anus. Superiorly and laterally the incision should parallel the wing of the ilium to the anterior superior iliac spine. It then continues distally along the midpoint of the lateral aspect of the thigh to the junction of the lower and middle thirds of the thigh.

The medial incision courses 2 to 3 cm lateral to the anus, then anteriorly in the gluteal crease toward the pubic tubercle. It then continues along the midpoint of the thigh to the junction of the lower and middle thirds of the thigh. The two longitudinal incisions extending along the lateral and medial aspects of the thigh are connected by a transverse incision over the anterior aspect of the thigh. The location of this transverse incision determines the length of the myocutaneous flap. Hence it should be ascertained that the transverse incision is positioned so the tip of the flap will extend to the level of the iliac crest.

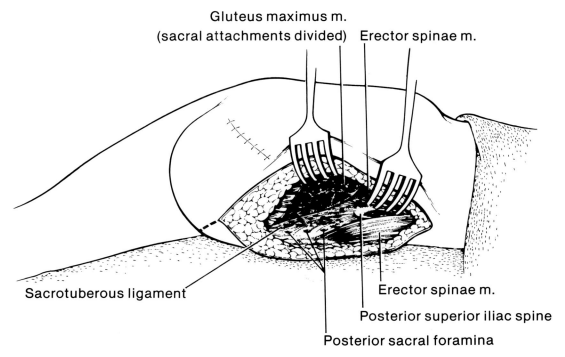

Gluteus maximus m.
(sacral attachments divided) Erector spinae m.

Sacrotuberous ligament

Erector spinae m.

Posterior superior iliac spine

Posterior sacral foramina

Figure 9–4. POSTERIOR INCISION TO DETERMINE OPERABILITY. In excision of buttock tumors the medial margin of the tumor is usually the closest one to the line of excision. Therefore the dissection should commence medial to the tumor to allow the surgeon to assess operability before completion of the amputation is required. The initial incision is made superficial to the sacrum in the midline, through fascia to the midsacral spines. A cuff of skin 2 to 3 cm in length should be preserved around the anus. The sacral attachments of the gluteus maximus and erector spinae muscles are divided from their origins between the midsacral spines and the dorsal sacral foramina. Biopsies from the medial margin of resection are secured. By removing the outer table from the sacrum, biopsies from sacral nerves may also be obtained if indicated. If by cryostat sectioning and histologic examination these biopsies are negative, the amputation may proceed.

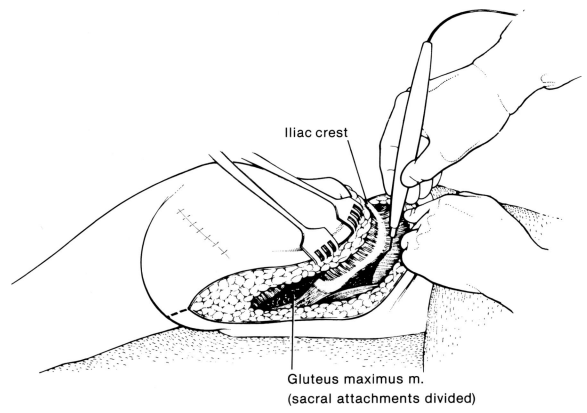

Iliac crest

Gluteus maximus m.
(sacral attachments divided)

Figure 9–5. RELEASE OF BACK MUSCLES FROM THE ILIAC CREST. Abdominal and back muscles that arise on the sacrum and the iliac crest are incised in the plane of attachment of muscle to bone to minimize blood loss. The muscles to be severed include the external oblique, erector spinae, latissimus dorsi, and quadratus lumborum.

141

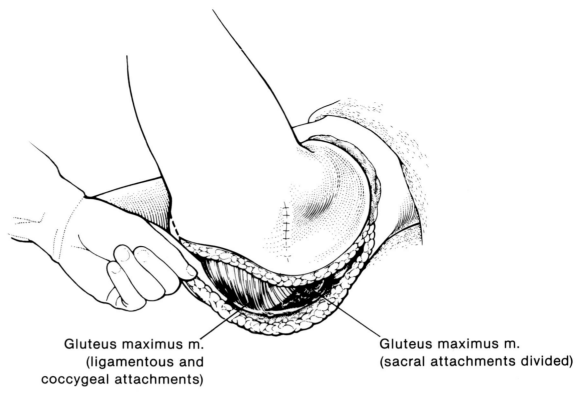

**Gluteus maximus m.
(ligamentous and
coccygeal attachments)**

**Gluteus maximus m.
(sacral attachments divided)**

Figure 9–6.   POSTERIOR DISSECTION IN THE ISCHIORECTAL SPACE. The extremity is flexed at the hip to place the tissues in the area of the gluteal crease under tension. The perianal incision is extended toward the pubic tubercle along the gluteal crease. The deep dissection is continued lateral to the rectum into the ischiorectal fossa. The remaining origins of the gluteus maximus muscle are now severed from the coccyx and sacrotuberous ligament.

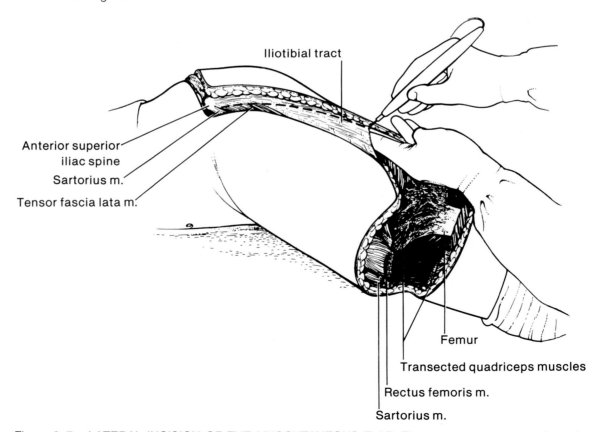

Iliotibial tract

Anterior superior
iliac spine

Sartorius m.

Tensor fascia lata m.

Femur

Transected quadriceps muscles

Rectus femoris m.

Sartorius m.

Figure 9–7.   LATERAL INCISION OF THE MYOCUTANEOUS FLAP. The surgeon now moves from the posterior to the anterior aspect of the patient. The anterior incision at the junction of the middle and lower thirds of the thigh is made and continued down to the femur, transecting the entire quadriceps muscle. Laterally, this incision is continued up toward the greater trochanter to the anterior superior iliac spine; the tensor fascia lata muscle is separated from its investing fascia so that it is included with the specimen.

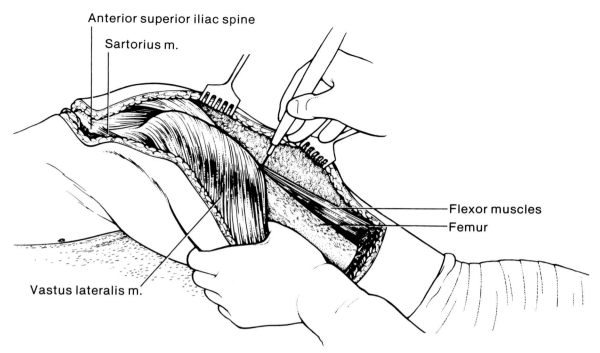

Anterior superior iliac spine

Sartorius m.

Flexor muscles
Femur

Vastus lateralis m.

Figure 9–8. RELEASE OF THE VASTUS LATERALIS FROM THE FEMUR. The fascial covering of the vastus lateralis of the quadriceps femoris muscle is dissected free of the flexor muscles and traced to its insertion on the femur. Then the vastus lateralis is severed from the femur using electrocautery. In performing the dissection from this point on, care must be taken not to separate muscle bundles of the myocutaneous flap from the overlying skin and subcutaneous tissue.

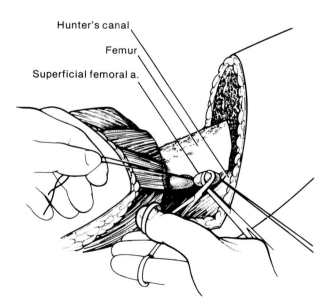

Hunter's canal

Femur

Superficial femoral a.

Figure 9–9. TRANSECTION OF SUPERFICIAL FEMORAL ARTERY. The medial skin incision is from the area of Hunter's canal to the pubic tubercle. The superficial femoral vessels are located at their point of entry into the adductor muscles, and are ligated and divided at this level. These vessels course along the deep margin of the myocutaneous flap, and in the subsequent dissection they are traced superiorly to the inguinal ligament. Multiple small branches from the superficial femoral vessels to the adductor muscles must be clamped, divided, and ligated.

143

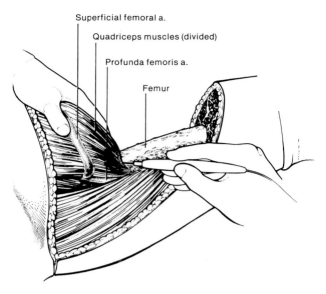

Superficial femoral a.

Quadriceps muscles (divided)

Profunda femoris a.

Femur

Figure 9–10. RELEASE OF THE QUADRICEPS MUSCLE FROM THE FEMUR. Vigorous upward traction on the myocutaneous flap allows the origins of the vastus intermedius and the vastus medialis to be severed from the femur. As the release of the myocutaneous flap continues up toward the pelvis, the profunda femoris vessels are identified. These vessels are ligated and divided at their origin from the common femoral artery.

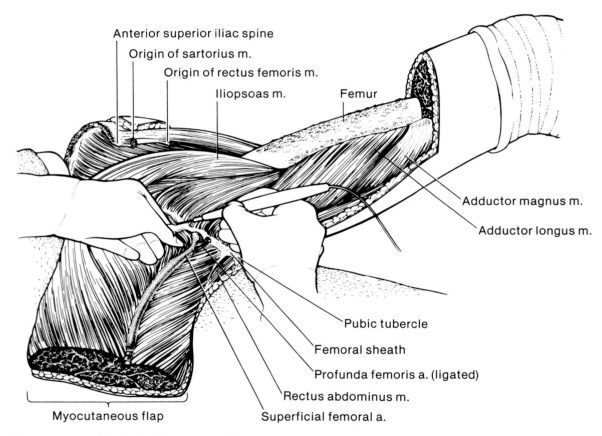

Anterior superior iliac spine

Origin of sartorius m.

Origin of rectus femoris m.

Iliopsoas m.

Femur

Adductor magnus m.

Adductor longus m.

Pubic tubercle

Femoral sheath

Profunda femoris a. (ligated)

Rectus abdominus m.

Superficial femoral a.

Myocutaneous flap

Figure 9–11. RELEASE OF THE MYOCUTANEOUS FLAP FROM THE PELVIS. The myocutaneous flap is freed from its pelvic attachments by the following procedure: the abdominal muscles and fascia are severed from the iliac crest; the sartorius muscle is transected at its origin on the anterior superior iliac spine; the rectus femoris is transected at its origin on the anterior inferior iliac spine; the femoral sheath overlying the hip joint is divided; and the left rectus abdominus muscle is released from the pubic bone. By retracting the myocutaneous flap medially, full access to the pelvis is achieved. Blunt dissection along the femoral nerve allows rapid dissection into the pelvis to expose the vessels and nerves to be transected in the subsequent phases of the procedure.

144

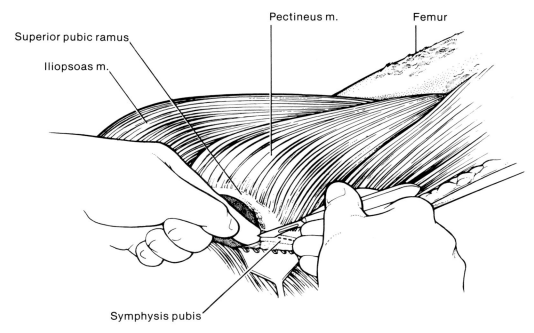

Figure 9–12.   DIVISION OF THE PUBIC SYMPHYSIS. To divide the pubic symphysis, the bladder and urethra are protected and a scalpel is used to locate and divide the cartilaginous joint.

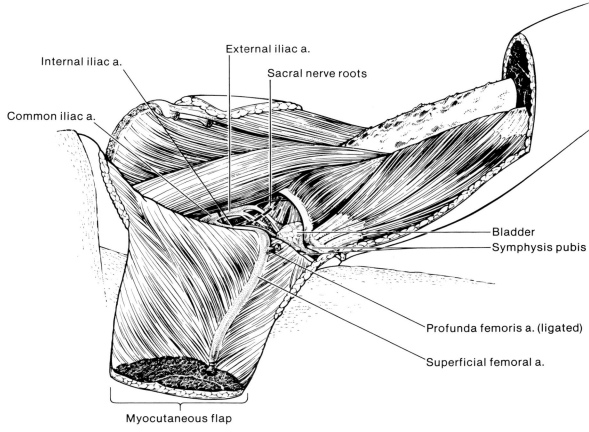

Figure 9–13.   TRANSECTION OF INTERNAL ILIAC VESSELS AND BRANCHES. The internal iliac artery and vein are divided at their point of origin from the common iliac vessels. Multiple visceral branches of the internal iliac vessels are divided in their course superficial to the sacral nerve roots. Strong medial traction on the viscera will help expose these vessels. When this phase of the dissection is completed, the nerve roots should be clearly visualized throughout their course in the pelvis.

It should be noted that the common iliac lymph nodes remain with the patient in this procedure, in contrast to a standard hemipelvectomy in which they are removed.

145

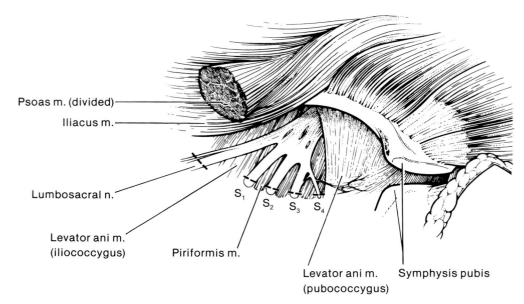

Psoas m. (divided)

Iliacus m.

Lumbosacral n.

Levator ani m.
(iliococcygus)

Piriformis m.

S₁ S₂ S₃ S₄

Levator ani m.
(pubococcygus)

Symphysis pubis

Figure 9–14. DIVISION OF THE PSOAS MUSCLE AND NERVE ROOTS. The psoas muscle is divided near its junction with the iliacus muscle. The obturator nerve deep to the muscle is also divided. Care is taken to preserve the femoral nerve coursing into the myocutaneous flap. The lumbosacral and sacral nerve roots are ligated and divided close to the ventral sacral foramina.

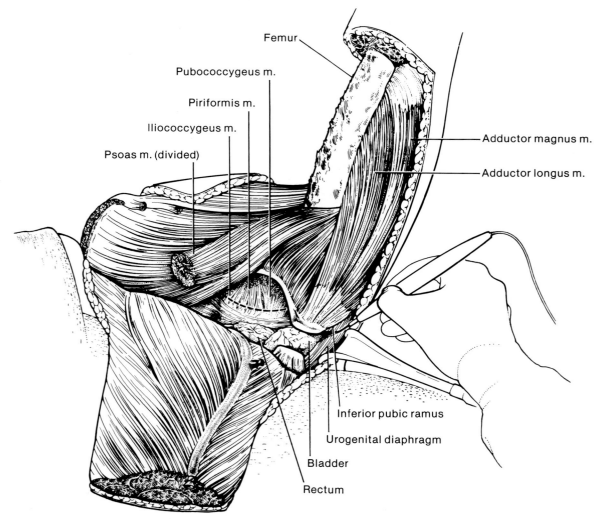

Femur

Pubococcygeus m.

Piriformis m.

Iliococcygeus m.

Psoas m. (divided)

Adductor magnus m.

Adductor longus m.

Inferior pubic ramus

Urogenital diaphragm

Bladder

Rectum

Figure 9–15. DIVISION OF THE PELVIC DIAPHRAGM. The leg is elevated to place under tension the individual muscles that constitute the pelvic diaphragm. Take care to protect the urethra, bladder, and rectum. The urogenital diaphragm, levator ani, and piriformis muscles are divided. These muscles are transected near their pelvic attachments.

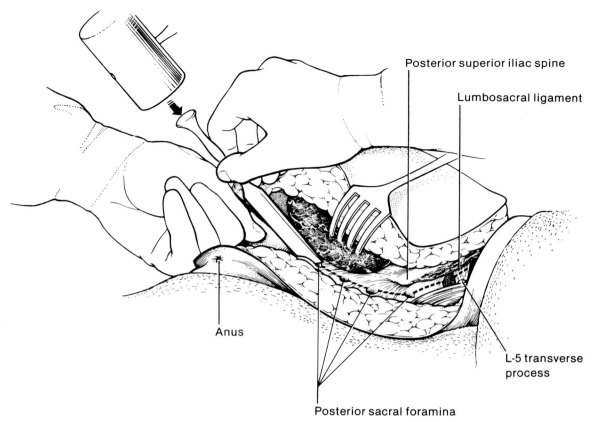

Posterior superior iliac spine

Lumbosacral ligament

Anus

L-5 transverse process

Posterior sacral foramina

Figure 9–16.   DIVISION OF THE SACRUM. The surgeon should again change orientation and move back to the posterior aspect of the patient. Using an osteotome and commencing at the tip of the coccyx, the coccyx and sacrum are divided in a plane that bisects the sacral foramina. Initially, the course of the osteotome should parallel the midsacral spines. The surgeon, being posterior to the patient, reaches around the coccyx with the left hand to locate the S-5 neural foramina from within the sacrum. This is at the junction of the sacrum and the coccyx. By holding the osteotome with the right hand, the direction for bone transection can be precisely determined. The assistant drives the osteotome through the bone with the mallet. At the upper portion of the sacrum, care must be taken not to fracture inadvertently through the bone. The lumbosacral ligament is divided to release the specimen.

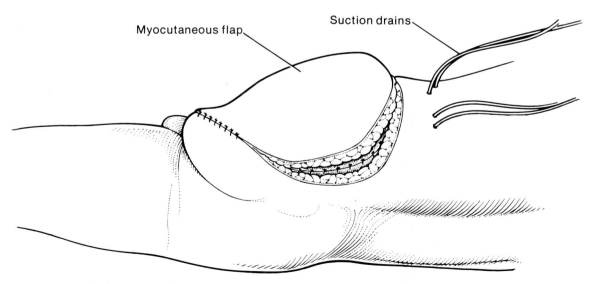

Myocutaneous flap

Suction drains

Figure 9–17.   CLOSURE. The operative site and myocutaneous flap are copiously irrigated and bleeding points are secured. The myocutaneous flap is folded posteriorly into the operative defect over two sets of suction drains. The fascia of the quadriceps femoris is sutured to the musculature of the anterior abdominal wall, to the back muscle, to the sacrum, and to the muscles of the pelvic diaphragm. The skin is closed with interrupted sutures.

If the patient is hemodynamically stable, ambulation may begin on the first postoperative day. The Foley catheter is removed at one week, and the suction drains are removed when the serous drainage is substantially reduced.

DISCUSSION

Patients with extensive soft tissue sarcoma in the buttock or patients with osteosarcoma of the pelvis extending posteriorly have previously been thought incurable by amputation. Hemipelvectomy procedures formerly described required a flap of buttock skin to cover the surgical defect. Anterior flap hemipelvectomy allows sacrifice of the entire buttock and all the overlying skin and soft tissue to the midline. Even patients who have a tumor-contaminated buttock to the midline may have a potentially curative procedure.

If at all possible, tumors in this area, especially those of low histologic grade, should be treated with an excision of the gluteus maximus muscle (buttockectomy).[3] However, if tumor extends through the gluteus maximus muscle to involve the gluteus medius or minimus, if tumor encases the sciatic nerve, or if tumor is directly adjacent to the pelvic bones, a radical amputation utilizing an anterior myocutaneous flap is indicated.[2,4]

Early postoperative complications with this procedure have not occurred to date. The serious problem of skin flap ischemia seen in nearly one quarter of patients undergoing a standard posterior flap hemipelvectomy has not been observed.[5] The numerous muscular branches of the superficial femoral vessels to the quadriceps mechanism provide excellent blood supply to the preserved quadriceps muscles and to overlying skin and subcutaneous tissue. Care should be taken during the dissection not to shear overlying skin and subcutaneous tissue from the muscle mass; if this occurs, skin blood supply will be compromised.

The potential for rehabilitation with this procedure is excellent. The patients who are free of disease use a prothesis regularly. Patients walk with the prosthesis without the use of crutches or cane. The large mass of quadriceps muscle provides a cushion of viable tissue on the sacrum on which a prosthesis may comfortably rest without traumatizing the overlying skin. Figure 9–18 shows the tissue mass created by the transplanted muscle that can be used to bear the weight required with use of a prosthesis.

The most bothersome long-term postoperative problem with this procedure (as with a standard hemipelvectomy) is phantom limb pain. Approximately 20% of patients currently surviving have severe phantom limb pain requiring narcotic analgesic on a daily basis. However, this incidence of phantom limb pain is not noticeably different from that seen with standard hemipelvectomy.[6,7]

Occasionally, tumor tissue or heavily irradiated skin overlying the superficial femoral artery may require sacrifice of the skin pedicle. In this instance the island myocutaneous flap described by Lotze should be utilized.[8]

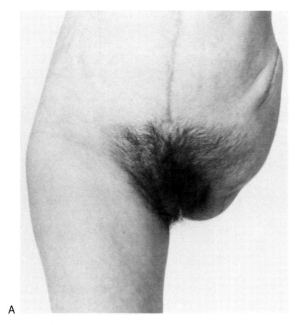

A

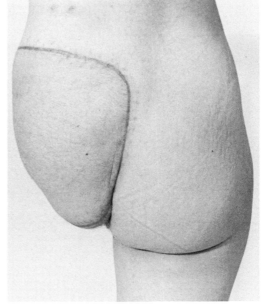

B

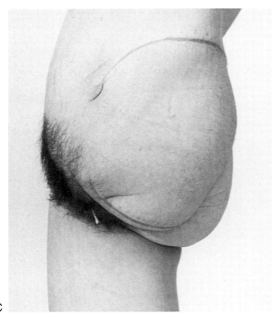

C

Figure 9–18. (A) Anterior, (B) posterior, and (C) lateral views of the completed amputation. The transplanted quadriceps muscle mass fills the defect created by the hemipelvectomy. This tissue mass can comfortably bear the weight required to use a prosthesis successfully. The quadriceps femoris muscle of the thigh is fully innervated.

REFERENCES

1. Bowden L, Booher RJ: Surgical considerations in the treatment of sarcoma of the buttock. *Cancer* 1953;6:89–99.
2. Frey C, Matthews LS, Benjamin H, et al: A new technique for hemipelvectomy. *Surg Gynecol Obstet* 1976;143:753–756.
3. Sugarbaker, PH, Chretien PB: A surgical technique for buttockectomy. *Surgery* 1982;91:104–107.
4. Mnaymneh W, Temple W: Modified hemipelvectomy utilizing a long vascular myocutaneous thigh flap. *J Bone Joint Surg* 1980;62:1013–1015.
5. Higinbotham NL, Marcove RC, Casson P: Hemipelvectomy: A clinical study of 100 cases with five year follow-up on 60 patients. *Surgery* 1966;59:706–708.
6. Douglas, HO, Razack M, Holyoke D: Hemipelvectomy. *Arch Surg* 1975;110:82–85.
7. Roth YF, Sugarbaker PH: Natural history of post-amputation pains and sensations: Late assessment following elective amputation. Abstract presentation, American Association Physical Medicine, 1980.
8. Lotze MT, Sugarbaker PH: Femoral artery based myocutaneous flap for hemipelvectomy closure: Amputation after failed limb sparing surgery and radiotherapy. *Am J Surg* 1985;150:625–630.

10

Internal Hemi-pelvectomy

CONSTANTINE P. KARAKOUSIS,
M.D., Ph.D.

OVERVIEW

This procedure involves the resection of the entire hemipelvis (innominate bone) with preservation of the ipsilateral extremity. Careful patient selection is required in order to minimize the incidence of local recurrence. It is indicated for malignant tumors involving the innominate bone without extension into soft tissue or with minimal or moderate extension into soft tissue such that would permit an en bloc resection through clean planes and allow preservation of the major nerves and vessels for the ipsilateral extremity. To do this, one must separate the sacroiliac joint and pubic symphysis. The sacrotuberous and sacrospinous ligaments must be divided along with the muscle groups that attach to the innominate bone. To do this without excessive blood loss, generous exposure is gained through a long incision extending from the posterior inferior iliac spine along the iliac crest to the anterior superior iliac spine, then along the inguinal ligament to the pubic symphysis; this is further opened by a generous T incision from the anterior superior iliac spine to behind the greater trochanter. Femoral and sciatic nerves are preserved, but the obturator nerve remains with the specimen. After division of the inferior epigastric vessels, the inguinal ligament is mobilized with the anterior abdominal wall, and the pubic symphysis is exposed and separated. The iliac vessels and muscular attachments are dissected free of the ilium, ischium, and pubis. When the sacroiliac joint is exposed, it is separated to allow removal of the specimen.

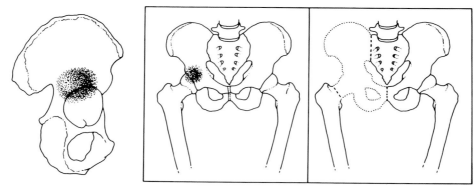

Figure 10–1. Internal hemipelvectomy involves complete resection of the innominate bone and head of the femur. The divided neck of the femur migrates cephalad postoperatively by 3 to 4 cm and may come to rest against a remaining portion of the ilium; an allograft or other form of internal fixation may be used to stabilize the neck of the femur against the proximal ilium or sacral ala. When no reconstruction is performed the neck of the femur after a period of 4 to 6 months is surrounded by dense fibrous tissue, which permits full weight bearing on this leg without further cephalad migration of the neck after the original one of about 4 cm.

INTRODUCTION

Steel reported his experience with this procedure and emphasized the need for proper patient selection. He utilized this procedure for chondrosarcoma of the acetabulum.[1–2] Enneking and Dunham[3] and Eilber and colleagues have presented their experience with complete removal of the hemipelvis.[3–5] In this book internal hemipelvectomy refers to the complete removal of ilium, ischium, and pubis plus the head of the femur (Fig. 10–1). Partial removal of major portions of the pelvic bones is discussed in chapter 13.

INDICATIONS

Tumors treatable by internal hemipelvectomy include osteosarcoma, chondrosarcoma, and soft tissue sarcoma that are closely related to the pelvic bones. Tumors located near the sacroiliac joints or pubic symphysis present a special problem in that positive margins of resection may occur unless the procedure is extended to the sacral ala or the contralateral side of the symphysis, respectively. Also, lesions medial to the pelvic bones may be adjacent to the neurovascular bundle and result in positive margins of excision. Induction chemotherapy may be useful to shrink these tumors prior to their surgical removal and thereby facilitate removal with more adequate resection margins.

A major complicating feature of these tumors may involve *tumor spill with biopsy* or an incomplete resection. Also, local hemorrhage and *tumor-contaminated hematoma* may make local control improbable. If *infection* occurs as a result of the biopsy, the early use of an internal stent may be impossible. Of course, *disseminated disease* to systemic sites or direct spread to intra-abdominal organs are contraindications to this procedure.

PROCEDURE

In order to resect the entire innominate bone, one has to separate the sacroiliac joint and pubic symphysis; also one has to divide the major ligaments (sacrotuberous and sacrospinous ligaments) connecting this bone (ischial tuberosity and ischial spine respectively) to the side of the sacrum. The incision to be used should provide access to these three bony landmarks, ie, pubic symphysis, sacroiliac joint, and ischial tuberosity. Furthermore, it should provide exposure for the dissection and preservation of the iliofemoral vessels and the sciatic and femoral nerves.

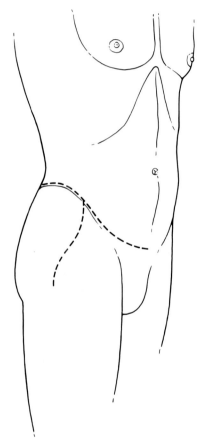

Figure 10–2. INCISION. The patient is placed in a supine position with the involved extremity draped free.
From the coinsideration of the needs for exposure, the incision to be used becomes fairly obvious. An incision is made from the posterior inferior iliac spine near the sacroiliac joint, carried along the iliac crest to the anterior superior iliac spine, then along the inguinal ligament to the pubic tubercle, and then along the pubic crest to the pubic symphysis. This incision provides exposure of the sacroiliac joint posteriorly and the pubic symphysis anteriorly. Following division of the inferior epigastric vessels the inguinal ligament is detached from the pubic tubercle and the anterior superior iliac spine; the anterior rectus sheath and muscle are divided off the pubic crest, and the anterolateral abdominal wall muscles off the iliac crest. This allows exposure of the iliac fossa, the iliac vessels, and the femoral nerve. If the tumor is confined to the bone or extends medially only, then one can detach laterally with the use of the osteotome the muscle fibers of gluteus medius and minimus (and a small portion of the gluteus maximus posteriorly) off the iliac bone to the greater sciatic notch, to allow proximal division of this bone. There is no risk of injury to the sciatic nerve, which need not be visualized in this approach since it courses deep to piriformis muscle. However, when the tumor involves the lateral surface of the iliac bone and/or the adjacent glutei, then it is obvious that these muscles must be resected en bloc with the bone, and greater exposure, permitting the dissection and preservation of the sciatic nerve, will be required. With another incision from the anterior superior iliac spine to behind the greater trochanter, a flap can be now developed that provides unhampered exposure of the sciatic nerve. The complete incision viewed from the feet of the patient resembles a reverse Y.
It is best to start with the long curvilinear incision along the iliac crest. If a previous biopsy incision has been made, it is important to encompass it through an elliptical incision and modify the overall design of the incision so that an en bloc resection of the biopsy track with the tumor will be possible.

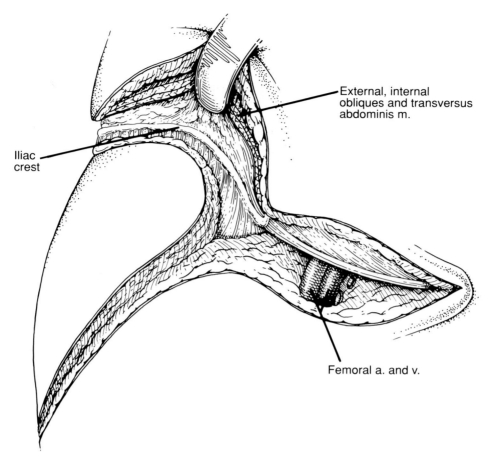

Iliac crest

External, internal obliques and transversus abdominis m.

Femoral a. and v.

Figure 10–3. EXPOSURE OF BONY PROMINENCES AND DEEP FASCIA. The incision is deepened through the subcutaneous fat to the surface of the external oblique aponeurosis. The latter is divided as well as the internal oblique, transversus abdominis muscles and transversalis fascia close to the iliac crest.

153

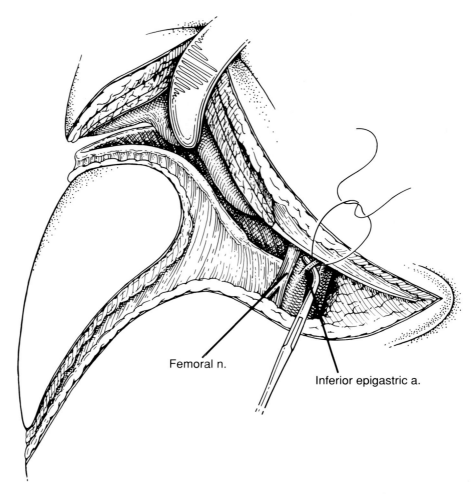

Femoral n.

Inferior epigastric a.

Figure 10–4.   EXPOSURE OF FEMORAL VESSELS AND LIGATION OF INFERIOR EPIGASTRIC ARTERY AND VEIN. Anteriorly the femoral vessels are exposed below the inguinal ligament. The retroperitoneal space is entered, and the peritoneum is displaced medially. The inguinal ligament is divided at the attachment to the anterior superior iliac spine, and its lateral third is dissected off the iliac fascia to which it is fused. At the junction of the lateral and middle thirds these two structures diverge, the inguinal ligament extending in front of, and the iliac fascia behind, the femoral vessels. As the free lateral portion of the inguinal ligament is retracted, the inferior epigastric artery and vein are serially encountered, ligated, and divided. The identification, ligation, and division of the inferior epigastric vessels are key operative maneuvers not only in this operation but also in the abdominoinguinal incision and the radical groin dissection. In standard hemipelvectomy the incision along the iliac crest may be continued (it is actually simpler to do so) above the inguinal ligament, ie, leaving the latter with the extremity to be removed. The iliofemoral vessels course between the inguinal ligament in front of the iliopsoas muscle and the corresponding portion of the innominate bone underneath. Therefore to perform internal hemipelvectomy, the inguinal ligament has to be divided at least at one point of attachment to allow the extrication, and therefore the preservation, of the vessels and the extremity.

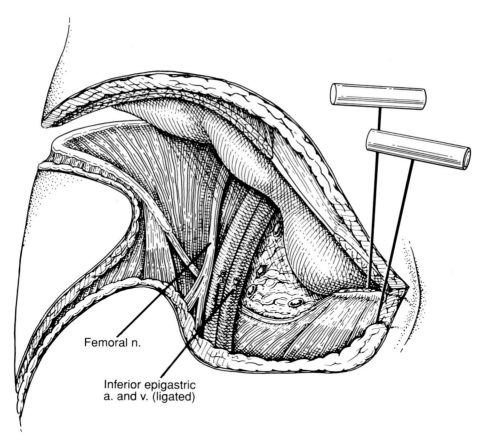

Femoral n.

Inferior epigastric
a. and v. (ligated)

Figure 10–5. **DIVISION OF THE INGUINAL LIGAMENT AND PUBIC SYMPHYSIS.** The inguinal ligament is divided also at its insertion to the pubic tubercle, and the anterior rectus abdominis sheath and muscle are divided close to the pubic crest until the midline is reached. With blunt, finger dissection in the prevesical space along the posterior surface of the pubic symphysis, the posterior arch of the symphysis is felt. With sharp dissection the anterior surface of the symphysis is exposed until again its arch is felt. A right-angle clamp is passed around the symphysis and then a Gigli saw, with which the symphysis is divided.

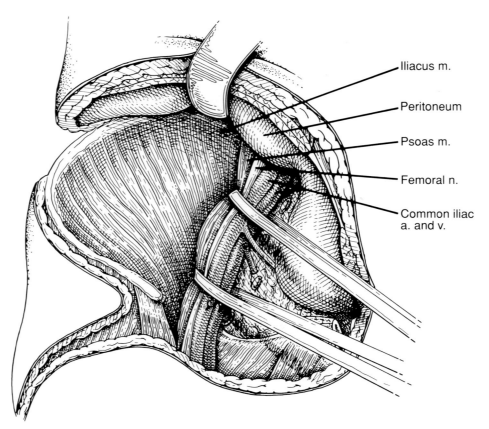

Iliacus m.

Peritoneum

Psoas m.

Femoral n.

Common iliac
a. and v.

Figure 10–6. MOBILIZATION OF COMMON FEMORAL VESSELS, FEMORAL NERVE, AND PSOAS MUSCLE. In the iliac fossa the common iliac vessels are exposed, and a tape is passed around them. Lateral and medial branches from the common femoral vessels (superficial iliac and external pudendal) are ligated and divided close to their origin to allow the mobilization of the femoral vessels, which are encircled with a tape.

Lateral and posterior to the femoral artery the iliac fascia is incised and the femoral nerve, about 1 cm or less lateral to the artery, is exposed. The nerve is traced proximally as it lies in the groove between psoas and iliacus muscle. The latter muscle may be left on the inner surface of the iliac bone from which it originates. Even when that surface is intact and uninvolved by the tumor it is not helpful to try to preserve the iliacus since it is defunctionalized by removing the bone to which its origin is attached. It provides an extra layer of muscle around the tumor if it is not removed. When the psoas muscle is not involved, it may be retained since its origin and insertion from the lower lumbar area to the lesser trochanter, respectively, may be preserved along with its innervation from the femoral nerve. The tapes are then revised to pass around the neurovascular bundle and the psoas so that these structures may be retracted as one unit. If there is a question of proximity to the tumor, the psoas muscle is divided proximally and distally to be removed en bloc with the specimen.

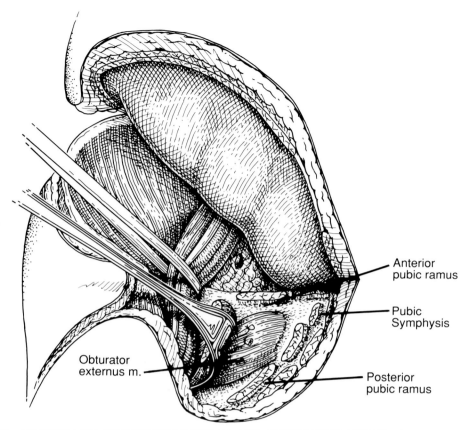

Anterior
pubic ramus

Pubic
Symphysis

Obturator
externus m.

Posterior
pubic ramus

Figure 10–7. DIVISION OF ADDUCTOR MUSCLES AND OBTURATOR NERVE. The dissection then is continued along and just below the pubic crest, pubic tubercle, and pectineal line (on which Cooper's ligament extends) dividing the origin of the adductor group of muscles. The gracilis is medial, and the adductor longus and pectineus are anterior. The adductor brevis is in the middle of these attachments and adductor magnus posteriorly. All are divided near the corresponding pubic ramus. The anterior and posterior branches of the obturator nerve and vessels lying respectively anterior and posterior to the adductor brevis are divided also. It is not possible to preserve this nerve traversing the obturator foramen if the pubic bone is removed in its entirety. If one were to remove the iliac bone and acetabulum and divide just medial to the latter the anterior and posterior pubic rami, the obturator nerve can be preserved; in this case, of course, the adductor muscles retain both origin and insertion intact and it makes sense to try to preserve their innervation (see chapter 13). The obturator nerve (L2–4 roots) coursing behind or through the fibers of psoas muscle, then goes behind the iliac vessels, and emerges lateral to the internal iliac vessels about 5 cm posterior to the external iliac vein. Then, accompanied by the obturator vessels, it courses close to the fascia covering the obturator internus until it exits through the obturator foramen.

Following division of the origin of the adductor muscles from the pubic bone the inferior surface of obturator externus muscle is exposed. The obturator externus muscle is left on the specimen. The most lateral portion of the origin of the adductor magnus extending to the ischial tuberosity will be divided later in the operation through a lateral approach.

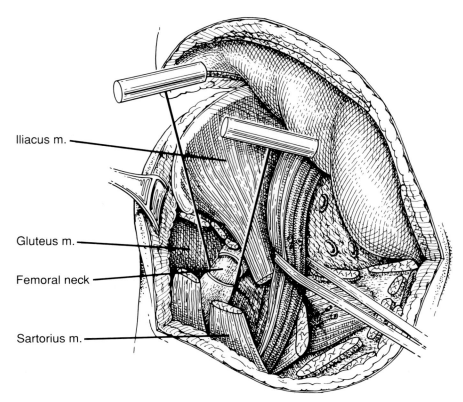

Iliacus m.

Gluteus m.

Femoral neck

Sartorius m.

Figure 10–8. DIVISION OF ORIGINS OF ANTERIOR THIGH MUSCLES AND FEMORAL NECK. The tensor fascia lata and sartorius muscle are divided below their origin, and the straight and reflected heads of the rectus femoris muscle are divided off their origin from the anterior inferior iliac spine and the rim of the acetabulum, respectively. The capsule of the hip joint is then transversely incised, exposing the neck of the femur. The latter is divided with a Gigli saw; alternatively, the femur may be disarticulated by retracting the extremity inferolaterally and dividing the ligamentum teres, which attaches the head of the femur to the acetabulum. The posterior portion of the capsule is then divided. The inferolateral extension of the reverse Y is then made, if not done already. It is preferable to wait until this moment to make this portion of the incision because unnecessary blood loss is thus avoided.

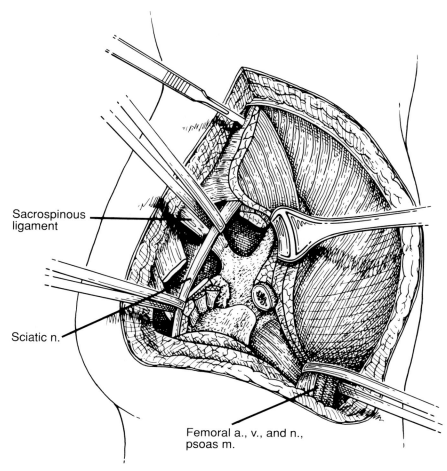

Sacrospinous ligament

Sciatic n.

Femoral a., v., and n., psoas m.

Figure 10–9. **EXPOSURE OF SACROILIAC JOINT, MOBILIZATION OF SCIATIC NERVE, AND INCISION OF POSTERIOR ATTACHMENTS OF ISCHIUM.** The inferolateral incision extends from the anterior superior iliac spine in continuity with the curvilinear incision, to behind the greater trochanter. It is deepened to the surface of fascia lata. The posterolateral flap is then developed by dissecting on top of the fascia covering the gluteus minimus and medius, but then further laterally through the fascia and deep to the gluteus maximus muscle if the latter is not involved by the tumor. It will be recalled that the gluteus maximus arises from a small area on the lateral surface of the iliac bone close to the sacroiliac joint, but mostly from the surface of the lateral edge of the sacrum. The origin arising from the iliac bone may be detached with the use of a periosteal elevator in order to expose the sacroiliac joint. It is important that the gluteus maximus remain attached to the posterolateral flap in order to avoid necrosis of the tip of this flap. Necrosis may result if the entire gluteus maximus muscle is dissected off the posterior skin flap.

The fascia lata, to which the gluteus maximus inserts, is incised just anterior to the greater trochanter, a maneuver permitting entrance into a plane anterior to gluteus maximus. The insertion of the gluteus maximus into the gluteal tuberosity of the femur may be divided for additional exposure. The sciatic nerve is surrounded with vessel loops and dissected to the greater sciatic notch. The piriformis muscle is divided. The ischial tuberosity is exposed, and the origin of the hamstring muscles is divided. Further along the inferior aspect of the ischium the remaining attachment of adductor magnus to the inferior ramus is divided. The sacrotuberous ligament (spanning between the sacrum and the ischial tuberosity) is divided close to the ischial tuberosity. This permits entrance into the ischiorectal fossa. With blunt dissection through an anterior and posterior approach, the bladder and rectum are separated from the surface of obturator internus. The sacrospinous ligament is divided at this point or following division of the sacroiliac joint. The sacroiliac joint is exposed both anteriorly and posteriorly and divided with an osteotome or a knife. The joint may be approached through its posterior surface when the patient is in a lateral position. When the patient has been placed in a supine, or semilateral, position the joint is approached from its medial surface or its superior border. It is always helpful if one feels the other side of the joint periodically as it is divided so that the appropriate orientation to the osteotome is given.

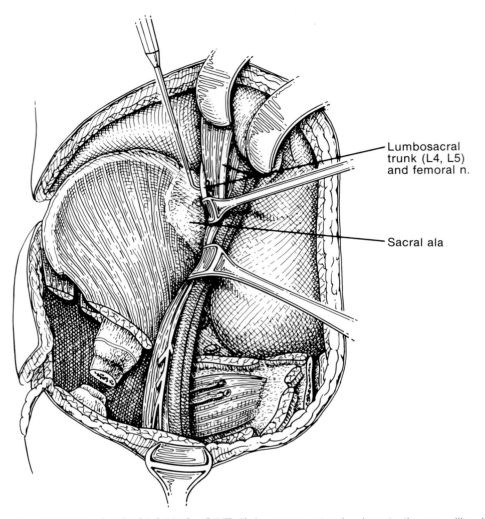

Lumbosacral trunk (L4, L5) and femoral n.

Sacral ala

Figure 10–10. DIVISION OF SACROILIAC JOINT. If the tumor extends close to the sacroiliac joint, the division of the bone is carried out medial to the joint through the sacral neural foramina. It is important to remember that the lumbosacral trunk (composed of L4–L5 roots), en route to joining S1–S3 roots and thus forming the sciatic nerve, courses in front of the sacral ala. This trunk should be identified and retracted medially, before the osteotomy is begun.

The specimen should be almost free now, and by retracting it any remaining muscular and ligamentous attachments can be divided. If they have not been divided previously, the insertions of gluteus minimus, medius, piriformis, obturator internus and externus, and gemelli and quadratus femoris to the greater trochanter are transected. Obviously, one does not need to recognize and name all the anatomic structures involved in this operation. It is important, however, to be familiar with the dissection around the iliofemoral vessels and the femoral and sciatic nerves; in the remainder of the dissection one follows the borders of the bone to be removed or the palpable extent of the tumor in dividing muscular and tendinous attachments.

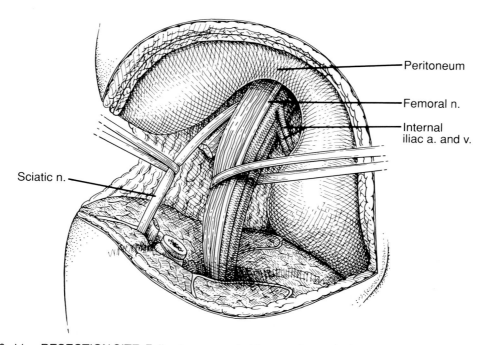

Figure 10–11.   RESECTION SITE. Following removal of the specimen, the lower extremity is connected to the trunk by the iliofemoral vessels, the femoral and sciatic nerves, possibly the psoas muscle (if preserved), and the undivided posteromedial portion of the skin and subcutaneous tissue at the root of the thigh.

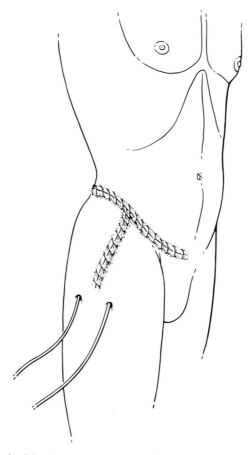

Figure 10–12.   CLOSURE. The incision is closed by approximating the fascia, when possible, or subcutaneous fat and then the skin. Suction drains are placed in the wound. A Steinman pin is placed through the tibial tuberosity, and the extremity is placed in traction with 4–6 lb of weight for two to three weeks.

161

POSTOPERATIVE COURSE AND REHABILITATION

The patient remains on bed rest for two to three weeks after this operation. An overhead trapeze is helpful in lifting the body for the use of the bedpan or in changing position and by periodically relieving the pressure on the back in avoiding bedsores. Systemic anticoagulation or aspirin treatment may be advisable in reducing the incidence of thrombophlebitis.

Physical therapy is started immediately with muscle-strengthening exercises for the arms. The patient is allowed non-weight bearing at three weeks, partial weight bearing at two to three months, and unlimited weight bearing with crutches or a cane on the operated side at four to six months.

With resection of the innominate bone a 3–5-cm shortening of the ipsilateral extremity occurs (Fig. 10–13). The patient has normal function at the ankle and knee joints, but no function at the hip area. As a result, these patients usually require the use of crutches on a permanent basis. Younger patients manage to walk easily on a flat surface, but they can also go up and down stairs.

An alternative approach for static suspension of the lower extremity across the excised ilium involves a stent between the femoral neck and sacrum. This custom-made prosthesis involves the coupling of a screw plate on the sacrum and a femoral rod. Continued experience with this prosthesis suggests that it may improve and hasten mobility.

DISCUSSION

Internal hemipelvectomy signifies, as the term suggests, the removal of the entire hemipelvis with preservation of the extremity. It is performed for primary malignant tumors of the innominate bone or for cancers involving this bone by direct extension.

The operation may be performed in a supine position with a sandbag under the proximal portion of the buttock, and the extremity prepped and draped so that it can be manipulated freely during the operation. For a tumor extending into the gluteal muscles a lateral position may be preferable, particularly if the tumor extends to the sacroiliac joint. A semilateral, 45° position is often a useful compromise that allows good exposure both for the anterior and posterior exposure.

Steel has used an incision from the posterior inferior iliac spine along the iliac crest, over the inguinal ligament and pubic crest to the pubic symphysis, which is then continued over the inferior pubic ramus and the subnatal crease to the greater trochanter.[1,2] Enneking et al have used an incision that starts from the posterior inferior iliac spine, runs along the iliac crest and lateral half of the inguinal ligament, where over the femoral vessels it turns distally along the rectus femoris for 5–7 cm, and then curves laterally to the junction of the proximal and middle thirds of the thigh; this incision permits the development of a large flap exposing the entire buttock while access to the pubic symphysis is accom-

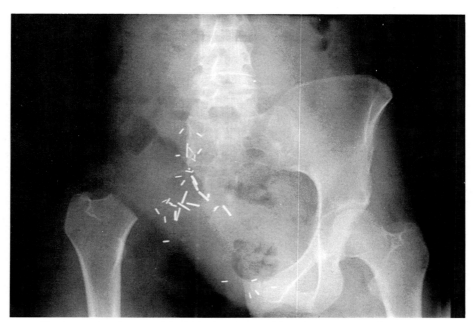

Figure 10–13. Radiograph of the pelvis following internal hemipelvectomy. A 3–5-cm shortening of the ipsilateral extremity occurs.

plished through supplementary incision along the medial half of the inguinal ligament to the pubic symphysis.[3] Eilber et al have used a similar incision[4,5] to that described by Enneking.

Both Enneking and Steel emphasize the preservation of the head of the femur and any portion of the proximal iliac bone when the location of the tumor permits, because abutment of these structures as the extremity shortens and development of callus allow a greater degree of stability.[1–3]

Since the loss of the hip joint function is a sufficiently severe impairment in itself, it is generally believed that involvement by the tumor of one of the major nerves, ie, sciatic or femoral, requiring its sacrifice, should revise the operative plan to that of a standard hemipelvectomy. Of course, such an eventuality should be explained beforehand to the patient, and the appropriate consent should be obtained.

At present, there is no satisfactory or easy replacement of the innominate bone. Abutment of the trochanter and sacrum and the development of scar tissue later provide a measure of stability. Although the appropriate size allograft or hemipelvis prosthesis may be used and fixed into position at the time of resection, the risk and consequences of infection increase with the use of a foreign body.

In our experience, internal hemipelvectomy is, when the appropriate indications are applied, a procedure definitely superior to hindquarter amputation both functionally and cosmetically, particularly for younger patients motivated and capable of undergoing extensive physical rehabilitation.

REFERENCES

1. Steel HH: Partial or complete resection of the hemipelvis. An alternative to hindquarter amputation for periacetabular chondrosarcoma of the pelvis. *J Bone Joint Surg* 1978;60A:719–730.
2. Steel HH: Resection of the hemipelvis for malignant disease: An alternative to hindquarter amputation for periacetabular chondrosarcoma of the pelvis. *Sem Oncol* 1981;8:222–228.
3. Enneking WF, Dunham WK: Resection and reconstruction for primary neoplasms involving the innominate bone. *J Bone Joint Surg* 1978;60A:731–746.
4. Eilber FR, Grant TT, Sakai D, et al: Internal hemipelvectomy—excision of the hemipelvis with limb preservation. *Cancer* 1979;43:806–809.
5. Huth JF, Eckardt JJ, Pignatti G, et al: Resection of malignant bone tumors of the pelvic girdle without extremity amputation. *Arch Surg* 1988;123:1121–1124.

11

The Abdomino-inguinal Incision for the Resection of Pelvic Tumors

CONSTANTINE P. KARAKOUSIS, M.D., Ph.D.

OVERVIEW

The abdominoinguinal incision allows a vast improvement in the exposure and resectability of tumors in the lower abdomen with fixation to the pelvic side wall. A midline abdominal incision is connected to a longitudinal inguinal incision across the inguinal ligament. The pelvic side wall is directly exposed by detachment of the rectus muscle from its origin on the pubic crest and by division of the inguinal canal along the spermatic cord. This exposure allows safe resections along the iliac vessels without tumor spillage. The abdominoinguinal incision should be part of the armamentarium of every surgeon willing to accept responsibility for pelvic and pelvic side wall malignancy.

INTRODUCTION

Pelvic tumors with lateral fixation present difficulties in their resection, primarily due to inadequate exposure through conventional abdominal incisions. The difficulty arises especially with tumors in the lower parts of the pelvis where the anterior abdominal wall converges with the retroperitoneal structures (eg, iliopsoas muscle, iliac vessels). In this area the inguinal ligament spanning between the anterior superior iliac spine and the pubic tubercle provides an obstacle to unhindered exposure.

A midline, paramedian, or oblique abdominal incision often does not provide adequate exposure for these tumors. These incisions render sufficient exposure for the dissection and control of the common iliac vessels proximally, below the bifurcation of the aorta, but do not afford exposure of the terminal portion of the external iliac vessels because the presence of tumor hinders further visibility. Often these tumors are considered unresectable or are managed with hemipelvectomy.

Queral and Elias reported a two-stage procedure for removal of a sarcoma localized in the right iliac fossa with involvement of the iliac vessels.[1] In the first operation a femorofemoral bypass was performed from the left side to the right, and the common femoral artery was proximally ligated and divided. In the second operation, through an abdominal incision the mass was resected with en bloc resection of a segment of the right iliac vessels, which were ligated and divided proximally. This example provides a solution to the distal control of the iliac vessels. But it requires two operations, and exposure at the time of resection of the tumor mass through an abdominal incision remains suboptimal.

What is needed for the resection of these tumors is an incision that would simultaneously provide an in-continuity exposure of the abdominal cavity and one or both groins so that both iliac and femoral vessels would be exposed in one field. For this incision, an abdominal component would be needed and an in-continuity inguinal component, ie, an abdominoinguinal incision. The inguinal ligament would have to be divided to allow uninterrupted exposure and control of the iliofemoral vessels.

A lower midline incision provides good exposure of the intrapelvic structures. An inguinal incision exposes the femoral vessels. A transverse incision connecting the two, by dividing the origin of the rectus abdominis from the pubic crest and the insertion of the inguinal ligament to the pubic tubercle, provides the necessary link that allows a single in-continuity field and optimizes exposure. Although in the preceding discussion we arrived at the abdominoinguinal incision deductively, in reality I stumbled upon variations of it in the first few cases in the process of designing an incision for a specific tumor.[2] Later I realized that this could be developed into a formal incision for exposure in the lower quadrants of the abdomen. The abdominoinguinal incision may function much in the same way that the thoracoabdominal incision is used for the upper quadrants of the abdomen.[3]

INDICATIONS

The indications for the abdominoinguinal incision are (1) abdominal or pelvic tumors extending over the iliac vessels, (2) tumors in the iliac fossa (Fig. 11–1), (3) primary tumors, possibly involving the iliac vessels or large iliac lymph node metastases, (4) tumors with fixation to the wall of the true pelvis or large obturator nodes, (5) tumors involving the pubic bone with or without extension to the pelvis or adductor group of muscles, and (6) tumors of the groin when they involve the vessels or the lower abdominal wall or extend in the retroperitoneal area.

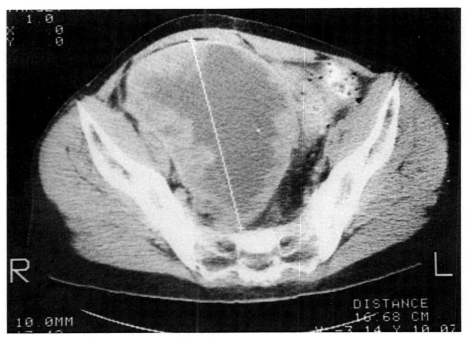

Figure 11–1. Computerized tomogram of the pelvis. A large soft tissue sarcoma closely adherent to the iliac fossa was resected with a clear margin of resection by using the abdominoinguinal incision.

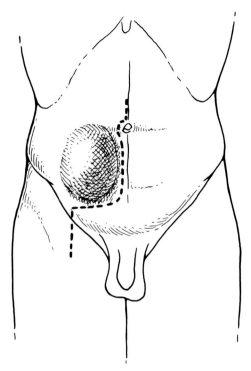

Figure 11–2.   **POSITION AND INCISION.** With the patient in the supine position, a lower midline abdominal incision is outlined from just above the umbilicus to the pubic symphysis. The peritoneal cavity is entered, and exploration is carried out to assess the extent of disease. Preliminary dissection between the tumor mass and midline pelvic structures may be carried out. Involvement of the latter does not necessarily mean unresectability, of course, since they can often be removed en bloc with the tumor. When there is a question of involvement of the iliac vessels distally, the common iliac vessels are dissected free and vessel loops are passed around them.

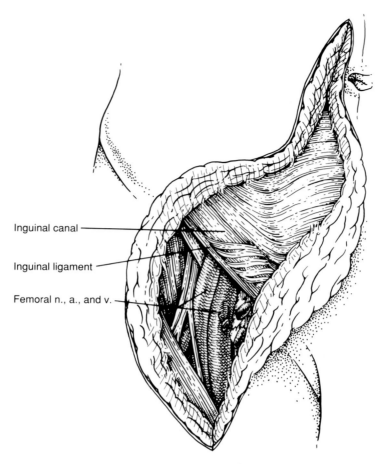

Inguinal canal

Inguinal ligament

Femoral n., a., and v.

Figure 11–3. INCISION THROUGH INGUINAL CANAL. If the decision is made to proceed with the resection, the lower end of the incision is extended transversely to the midinguinal point and then vertically, over the course of the femoral vessels, for a few centimeters. The vertical portion of the incision is deepened to expose the common femoral vessels.

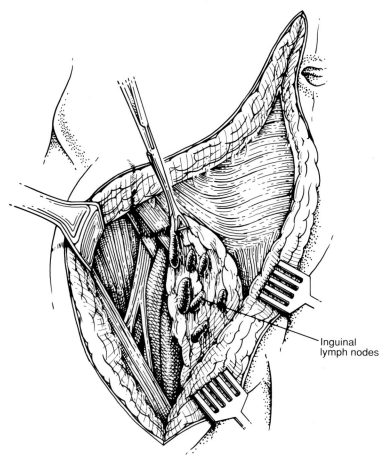

Inguinal
lymph nodes

Figure 11–4.   DISSECTION OF INGUINAL NODES. When the operation is performed for large iliac and/or obturator nodes or if there is clinical or potential microscopic involvement of the inguinal nodes, the vertical portion of the incision is made to extend to the apex of the femoral triangle, flaps are raised as in a groin dissection,[4] and the nodes are mobilized off the femoral vessels, but their proximal continuity with the deep nodes is preserved.

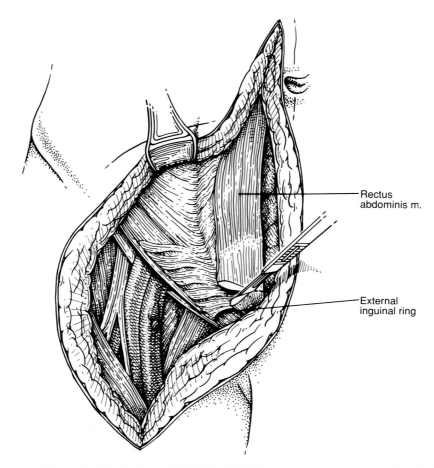

Figure 11–5. **DIVISION OF RECTUS ABDOMINIS MUSCLE.** The transverse portion of the incision is deepened to the surface of the anterior rectus sheath, which is divided, and the rectus abdominis muscle is transected a few millimeters from its origin on the pubic crest. This incision is through its tendinous portion.

Rectus abdominis m.

External inguinal ring

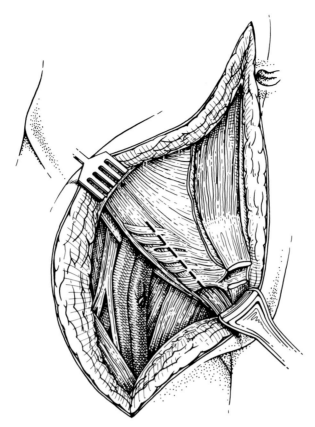

Figure 11–6. OPENING THE INGUINAL CANAL. The round ligament in women is divided over the pubic tubercle. In men, if the tumor is not too close to the internal inguinal ring, the spermatic cord can usually be preserved. The medial crus of the external inguinal ring is divided close to the pubic tubercle. The external oblique aponeurosis is split from the external inguinal ring lateral as in an inguinal herniorrhaphy.

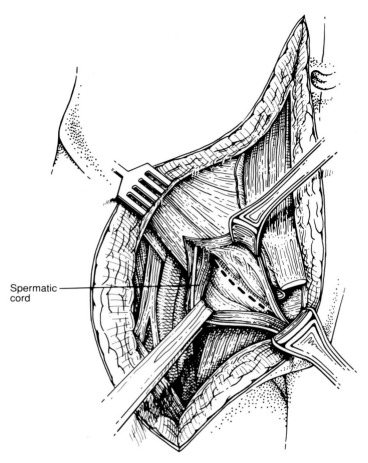

Spermatic cord

Figure 11–7.   INCISING THE FLOOR OF THE INGUINAL CANAL. The inguinal canal floor is divided in the same direction up to and including the medial border of the internal inguinal ring. In so doing, the spermatic cord is displaced medially. Alternatively, after division of the medial crus the inguinal floor may be incised from inside and the cord exposed from within the abdomen and extracted from the inguinal canal for medial displacement. Deep to the internal inguinal ring the structures of the cord deviate, the vas deferens coursing medially, and the internal spermatic vessels toward a lateral and cephalad direction. Depending on the location of the tumor, the internal spermatic vessels may have to be divided at this level; this maneuver usually leaves a viable ipsilateral testis. Division of the cord at the level of the external inguinal ring does not require ipsilateral orchiectomy but will be accompanied by testicular atrophy.

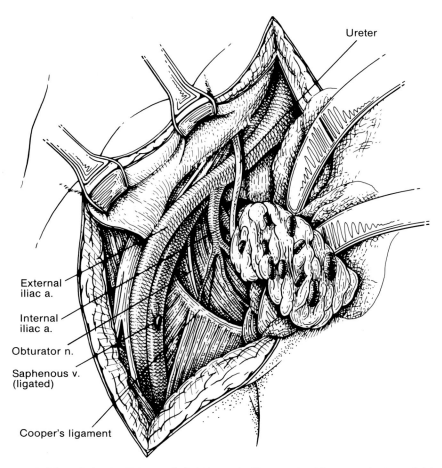

Ureter

External iliac a.

Internal iliac a.

Obturator n.

Saphenous v. (ligated)

Cooper's ligament

Figure 11–8. **EXPOSURE OF THE PELVIC SIDE WALL.** The inguinal ligament is then divided at the pubic tubercle and dissection carried on its undersurface until the inferior deep epigastric vein and artery are encountered, ligated, and divided. The lateral third of the inguinal ligament is then detached off the iliac fascia. This allows the completion of the abdominoinguinal incision and provides wide exposure of abdomen and pelvis.

Further dissection depends on the location of the tumor. If the tumor is simply a pelvic mass extending over and obscuring the iliac vessels, the improved exposure now makes easy the dissection of the mass off the vessels and safe ligation of any tumor-feeding branches. For large nodes the dissection is carried on the surface of the iliac vessels which are skeletonized. For a tumor located in the iliac fossa, the femoral nerve is located lateral to the femoral artery, immediately posterior to the continuation of the iliac fascia. A vessel loop is passed around it. Further cautious dissection along this nerve determines its relation to the tumor and whether it can be saved. If the tumor involves the vessels, proximal and distal control are secured and the dissection completed around the tumor mass, with any involved organs removed en bloc. When the specimen is held only by the attachment to the vessels, the patient is heparinized, vascular clamps are placed proximally and distally, the specimen is removed, and vascular reconstruction is performed.

When the iliofemoral vessels are to be resected, the profunda femoris branches may have to be divided at a distance from the tumor in order to allow the mobilization of the specimen.

For tumors attached to the wall of the lesser pelvis or the obturator fossa, the improved exposure usually allows their resection. For tumors involving the pubic bone, following the completion of the abdominoinguinal incision, the adductor muscles are divided off the pubic bone at an appropriate distance from the tumor, and the anterior and posterior pubic rami are exposed: the former just medial to the acetabulum and the latter medial to the ischial tuberosity. With the help of a right-angle clamp, a Gigli saw is passed around the pubic symphysis, which is divided along with the anterior and posterior pubic rami. The obturator nerve and vessels have to be divided proximally because they course through the obturator foramen. The defect may be replaced with a polypropylene mesh.

For a large tumor located in the groin, covering or involving the entire length of the common femoral vessels and possibly the lower abdominal wall, the abdominoinguinal incision provides incontinuity exposure of the iliofemoral vessels. In making the incision, flaps may have to be raised around the mass. If the lower abdominal wall and inguinal ligament are involved, following transection of the anterior rectus sheath and rectus abdominis muscle off the pubic crest, the incision is continued through the external oblique aponeurosis and internal oblique and transversus abdominis muscles at a sufficient distance from the tumor. The inguinal ligament is divided off the anterior superior iliac spine and the pubic tubercle, and thus the lower abdominal wall muscles and inguinal ligament are removed en bloc with the tumor. The inferior epigastric vessels are divided at the point they proceed behind the rectus muscle.

In the drawing above, the lateral third of the inguinal ligament has not been detached off the iliac fascia, a **173** step providing further exposure.

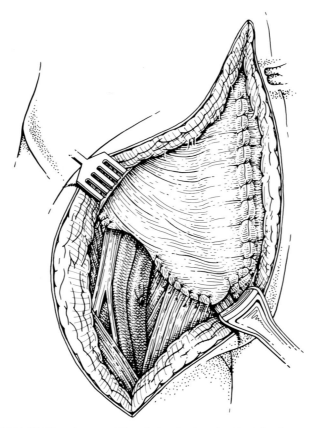

Figure 11–9. DEEP CLOSURE. The closure of the abdominoinguinal incision is uncomplicated. Lateral to the vessels the inguinal ligament is approximated to the iliac fascia and medial to the vessels to Cooper's ligament. The rectus sheath and muscle are approximated to their remnants on the pubic crest. A suction drain is placed in the inguinal portion of the incision. A subcutaneous layer of absorbable material may be used. The skin and the midline portion of the incision are closed in a routine fashion.

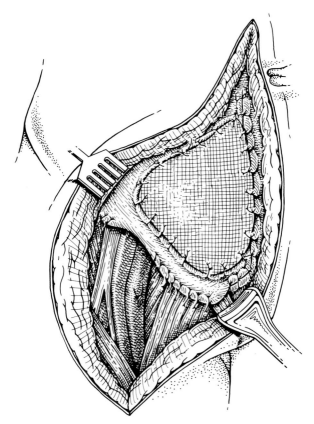

Figure 11–10.   DEEP CLOSURE REQUIRING MESH. When a defect in the fascia has been created, it may be covered with a plastic mesh, which also replaces the inguinal ligament. The mesh should not be in direct contact with the vessels. This can usually be done by dividing the sartorius muscle distally at the apex of the femoral triangle and mobilizing the distal end so that the vessels are covered, taking care to avoid devascularization of this muscle.

When the defect in the groin also involves the skin, we have used the contralateral rectus abdominis muscle, which is divided proximally and rotated with the posterior sheath attached to it, its blood supply deriving from the inferior epigastric vessels. The muscle is sutured to the defect and skin-grafted immediately.

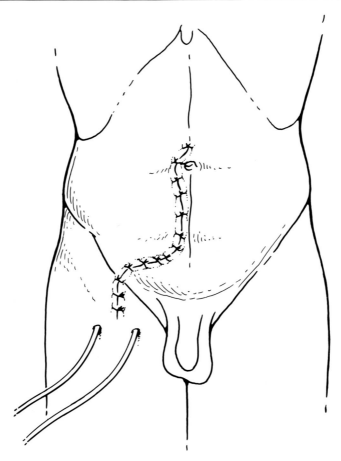

Figure 11–11. SKIN CLOSURE.

DISCUSSION

The abdominoinguinal incision has been used in over 50 patients with a variety of tumors, usually soft tissue sarcomas. One of these patients had adenocarcinoma of the sigmoid fixed to the iliac fascia. This tumor was thought to be unresectable at another hospital, but was successfully removed through this incision. The majority of the patients had been operated on once or twice elsewhere, and were found to be unresectable or thought to need a hemipelvectomy.

All these tumors, presenting with fixation to the soft tissues of the wall of the pelvis, were resected with the abdominoinguinal incision, with the exception of two patients. They required hemipelvectomy due to extensive nerve involvement. One patient required an abdominobiinguinal incision, ie, bilateral extension of abdominal inguinal the midline incision to the groins. Tumors involving the innominate bone, with the exception of the medial portion of the pubic bone, are resected best with the use of the techniques of internal hemipelvectomy[5] and, if necessary, hemipelvectomy.

The abdominoinguinal incision heals well without complications. In the event of a previous transverse incision in the lower quadrant, which may have interrupted the connection to the superior epigastric vessels and the distal portion of intercostal and lumbar branches, a small area of necrosis at the junction of the midline and transverse portions of the incision may occur, since this incision divides the inferior epigastric vessels. In two patients with this condition a small area of ischemic necrosis developed, which, following debridement, healed by secondary intention.

There was one death two weeks postoperatively, which resulted from erosion and hemorrhage of a previously heavily radiated external iliac artery that was in contact with a mesh used to replace a fascial defect. It is important therefore to cover the vessels with the sartorius or rectus femoris muscle (by dividing its origin from the anterior inferior iliac spine and displacing it medially) when a mesh is placed adjacent to the vessels or when there is concern about flap necrosis. No instances of postoperative incisional hernia have been noted.

The abdominoinguinal incision renders resectable the majority of pelvic tumors with lateral fixation to the soft tissues of the pelvis, and, through improvement in exposure, allows for a safe, deliberate dissection. It is the counterpart of the thoracoabdominal incision for the upper quadrants of the abdomen. The results from the use of this incision obviously depend on the histologic type and stage of the tumor and the expected margin of resection one can thus obtain. It should be used when appropriate and in the context of the biology of the tumor, the expected margin, and the possible use of adjuvant treatments.

In many situations in which the tumor is not laterally fixed, but when it is large and distal and pressing against the obturator foramen(s) or the obturator areas, one can obtain sufficient exposure with a unilateral or bilateral use of the transverse portion of the full incision. In other words, the lower end of the midline incision is extended transversely from the pubic symphysis to the pubic tubercle, and the ipsilateral rectus sheath and muscle are divided off the pubic crest.

REFERENCES

1. Queral LA, Elias EG: Femoro-femoral and venous bypasses in association with resection of a pelvic leiomyosarcoma, in General Surgery Motion Picture Session 10/24/84 of the American College of Surgeons, 1984 Clinical Congress.
2. Karakousis CP: Exposure and reconstruction in the lower portions of the retroperitoneum and abdominal wall. *Arch Surg* 1982;117:840–844.
3. Karakousis CP: The abdominoinguinal incision in limb salvage and resection of pelvic tumors. *Cancer* 1984;54:2543–2548.
4. Karakousis CP: Ilioinguinal lymph node dissection. *Am J Surg* 1981;141:299–303.
5. Karakousis CP: Internal hemipelvectomy. *Surg Gynecol Obstet* 1984;158:279–282.

12

Buttockectomy

PAUL H. SUGARBAKER, M.D.
PAUL B. CHRETIEN, M.D.

OVERVIEW

The buttockectomy is an en bloc resection of the gluteus maximus muscle. It is usually performed for low-grade malignancy tumors of the buttocks that are encompassed by the muscle excised. After the incision of the skin widely around the tumor, skin flaps are created to expose the entire gluteus maximus muscle; the inferior rolled edge of the muscle is identified and traced laterally to its insertion on the iliotibial tract. For a left buttockectomy the operator proceeds clockwise, first releasing the insertions of the muscle from the iliotibial tract and great trochanter and the origins from the crest of ilium and sacrum. For a right buttockectomy one proceeds counterclockwise, again starting at the inferior aspect of the gluteus maximus muscle. Care must be taken to avoid damage to the sciatic nerve and to secure the inferior and superior gluteal vessels before they are transected. Suction drainage is secured to remove serum and ensure adherence of skin flaps to the resection site. If the skin closure is tight, retention sutures may be needed.

In 1953 Bowden and Booher[1] described a surgical approach for treatment of tumors (usually soft tissue sarcomas) of the buttock. They reiterated an important principle of management: the narrowest margin of resection of a tumor may determine the surgical procedure. In many patients a tumor may clear the *medial* line of resection (the sacrum) by only a few millimeters of normal tissue. Therefore local extirpation of such tumors may give a margin of resection equal to that of hemipelvectomy. This principle was their rationale for radical local resection of the buttock. In their report, experience with nine patients with buttock sarcomas was presented. The indications they gave for hemipelvectomy rather than buttockectomy were involvement of the bony pelvis or the sciatic nerve.

Wanebo et al[2] extended the studies of Bowden and Booher to 71 patients with malignant soft tissue sarcomas of the buttock. They performed buttockectomy in 36 patients. Local recurrence developed in 14 of these 36 and in 7 of 11 patients who had to have portions of bone or sciatic nerve resected in addition to the gluteus maximus muscle and overlying soft tissue. They point out that the incidence of distant tumor metastases was doubled in patients experiencing local recurrence. The need for careful patient selection before electing this surgical procedure is well documented in their studies. The impact that radiation therapy and adjuvant systemic chemotherapy may have in decreasing the local recurrence rate is currently under study.[3]

INDICATIONS

Patients with malignant tumors optimally treated by buttockectomy alone are not encountered frequently. Most often the tumors selected for this procedure are benign or of low-grade malignancy so that little or no tissue margin is required. Grade II or greater soft tissue sarcomas must be quite small and confined to the gluteus maximus muscle or overlying fascia and subcutaneous tissue to be considered for curative resection by buttockectomy. Radiation therapy is sometimes added to the treatment regimen in an attempt to achieve local control for aggressive sarcomas, but the benefit of adjuvant therapy needs to be demonstrated by prospective clinical trials.

If tumor penetration of the deep margin of the muscle is observed during the dissection of the gluteus maximus muscle from the sciatic nerve and deep muscles of the buttock, a major amputation is usually recommended. The anterior myocutaneous flap hemipelvectomy may be the procedure of choice.[4] The alternative treatment to spare the lower extremity is high-dose radiation therapy to a large field following buttockectomy that removes the primary tumor.[3] This large field of high-dose irradiation plus surgery does not necessarily result in a better quality of life than does amputation.[5]

PROCEDURE

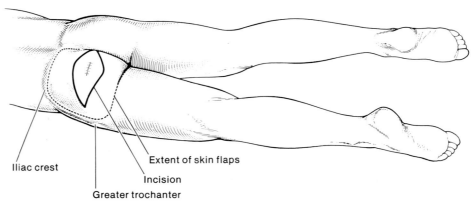

Iliac crest

Extent of skin flaps

Incision

Greater trochanter

Figure 12–1.   INCISION AND SKIN FLAPS. The patient is placed in the supine position with the legs slightly separated. The left leg need not be draped free, for if an anterior flap hemipelvectomy is indicated the patient must be turned to the lateral position, reprepared, and redraped. A generous incision encompassing the biopsy site and tumor is outlined; because of the excellent mobility of buttock skin allowed by the gluteal fold, up to half of the longitudinal extent of buttock skin may be sacrificed with the specimen.

It is helpful to mark on the skin the extent of dissection of the skin flaps. Superiorly, this is the crest of the ilium; medially, the midline; inferiorly, the gluteal fold; and laterally, the greater trochanter. The incision is made, and tapered skin flaps that are progressively thicker toward their base are constructed to spare as great a thickness of subcutaneous tissue as is possible. The gluteal fascia should be left on the specimen.

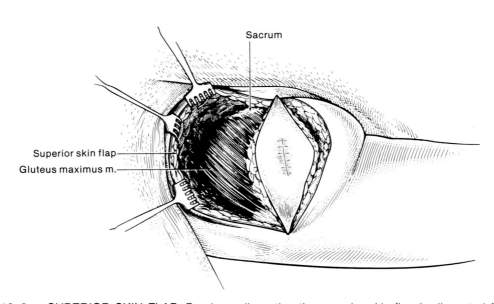

Sacrum

Superior skin flap
Gluteus maximus m.

Figure 12–2.   SUPERIOR SKIN FLAP. By sharp dissection the superior skin flap is dissected from the underlying muscle. Superiorly and laterally this flap extends to the crest of the ilium and medially to muscular insertions on the sacrum.

180

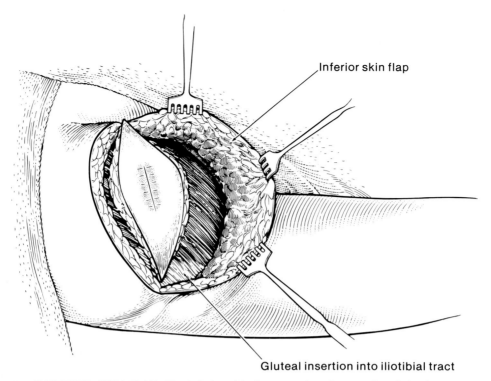

Inferior skin flap

Gluteal insertion into iliotibial tract

Figure 12–3. INFERIOR SKIN FLAP. The inferior skin flap must be dissected until the lower margin of the gluteus maximus muscle is defined in its entirety. Laterally, the skin flap is continued out to the greater trochanter.

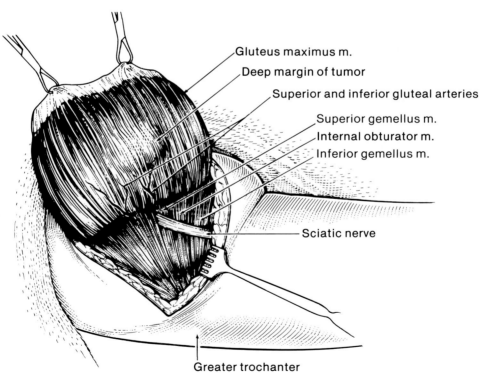

Gluteus maximus m.

Deep margin of tumor

Superior and inferior gluteal arteries

Superior gemellus m.

Internal obturator m.

Inferior gemellus m.

Sciatic nerve

Greater trochanter

Figure 12–4. RELEASE OF INSERTION OF GLUTEUS MAXIMUS MUSCLE. Commencing at the lower rolled edge of the gluteus maximus muscle, the dissection proceeds in a clockwise direction for left buttock tumors. The insertion of the muscle is released from the iliotibial tract and greater trochanter. This dissection exposes the deep margin of the muscle. Also, the sciatic nerve and inferior gluteal vessels exiting together beneath the inferior margin of the piriformis muscle can be well visualized. The inferior gluteal vessels may be exceptionally large if they exit from the overlying tumor. They should be clearly visualized then ligated in continuity before division. The fatty and fibroareolar tissue that covers the deep muscles of the buttock and surrounds the sciatic nerve should be preserved on the specimen to give the best margin possible. At this time careful examination of the deep margin of the specimen for tumor penetration should be performed. If the sciatic nerve, deep muscles of the buttock, or bony pelvis is involved by tumor, anterior flap hemipelvectomy should be considered. However, in some clinical settings adjuvant radiation therapy may be recommended.

181

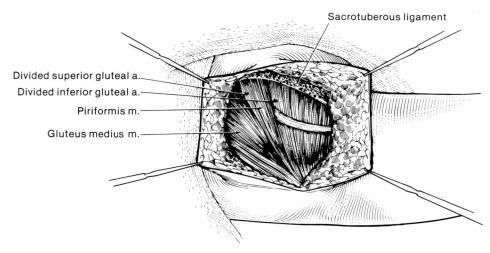

Figure 12–5. **RELEASE OF ORIGIN OF GLUTEUS MAXIMUS MUSCLE.** To complete the removal of the specimen, the origins of the gluteus maximus muscle on the crest of the ilium are divided by dissection from the lateral to the medial edge of the crest. The origins of the muscle on the sacrum are divided by dissecting from the superior origin inferiorly. The superior gluteal vessels must be visualized, ligated, and divided as they emerge from the superior aspect of the sacrotuberous ligament and piriformis muscle up into the gluteus maximus muscle.

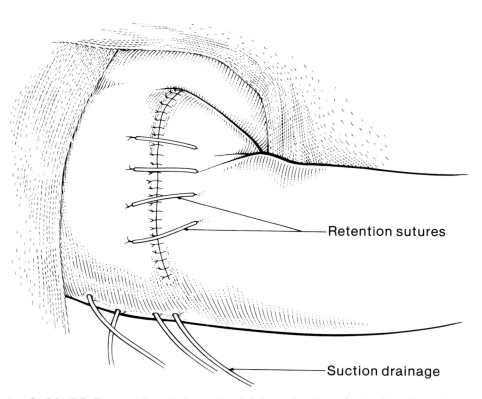

Figure 12–6. **CLOSURE.** The excision site is copiously irrigated and any further bleeding points secured. If the skin closure is tight, retention sutures are positioned. Generous suction drainage is secured. The subcutaneous tissue is approximated with absorbable suture and the skin closed with monofilament sutures. Retention sutures are recommended unless there is no tension on the skin flaps. They are used to avoid wound disruption should the patient inadvertently flex the hip before the incision is healed. Suction catheters are not removed until drainage has nearly ceased.

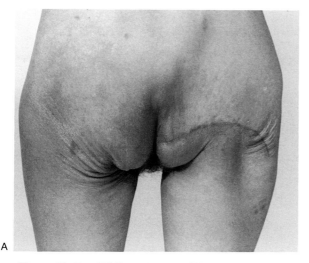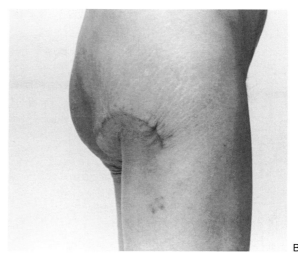

A   B

Figure 12–7.   (A) Posterior and (B) lateral views of patient after buttockectomy. The excess skin that normally forms the gluteal fold is absent on the operative side.

DISCUSSION

Buttockectomy in carefully selected patients gives good results in that postoperative morbidity is minimal and rehabilitation is generally complete (Fig. 12–7). A single postoperative misadventure that has occurred is dehiscence of the incision when activity is resumed. The patient should not be allowed to sit until the wound is securely healed. If the skin edges are under extreme tension because of sacrifice of skin over a tumor mass, retention sutures are indicated.

The most common problem with this procedure occurs because of an inadequate deep margin of resection. If tumor is found to border on bone or sciatic nerve, the buttockectomy procedure can be stopped and an anterior flap hemipelvectomy can be performed.

REFERENCES

1. Bowden L, Booher RJ: Surgical considerations in the treatment of sarcoma of the buttock. *Cancer* 1953;6:89–99.
2. Wanebo HJ, Shah J, Knapper W, et al: Reappraisal of surgical management of sarcoma of the buttock. *Cancer* 1973;31:97–104.
3. Rosenberg SA, Kent H, Costa J, et al: Prospective randomized evaluation of the role of limb-sparing surgery, radiation therapy, and adjuvant chemoimmunotherapy in the treatment of adult soft tissue sarcomas. *Surgery* 1978;84:62–69.
4. Sugarbaker PH, Chretien PA: Hemipelvectomy for buttock tumors utilizing an anterior myocutaneous flap of quadriceps femoris muscle. *Ann Surg* 1983;197:106–115.
5. Sugarbaker PH, Barofsky I, Rosenberg SA, et al: Quality of life assessment of patients in extremity sarcoma clinical trials. *Surgery* 1982;91:17–23.

13

Summary of Alternative Approaches to Hemi-pelvectomy

PAUL H. SUGARBAKER, M.D.
CONSTANTINE P. KARAKOUSIS, M.D., Ph.D.
MARTIN M. MALAWER, M.D.

OVERVIEW

A hindquarter amputation is the appropriate treatment for many patients with sarcoma of the upper thigh and buttock. In the standard *posterior flap hemipelvectomy*, surgical trauma is minimized by an extraperitoneal approach, by transection of the sacroiliac joint and pubic symphysis rather than bone, and by sparing autonomic nerves to the bladder and genitalia. Frequently, modifications of the standard procedure are indicated. With tumors of the adductor muscle group, conservation of tissue may be achieved by sparing much of the iliac bone. If the crest of the ilium is spared, the procedure is referred to as a *modified hemipelvectomy*. A more adequate tissue margin medially with buttock tumors may be gained by transecting the sacrum through the neural foramina. If sacral transection is through the neural foramina, the procedure is called an *extended hemipelvectomy*. If the tumor mass is located in the buttock or high in the posterior thigh and does not involve the femoral vessels, then an *anterior flap hemipelvectomy* should be performed. In this procedure the surgical defect created by resection of the hemipelvis is covered by a myocutaneous flap created from the quadriceps femoris muscle. Occasionally, an intrapelvic tumor may be approached more safely by entering the peritoneal cavity. If bladder, rectum, or female internal genitalia are invaded by tumor and removed with the hindquarter specimen, the procedure is referred to as a *compound hemipelvectomy*. The *abdominoinguinal incision* should be considered in these patients. With adequate exposure a local excision may be possible. *Internal hemipelvectomy* is a resection of the hemipelvis (entire innominate bone) with preservation of the extremity. Partial removal of the hemipelvis is classified as *Type I, II, and III innominate bone resections*. Occasionally, with low-grade tumors of the upper femur, prosthetic replacement allows preservation of the extremity. The types of resections vary with the anatomic location of the tumor, the biologic aggressiveness of the malignant process, and the response to induction chemotherapy.

INTRODUCTION

The alternative approaches to hemipelvectomy are listed below. These procedures differ in the position through which the sacrum is transected, in the skin coverage of the operative defect, and in the structures removed. With an internal hemipelvectomy, innominate bone resection, or prosthetic replacement of the upper femur, the extremity is preserved; however, careful patient selection is required to prevent local treatment failure with these approaches.

1. Posterior flap (with posterior buttock skin flap; chapter 8)
2. Modified (spares wing of ilium)
3. Extended (sacral osteotomy through neural foramina)
4. Anterior flap (a myocutaneous flap of quadriceps muscle covers the operative defect created by excision of a buttock tumor; chapter 9)
5. Intraperitoneal
6. Compound (excision of a viscus plus the hindquarter specimen)
7. Internal (excision of the hemipelvis with preservation of the extremity)
8. Innominate bone resection (excision of one or more parts of the innominate bone)

POSTERIOR FLAP HEMIPELVECTOMY

Indications

Indications for the standard posterior flap hemipelvectomy are high-grade soft tissue sarcomas of the anterior and lateral thigh and bony tumors of the upper femur and pelvis. In the standard hindquarter amputation a long posterior flap of buttock skin is used to cover the large defect created by removal of the lower extremity and its hemipelvis (Figs. 13–1 and 13–2).

MODIFIED HEMIPELVECTOMY

Indications

Large soft tissue sarcomas occurring high in the medial thigh are the most common indication for modified hemipelvectomy (Fig. 13–3). The tumor must not involve the sartorius muscle, because sarcomas may spread long distances along muscle groups. The origin of the sartorius (the anterior superior iliac spine) remains with the patient in a modified hemipelvectomy (Figs. 13–3—13–6). Soft

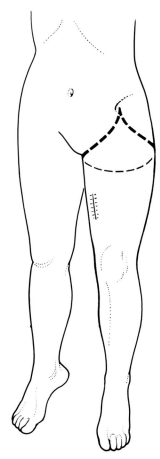

Figure 13–1. Skin incision. The skin incision allows adequate exposure and provides generous skin coverage of the operative defect. Ischemic complications with this skin coverage are not common. Karakousis has emphasized the need to preserve a portion of gluteus maximus muscle attached to the proximal portion of the skin flap. In his patients who had preservation of a portion of the gluteus muscle, flap necrosis did not occur.[1]

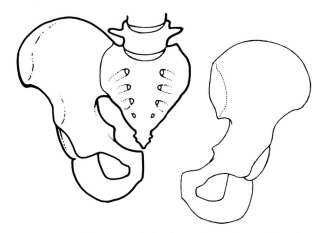

Figure 13–2. Release of the innominate bone. The bony portions of the specimen are released by the bloodless transection of the pubic symphysis and sacroiliac joint.

tissue sarcomas of the anterior or lateral thigh may spread along muscle bundles to involve muscular insertions on the ilium and should not be treated by the modified procedure. Large bony tumors of the upper femur with soft tissue extension should not be treated by modified hemipelvectomy, because the tumor may extend into the gluteus muscles and surrounding soft tissue. Small bony tumors of the upper femur with minimal soft tissue extension (osteosarcoma or chondrosarcoma) may be treated with modified hemipelvectomy. However, limb-sparing procedures with prosthetic bone replacements may occasionally be selected in this group of patients.

DISCUSSION

The major advantage to the patient of modified hemipelvectomy is cosmetic. With the wing of the ilium intact, the waistline remains normal, and clothes feel and fit better (Fig. 13–7). Some have claimed that a prosthesis can be fashioned in which weight is distributed on the transected iliac bone, but this is only occasionally of benefit. The major advantage of this approach is technical; in sparing the superior and inferior gluteal vessels along with the posterior portion of the gluteus maximus muscle, vascularity of the long posterior skin flap improves. The requirement to maintain longer posterior skin flap is a possible disadvantage of the procedure. This flap may have considerable tension exerted on it from the protruding anterior superior iliac spine, resulting in flap necrosis. Also, blood loss from bony

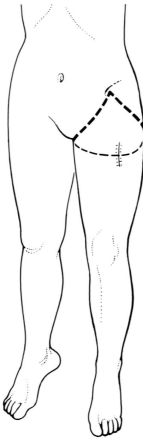

Figure 13–3.   Skin incision. The incision and early dissection of the skin flaps for a modified hemipelvectomy are similar to those described for the standard hemipelvectomy, except that less skin is sacrificed at the level of the anterior superior iliac spine and a longer posterior skin flap is required for closure.

Figure 13–4.   Division of the gluteus muscle, posterior view. During the procedure, when an imaginary line coursing between the anterior superior iliac spine and the tip of the coccyx is reached, cease dissection of the posterior skin flap off of the gluteus maximus muscle. After exposure of the iliac vessels and release of the pubic symphysis, the sciatic notch is identified from within the pelvis. This facilitates location of the sciatic notch posteriorly. It is at the lower edge of the gluteus muscles at their sacral origin. Transect gluteus muscles using electrocautery between the anterior superior iliac spine and the sciatic foramen posteriorly.

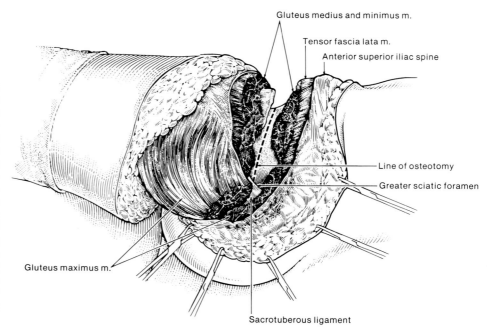

Gluteus medius and minimus m.

Tensor fascia lata m.

Anterior superior iliac spine

Line of osteotomy

Greater sciatic foramen

Gluteus maximus m.

Sacrotuberous ligament

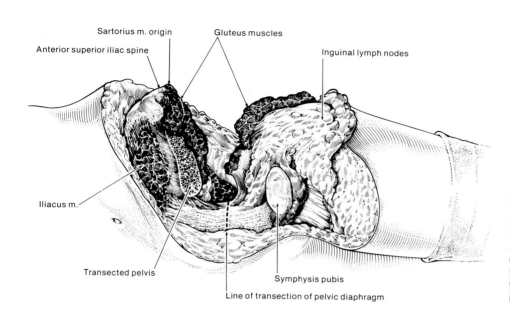

Sartorius m. origin

Gluteus muscles

Anterior superior iliac spine

Inguinal lymph nodes

Iliacus m.

Transected pelvis

Symphysis pubis

Line of transection of pelvic diaphragm

Figure 13–5. Osteotomy of the hemipelvis, anterior view. Move at this point to the anterior aspect of the patient. By blunt dissection expose the common iliac artery and vein. Release the ipsilateral rectus muscle from the superior pubic ramus and divide the pubic symphysis. Locate the greater sciatic foramen from both its anterior and posterior aspects. All the gluteus muscles between the anterior superior iliac spine and the greater sciatic foramen posteriorly should have been divided. Similarly, divide the iliacus muscle and psoas tendon anteriorly to expose the surface of the pelvis. The sartorius muscle is seen arising from the anterior superior iliac spine and is transected through its tendinous portion. Pass a Gigli saw through the greater sciatic foramen and use it to osteotomize the pelvis. The ischium and pubis are released from the ilium by an osteotomy from the sciatic notch to the indentation of bone between anterior superior and anterior inferior iliac spine.

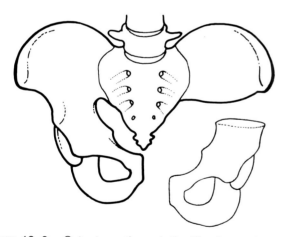

Figure 13–6. Osteotomy through the iliac bone above the acetabulum. Following transection of the pelvis, the extremity can be retracted caudally to widely expose the visceral branches of the internal iliac vessel. The superior vesical, obturator, and inferior vesical branches are severed, but blood supply to the gluteus muscles through the superior and inferior gluteal vessels remains intact. The sciatic nerve is divided at the same level at which muscles were transected. Transection of the urogenital diaphragm and levator ani muscle is accomplished with strong upward traction on the extremity so that a free plane above urethra, bladder, and rectum is clearly delineated. Wound drainage and closure are similar to standard hemipelvectomy. If one is careful to conserve skin overlying the anterior superior iliac spine, delayed wound healing from tension over the bony prominence should not occur.

transection through the ilium may be considerable, and postoperative hematoma may result. The modified hemipelvectomy results in less tissue resection; it should be performed if the adequacy of tissue margins on the tumor are not compromised.

EXTENDED HEMIPELVECTOMY, SACRAL OSTEOTOMY THROUGH THE NEURAL FORAMINA

Indications

Osteosarcoma of the ilium or ischium may extend up to the sacroiliac joint, but seldom invades through the cartilage that constitutes this joint. If a standard hemipelvectomy is performed with division of the sacroiliac joint, tumor spillage and dissemination may occur. More proximal transection of bone through the sacral foramina may prevent this catastrophe. Also, buttock tumors located within the gluteus muscles may expand to but not through the gluteal fascia. If the origins of the gluteus maximus and medius muscles and the gluteal fascia between the posterior superior and the posterior inferior iliac spine are not transected, tumor spillage may be avoided and a more adequate tissue margin obtained. Finally, some soft tissue sarcomas, usually of neural origin, may extend for great distances along

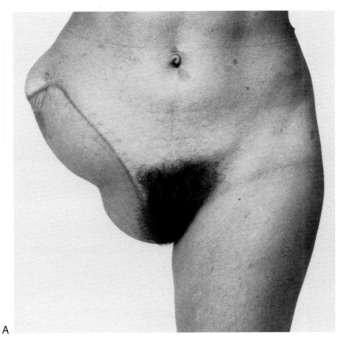

A

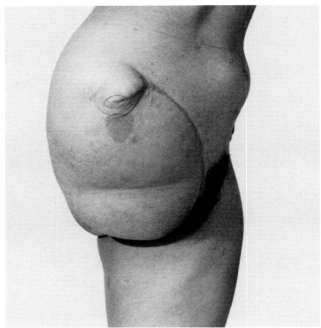

B

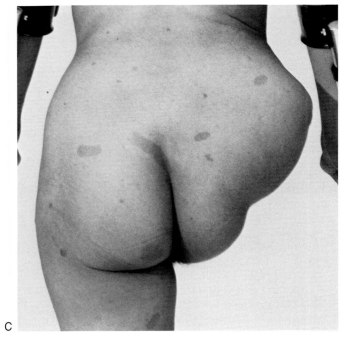

C

Figure 13–7. (**A**) Anterior, (**B**) lateral, and (**C**) posterior views of a patient who underwent modified hemipelvectomy. Note the more normal body contour at the hips. The patient has von Recklinghausen's disease with numerous café au lait spots.

nerve sheaths. A more proximal margin on sacral nerves may be obtained by dividing the nerve roots within the sacrum (Figs. 13–8 and 13–9).

ANTERIOR FLAP HEMIPELVECTOMY

Indications

Small buttock tumors are removed by using wide local excision or the buttockectomy procedure. If

involvement by a buttock tumor of the pelvic bones, upper femur, or sciatic nerve is documented, amputation utilizing the anterior flap hemipelvectomy procedure is indicated. The margin of excision most likely to be compromised is the one on the sacrum. To avoid the disaster of a stump recurrence, the sacral ostomy is usually performed through the neural foramina (Fig. 13–8).

If the anterior flap hemipelvectomy can be utilized without compromise of the margins, then it is the preferred procedure over the posterior flap hemipel-

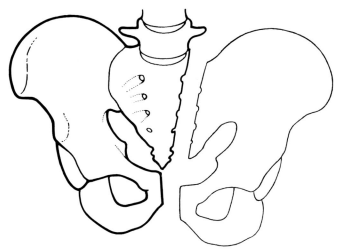

Figure 13–8. Sacral osteotomy for extended hemipelvectomy. Instead of disarticulating the sacroiliac joint as in a standard hemipelvectomy, the line of bone transection extends through the sacral foramina up to the narrow angle between the sacrum and the transverse process of the fifth lumbar vertebra. If performing a hemipelvectomy utilizing a posterior skin flap, this flap must be dissected back to the midsacral spines. This allows for accurate localization of the dorsal foramina. If an anterior flap hemipelvectomy is performed, the medial skin incision should be over the midsacral spines. This will allow the dorsal sacral foramina to be visualized. Anteriorly, a meticulous dissection of all branches of the internal iliac artery overlying the sacral nerve roots is required. If these vessels are not secured, considerable blood will be lost while the nerve roots and sacrum are transected.

vectomy. Filling the operative defect with a large muscle mass fills out the contours of the pelvis (Figs. 13–10 and 13–11). The cushioning effect of the muscle mass over bony prominences allows more comfortable sitting. Also the cosmetic appearance is considerably improved. Most importantly, the bulky anterior flap rarely manifests wound-healing problems. Slow wound healing and flap necrosis are, unfortunately, seen with the long buttock skin flap needed for the posterior flap hemipelvectomy.

INTRAPERITONEAL APPROACH TO HEMIPELVECTOMY

There may be several advantages to an intraperitoneal approach to hemipelvectomy. First, this procedure is usually performed for large tumors that extend into the pelvis and may be of questionable resectability. Opening the peritoneal cavity early in the dissection allows a thorough abdominal exploration to rule out disseminated disease. Second, for tumors in the pelvic fossa, it may be difficult (or impossible) to secure the iliac vessels when working over the top of a large tumor from an extraperitoneal approach. An intraperitoneal approach with ligation of the common iliac vessels at the bifurcation of the

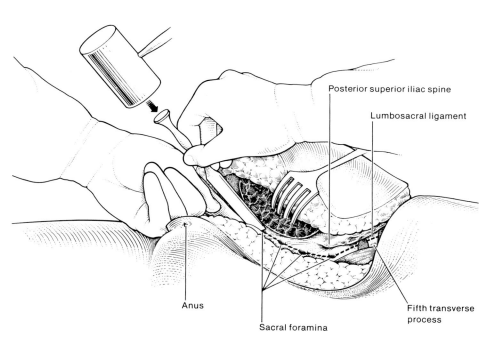

Figure 13–9. Technique for sacral osteotomy. The surgeon should be oriented at the posterior aspect of the patient. Commencing near the tip of the coccyx, use an osteotome to divide the coccyx and sacrum in a plane that bisects the sacral foramina. Initially, the course of the osteotome should parallel the midsacral spines. The surgeon, being posterior to the patient, reaches around the coccyx with the left hand to locate the S-5 neural foramina from within the sacrum. One should use the surgical principle of "going from the known to the unknown" in dividing the sacrum. That is, start at the coccyx below S-5 and work superiorly, progressing from foramina to foramina. Holding the osteotome with the right hand, the direction for bone transection can be guided precisely by the left hand, which has located the next-highest foramina. The assistant drives the osteotome through the bone with the mallet. At the upper portion of the sacrum, care must be taken not to fracture inadvertently through the bone. The lumbosacral ligament is divided to release the specimen.

Labels in figure: Posterior superior iliac spine, Lumbosacral ligament, Anus, Sacral foramina, Fifth transverse process

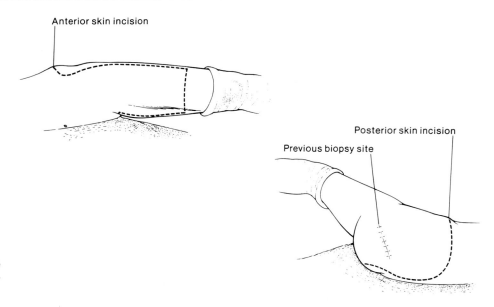

Figure 13–10. Skin incisions for the anterior flap hemipelvectomy procedure.

aorta may prevent much blood loss and lessen the danger of disrupting the tumor capsule and causing tumor contamination of the operative field. Third, with the intraperitoneal approach and a high ligation of common iliac vessels, lymph node dissection is more adequate. The deep iliac nodes need not be separated from the specimen for their complete removal. If needed, a complete para-aortic node dissection may be performed. Fourth, the psoas muscle may be taken many inches higher by opening the peritoneum. Finally, if the ureter is bound down in tumor that is otherwise resectable, division of the ureter well above the tumor and a cross ureter-oureterostomy to the opposite side of the abdomen may be safely accomplished (Fig. 13–12).

COMPOUND HEMIPELVECTOMY

Occasionally, pelvic tumors will involve the bladder, the rectum, female internal genitalia, or other viscera. Excision of these structures along with the hemipelvis may be indicated in carefully selected patients. Patients with locally aggressive tumors that are of low-grade malignancy may be the best candidates for compound procedures.

INTERNAL HEMIPELVECTOMY

Karakousis in this volume and Eilber and colleagues have described an extensive innominate bone resec-

tion. In this procedure the entire hemipelvis and hip are resected, but the neurovascular bundle is preserved (Fig. 13–13).[3] Partial weightbearing by the affected extremity may become possible because of fibrous union across the resection site. In other patients with a partial resection of the innominate bone, a stent may properly space and stabilize the defect between torso and femur (Fig. 13–14).

PARTIAL RESECTIONS OF THE INNOMINATE BONE

In carefully selected patients, major resections of the pelvis can be performed without sacrificing the extremity (Fig. 13–15).[1–9] Enneking and Dunham have described the partial resections of the innominate bone that can be performed and the methods of reconstruction that have been attempted. These partial excisions of the hemipelvis are indicated for small tumors of high histologic grade and occasionally for large tumors of low-grade malignancy.[2] Enneking and Dunham emphasize that spread of tumor along tissue planes by hematoma resulting from the biopsy may exclude a patient from limb salvage by internal hemipelvectomy.

RESECTION OF THE ILIAC BONE

When resection of the iliac bone only is expected, the incision may be carried along the entire length of the

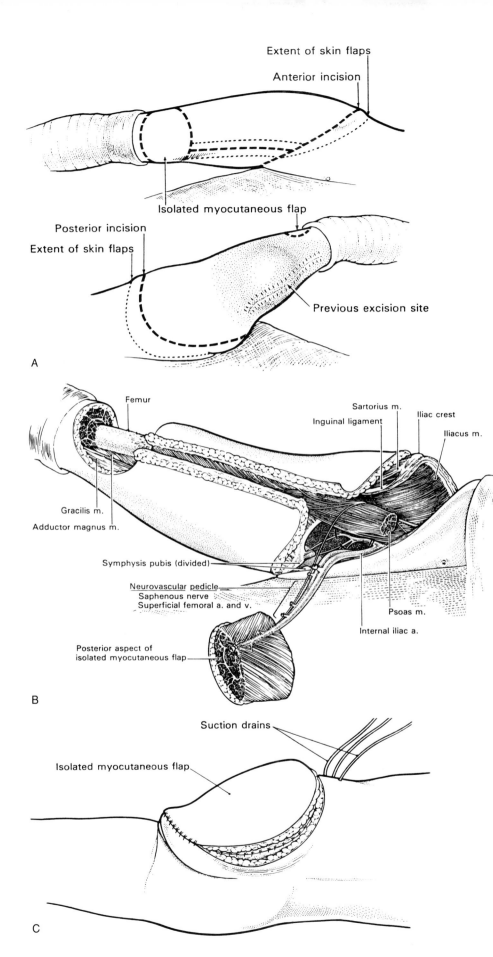

Extent of skin flaps

Anterior incision

Isolated myocutaneous flap

Posterior incision

Extent of skin flaps

Previous excision site

A

Femur

Sartorius m.

Inguinal ligament

Iliac crest

Iliacus m.

Gracilis m.

Adductor magnus m.

Symphysis pubis (divided)

Neurovascular pedicle
Saphenous nerve
Superficial femoral a. and v.

Psoas m.

Internal iliac a.

Posterior aspect of
isolated myocutaneous flap

B

Suction drains

Isolated myocutaneous flap

C

Figure 13–11. Anterior flap hemi-pelvectomy procedure utilizing an island of distal thigh skin and underlying quadriceps muscle to cover the resection site. **(A)** Usually the massive bony and soft tissue defect created by resection of the hemipelvis is covered by a myocutaneous flap of quadriceps femoris muscle.[10] **(B)** The blood supply is through the superficial femoral artery and vein along a skin pedicle at the groin. The skin bridge at the groin may be left intact, or an island pedicle flap of anterior thigh skin and quadriceps muscle may be utilized.[2] **(C)** Closure of the circular defect over suction drains.

191

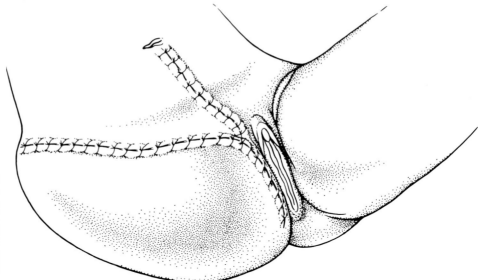

Figure 13–12. Low midline incision used for proximal exposure combined with a posterior flap hemipelvectomy incision. A combination of lower midline abdominal incision and a posterior flap hemipelvectomy incision affords proximal exposure within the abdominal cavity and heals well.[1]

iliac crest and then over the inguinal ligament to the pubic tubercle (Fig. 13–16). It will still be necessary to divide the lateral attachment of inguinal ligament and the inferior epigastric vessels. The iliacus portion of the iliopsoas muscle is divided as it courses behind the inguinal ligament, and with a periosteal elevator the anterior surface of the iliac bone is

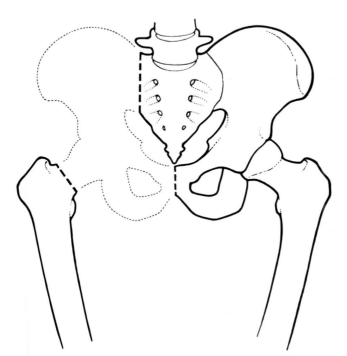

Figure 13–13. Internal hemipelvectomy. Complete resection of the hemipelvis with limb preservation (modified from Eilber et al[1]).

exposed at this level. The origins of the sartorius, tensor fascia lata, and rectus femoris muscles are divided. Then with blunt dissection aiming posteriorly, both on the medial and lateral aspects of the iliac bone immediately above the acetabulum, one reaches the greater sciatic notch. A Gigli saw is passed around, and the bone is divided from the greater sciatic notch toward the anterior inferior iliac spine. With this maneuver one is certain to be just above the acetabulum. This technique, a short-cut to the greater sciatic notch, has been described previously by Ariel and Shah in a modification of conservative hemipelvectomy.[9]

Whether the inferolateral extension of the internal hemipelvectomy incision toward the greater trochanter is required depends on the location and extent of tumor (see chapter 10).

If the tumor is not extending through the lateral surface of the iliac bone or around the greater sciatic notch into the gluteal muscles, it is much easier and preferable to use only the curvilinear portion of the incision along the iliac crest–inguinal ligament–pubic crest. Medial to the iliac crest the anterolateral abdominal wall muscles are divided to enter the retroperitoneal space as described before. Lateral and adjacent to the crest, the fascia and muscles are divided to expose the lateral surface of the iliac bone. With the periosteal elevator the origins of the gluteal muscles are stripped off the iliac bone until the greater sciatic notch in the middle, the sacroiliac joint posteriorly, and the neck of the femur anteriorly are exposed. With this technique the sciatic nerve is not exposed, but there is no risk of injuring it with the use of blunt instruments because it is covered at the

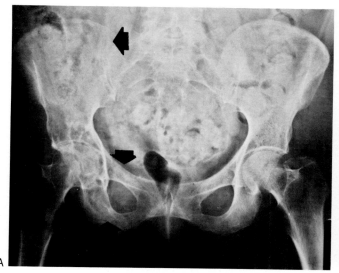
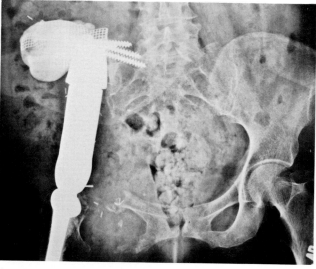

Figure 13–14.   Combined types I, II, III (partial); internal hemipelvectomy. (A) Chondrosarcoma involving the entire ilium and periacetabulum (arrows) treated by an internal hemipelvectomy, resection of the ilium, acetabulum, and most of the pelvic floor. (B) The defect was reconstructed with a custom pelvic, saddle prosthesis (W. Link, Hamburg, Germany). Plain radiograph at 14 months. Note the sacral articulation constructed with polymethylmethracrylate (PMMA), screws, and wire mesh fixed to the remaining sacrum.

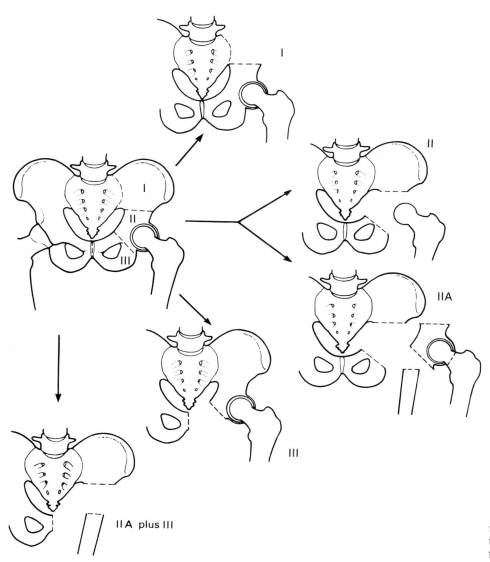

Figure 13–15.   Innominate bone resections. Types I, II, and III resections of the hemipelvis with preservation of the lower extremity (modified from Enneking WF, Dunham WK[2]).

193

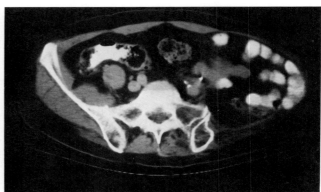

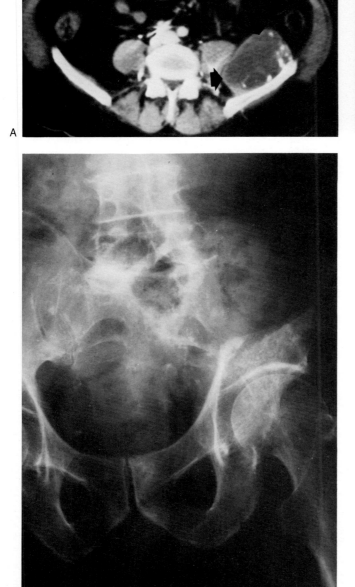

Figure 13–16. Type I pelvic resection. A large chondrosarcoma (arrows) arising from the iliac wing treated by resection of the ilium and adjacent iliacus muscle. (**A**) Preoperative CT showing a large tumor arising from the ilium with displacement of the psoas major. Note the calcification within the lesion, denoting a cartilage tumor. (**B**) Postoperative CT following resection of the ilium (Type I) and (**C**) the corresponding plain radiograph. Note the preservation of the acetabulum. The patient was free of tumor eight years later.

level of the greater sciatic notch by the piriformis muscle. On the medial aspect of the bone, the lumbosacral trunk and sacral roots of the nerve are visualized and protected.

The pubic bone may be removed with the use of the abdominoinguinal incision, described in chapter 11. The ischiac bone requires a posterior incision, although for a large tumor extending into the pelvis a combination of a posterior and an anterior incision may be required (Figs. 13–17 and 13–18).

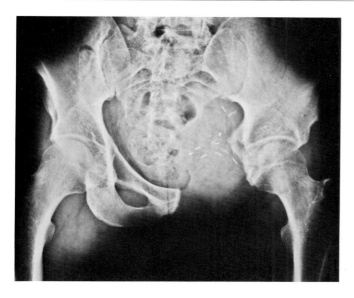

Figure 13–17. Type III resection, pelvic floor resection. Postoperative radiograph following resection of the entire pelvic floor for a large chondrosarcoma arising from the pubic rami. Note a portion of the medial wall of the acetabulum was also removed.

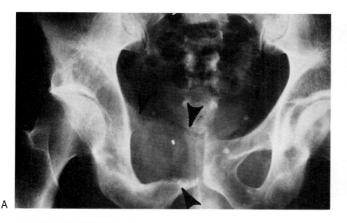

A

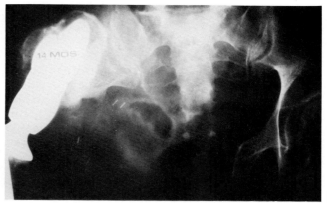

B

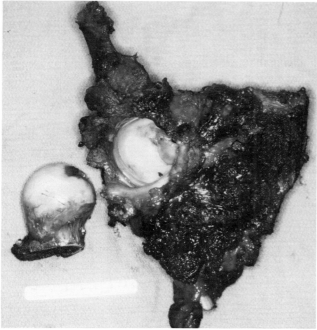

C

Figure 13–18. Types II and III pelvic resection; partial internal hemipelvectomy. (**A**) A high-grade MFH (arrows) arising from the pubic rami and pelvic floor involving the periacetabulum and lower ilium. The patient was treated by a limb-sparing resection following two courses of intra-arterial chemotherapy. (**B**) Gross specimen following resection. Note the pelvic floor, acetabulum, and lower ilium along with the femoral head were resected. (**C**) Plain radiograph demonstrating the reconstruction with a custom pelvic, saddle prosthesis (W. Link, Hamburg, Germany) at 14 months.

POSTOPERATIVE CARE FOR PARTIAL RESECTIONS OF THE INNOMINATE BONE

With partial resections of the innominate bone not involving the acetabulum, no traction is required and the patients are mobilized within two to three days after the operation.

With resections of the iliac bone preserving the acetabulum, partial weightbearing is allowed immediately. The patients use crutches for a variable period of time, depending on age and physical condition, advance to support by cane only, and finally walk, at least the younger ones, without any support. Due to loss of the support to the acetabulum provided by the proximal iliac bone, some cephalad migration of the acetabulum occurs, the latter often coming to impinge upon the sacral ala. The patient requires a modest shoe lift.

With resections of the pubic bone the patient is mobilized immediately and full weightbearing is allowed; ambulation without any support progresses rapidly within one to four weeks with no apparent residual disability.

If the acetabulum has been removed with or without the head of the femur, the hip joint is destabilized. The proximal portion of the femur may be fixed to the ischial tuberosity if it is intact. Alternatively, an internal prosthesis may give static support to the lower extremity and allow limited motion at the hip.

REFERENCES

1. Eilber FR, Grant TT, Sakai D, et al: Internal hemipelvectomy—excision of the hemipelvis with limb preservation. *Cancer* 1979;43:806–809.
2. Enneking WF, Dunham WK: Resection and reconstruction for primary neoplasms involving the innominate bone. *J Bone Joint Surg* 1978;60A:731–746.
3. Johnson JTH: Reconstruction of the pelvic ring following tumor resection. *J Bone Joint Surg* 1978;60A:747–751.
4. Papaioannou AN, Critselis AN, Volk H: Long-term survival after compound hemipelvectomy. *Surg Gynecol Obstet* 1977;144:175–178.
5. Sim FH, Chao EY, Peterson LFA: Reconstruction following segmental resection of primary bone tumors of the hip, in *Proceedings of the Third Open Scientific Meeting of the Hip Society.* St Louis, CV Mosby, 1975.
6. Sim FH, Chao EYS: Segmental prosthetic replacement of the hip and knee, in Chao EYS, Ivins JC (eds): *Tumor Prosthesis for Bone and Joint Reconstruction: The Design and Applications.* Stuttgart, Georg Thieme Verlag, 1983.
7. Steel HH: Partial or complete resection of the hemipelvis. *J Bone Joint Surg* 1978;60A:719–730.
8. Karakousis C, Emrich L, Driscoll DL: Variants of hemipelvectomy and their complications. *Am J Surg* 1989;158:404–408.
9. Ariel IM, Shah GP: The conservative hemipelvectomy. *Surg Gynecol Obst* 1977;144:406–413.
10. Lotze MT, Sugarbaker PH: Femoral artery based myocutaneous flap for hemipelvectomy closure: Amputation after failed limb sparing surgery and radiotherapy. *Am J Surg* 1985;150:625–630.

14

Hip Disarticulation

PAUL H. SUGARBAKER, M.D.
PAUL B. CHRETIEN, M.D.

OVERVIEW

Hip disarticulation is usually elected for malignant bony and soft tissue tumors below the lesser trochanter of the femur. The operation is performed with the patient in a posterolateral position; in the first phase of the procedure the surgeon stands anterior to the patient. After incision of the skin and division of the femoral vessels and nerve, muscles of the anterior thigh are transected off the pelvic bone from lateral to medial, starting with the sartorius and finishing with the adductor magnus. Muscles are divided at their origin except for the iliopsoas and obturator externus, which are divided at their insertion on the lesser trochanter of the femur. The quadratus femoris muscle is identified and preserved; then the flexor muscles are transected at their site of origin from the ischial tuberosity. During the next phase the surgeon is posterior to the patient, and the pelvis is rotated from the posterolateral position to the anterolateral position. After completion of the skin incision, the gluteal fascia, tensor fascia lata, and the gluteus maximus muscles are divided and dissected free of their posterior attachments to expose the muscles inserting by way of a common tendon onto the greater trochanter. These muscles are then transected at their insertion on the bone. The posterior aspect of the joint capsule is then exposed and transected. Finally, the sciatic nerve is divided and allowed to retract beneath the piriformis muscle. To close the wound, the preserved muscles are approximated over the joint capsule and the gluteal fascia is secured to the inguinal ligament over suction drains. The skin is closed with interrupted sutures.

INTRODUCTION

Evolution of the technique of hip joint disarticulation commonly used can be traced to the report of Kirk,[1] who, in 1943 described his experience with amputations through the hip joint. All muscles except those normally belonging in the buttock were removed from the stump, except one muscle flap that was conserved to fill up the acetabulum. In general, nearly all of the muscles were transected at their origins. Improvements in the technique were presented by Boyd,[2] who, in 1947 described an "anatomic disarticulation of the hip" designed to reduce blood loss by dividing all muscles at either their origin on the pelvis or at their insertion on the femur. Muscles (other than those of the buttock) that remained attached to the pelvis were the iliopsoas and the obturator externus. Slocum,[3] in his *Atlas of Amputations*, published in 1949, described a technique in which a long posterior skin flap was used to resurface the operative site. If a prosthesis were to be used, weightbearing was on the posterior myocutaneous flap rather than on a suture line. Slocum also emphasized high ligation of the femoral, obturator, and sciatic nerves so that they would retract out of the weight-bearing areas. An elastic bandage was used to provide compression and thereby minimize postoperative hematoma. Bickel and Koch[4] described a technique for hip disarticulation but did not amplify previously described techniques.

This description of hip disarticulation incorporates the concepts that have developed over the last four decades. A surgical plan is presented whereby

1. The sequence of steps allows for systematic completion of the dissection.
2. The incision does not lie over bony prominences or weight-bearing areas so that local pain with use of a prosthesis should be minimized.
3. All muscles are transected at either their origin or insertion to minimize blood loss and postoperative wound complications.
4. Viable musculature is preserved for use as a myodesis to cover the protruding acetabulum.

GENERAL INDICATIONS FOR HIP DISARTICULATION

This procedure is indicated for malignant, bony tumors, usually osteosarcoma of the femur below the lesser trochanter (Fig. 14-1). It is the procedure of choice in osteosarcoma of the distal femur with "skip metastases" within the marrow of the femur. Also malignant soft tissue tumors of the middle and lower

thigh may be appropriately treated with hip disarticulation. Similar to shoulder disarticulation, it is not performed as frequently as other thigh or hip amputations. Sarcomas of the medial aspect of the thigh more frequently require amputation because of *encasement of the superficial femoral artery.* Posterior tumors may intimately involve the *sciatic nerve;* not infrequently the nerve can be delicately dissected free of a tumor mass in the posterior compartment, and a limb-sparing approach can become a success (chapter 22).

If the sciatic nerve is encased or is the origin of the malignancy (neurosarcoma), the posterior compartment and sciatic nerve may be removed en bloc as a muscle group excision and the extremity spared. More frequently, questionable or positive margins make hip disarticulation the preferred operation.

Extensive soft tissue contamination by tumor can make a negative margin of resection impossible to achieve. This can result from extensive bleeding from a biopsy site, from spontaneous rupture of a tumor mass, or from a pathologic fracture. Infection may make local resection impossible.

Skeletal immaturity may result in marked leg-length discrepancy if wide excision plus radiation therapy is used to treat cancers adjacent to the proximal femoral epiphysis. Approximately 70% of the growth of the femur is from the proximal epiphysis. If marked leg-length discrepancy is predictable, then hip disarticulation should be recommended. Small osteosarcomas of the distal femoral epiphysis without skip osseous metastases can be managed by high above-knee amputation. Osteosarcomas at or above the lesser trochanter that are well developed in either bone or soft tissue must be treated by hemipelvectomy in order to eliminate the risk of local recurrence.

CLINICAL CONSIDERATIONS FOR HIP JOINT DISARTICULATION

The timing for this major surgical procedure is important. Physiological factors must be optimized. If the patient has received preoperative chemotherapy, it is essential that both leukocytes and platelets be permitted to return to normal. Significant deficits in red blood cell mass should be corrected by preoperative transfusion. Although vascular insufficiency is rarely a complicating factor of hip disarticulation, suboptimal wound healing may be a problem in patients who have received high-dose regional or systemic chemotherapy. Also, associated poor nutrition from nausea and vomiting induced by preoperative chemotherapy may further compound the

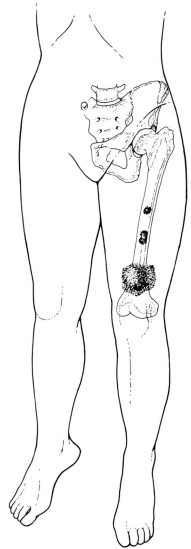

Figure 14–1. Hip disarticulation is indicated for malignant bony and soft tissue tumors below the lesser trochanter of the femur.

wound-healing problem. Because of potential wound-healing difficulties, flap closure must be secure and meticulous. Hematoma and seroma must be avoided by the use of adequate closed-suction drainage. One should defer removal of skin sutures for at least three weeks.

REHABILITATION AND EMOTIONAL SUPPORT

The cancer patient faces unique psychological problems. Not only is there a loss of the lower extremity but also a threat to life itself. Rehabilitation of a patient undergoing a hip disarticulation begins at the time of the staging studies. The entire health care team must develop an honest and caring relationship with the patient and include him or her in the early stages of all decision making. Based on this trust, the patient will be better able to accept the amputation and set realistic goals.

All patients undergoing an amputation will experience some phantom sensation. This may be severe in patients with hip disarticulation. It should be discussed with the patient prior to surgery. The patient needs to understand that this is to be expected, that it can be treated with analgesics, and that it will subside in its severity over time.

Although successful rehabilitation depends to a great extent on the patient's attitude, the surgical team can help tremendously in these efforts. A *positive attitude* toward functional recovery augmented by early or immediate postoperative ambulation will help the patient move rapidly toward rehabilitation goals. A positive attitude is amplified by contacts with other patients who have successfully met some of the rehabilitative challenges. This can provide an immeasurable psychological boost to the patient. The oncologist, rehabilitation therapist, and others involved in the postoperative care must coordinate their efforts carefully, yet realizing the possibility of conflicting demands on the patient's time. Also a different interpretation of the same clinical information may be perceived by the patient and family in talking with different caregivers.

RADIOLOGIC STUDIES

Preoperative chest computerized tomography and abdominal and pelvic CT are performed. The CT of the chest is to rule out metastases to the lungs. Retroperitoneal and deep iliac lymph node involvement can be ruled out by the abdominal and pelvic CT scan. CT scan, MRI, and bone scans should be used to determine that there will be a clean margin of excision. Tumors that encroach upon the hip joint itself should be treated wth hemipelvectomy rather than a hip disarticulation procedure.

PROCEDURE

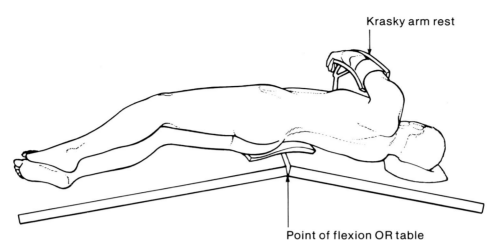

Krasky arm rest

Point of flexion OR table

Figure 14–2. PATIENT POSITION. Before preparation of the operative site a Foley catheter is placed in the bladder, and the opposite lower extremity is covered by an elastic wrap to prevent venous pooling. The patient is placed in a lateral position, and the position secured with pads anterior and posterior to the torso; there should be a slight posterior tilt. The skin is prepared from midchest to midcalf and the leg draped free.

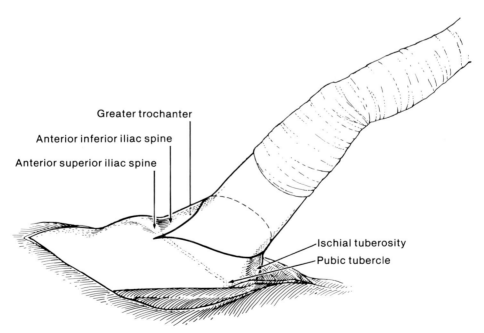

Greater trochanter

Anterior inferior iliac spine

Anterior superior iliac spine

Ischial tuberosity

Pubic tubercle

Figure 14–3. INCISION. Bony landmarks to be identified include the pubic tubercle, anterior superior iliac spine, anterior inferior iliac spine, ischial tuberosity, and greater trochanter. The anterior portion of the incision commences one fingerbreadth medial to the anterior superior iliac spine. It descends to the pubic tubercle and then over the pubic bone to two fingerbreadths distal to the ischial tuberosity and gluteal crease. If the buttock flap is extremely thick, the anterior portion of the incision should be moved laterally. The posterior portion of the incision extends two fingerbreadths anterior to the greater trochanter and then around the back of the leg distal to the gluteal crease. The distance the incision is beyond the gluteal crease is directly proportional to the anterior-posterior diameter of the patient's pelvis.

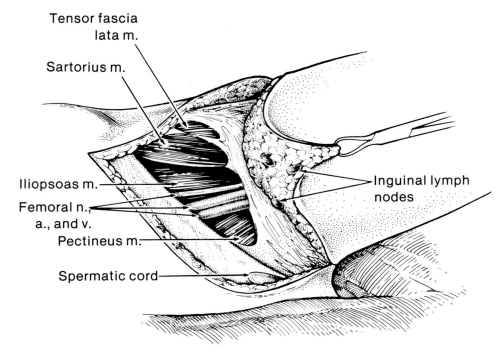

Tensor fascia lata m.

Sartorius m.

Iliopsoas m.

Femoral n., a., and v.

Pectineus m.

Spermatic cord

Inguinal lymph nodes

Figure 14–4. **EXPOSURE OF FEMORAL TRIANGLE.** The skin is incised, and the dissection is extended through subcutaneous fat and Scarpa's fascia until the external oblique aponeurosis is seen. Multiple venous bleeding points from branches of the saphenous vein are clamped, divided, and ligated. A moderate-sized artery, the superficial epigastric, and multiple branches of the external pudendal vessels must be secured. The superficial inguinal lymph nodes should be moved laterally with the specimen, and the round ligament in the woman or the spermatic cord in the man is exposed but not included in the specimen.

An Adair clamp is placed securely on the apex of the skin specimen for traction. By making an incision just below the inguinal ligament into the fossa ovalis, the femoral vein, artery, and nerve are widely exposed below the inguinal ligament.

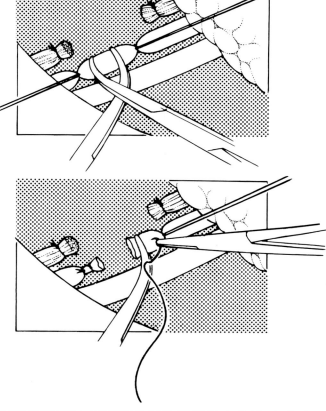

Figure 14–5. DIVISION OF FEMORAL VESSELS AND NERVE. Individual silk ties are placed around the femoral vessels; first the artery and then the vein are tied in continuity. Right-angle clamps are placed between the ties, and the vessels are severed. The proximal ends of the vessels are further secured by a silk suture ligature placed proximal to the right-angle clamps. The femoral nerve is placed on gentle traction and ligated at its point of exit from beneath the inguinal ligament. When the femoral nerve is severed, it retracts beneath the external oblique aponeurosis, so that if a neuroma forms it will not be in a weight-bearing portion of the stump.

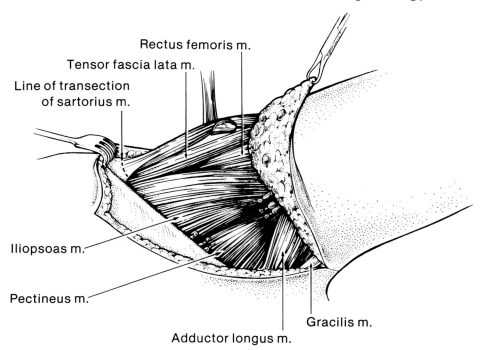

Rectus femoris m.

Tensor fascia lata m.

Line of transection
of sartorius m.

Iliopsoas m.

Pectineus m.

Adductor longus m.

Gracilis m.

Figure 14–6. DIVISION OF SARTORIUS MUSCLE AND FEMORAL SHEATH. The sartorius muscle is located as it arises from the anterior superior iliac spine. It is dissected free from the surrounding fascia and then transected from its origin on the spine by electrocautery. The femoral sheath and fibroareolar tissue posterior to the femoral vessels are also incised by electrocautery. This dissection exposes the hip joint capsule.

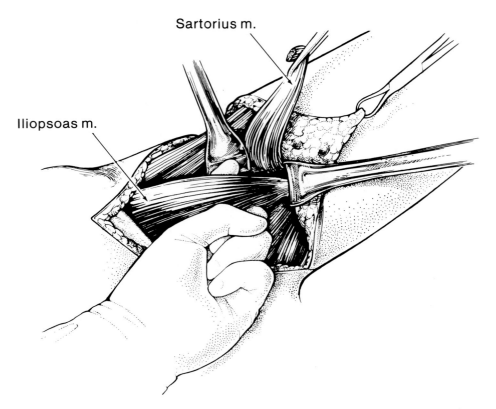

Sartorius m.

Iliopsoas m.

Figure 14–7.   DIVISION OF ILIOPSOAS MUSCLE AT ITS INSERTION. The hip is flexed slightly to relax the iliopsoas muscle. It is then possible to pass a finger around the iliopsoas muscle in a medial-to-lateral blunt dissection. If an attempt is made to pass the finger beneath the muscle from lateral to medial, the very intimate attachments between the iliopsoas muscle and the rectus femoris muscle prevent this from being easily done. By sharp and blunt dissection, the entire iliopsoas muscle is dissected until its insertion on the lesser trochanter is clearly defined. Several vessels of prominent size pass from the anterior surface of this muscle, and care should be taken to secure these vessels prior to their division. The iliopsoas muscle is severed at the level of its insertion onto the lesser trochanter.

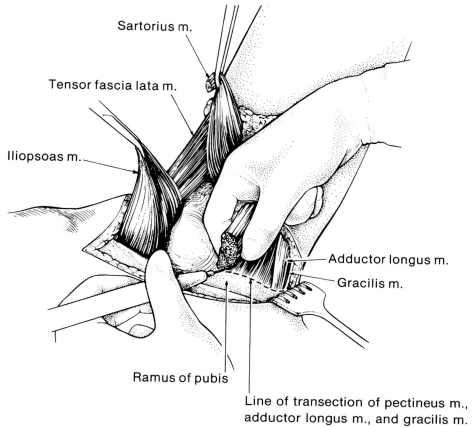

Sartorius m.

Tensor fascia lata m.

Iliopsoas m.

Adductor longus m.

Gracilis m.

Ramus of pubis

Line of transection of pectineus m.,
adductor longus m., and gracilis m.

Figure 14–8. **TRANSECTION OF PECTINEUS MUSCLE AT ITS ORIGIN.** Now attention is turned to the adductor muscles and their release from the pelvis. It is important to note that this dissection proceeds from lateral to medial around the extremity. To preserve the obturator externus muscle on the pelvis, locate its prominent tendon arising from the lesser trochanter. Locating this tendon identifies the plane between pectineus muscle and obturator externus; a difference in the direction of the muscle fibers of these two muscles is also apparent. A finger is passed beneath the pectineus muscle, and it is released at the level of its origin from the pubis by electrocautery. Beneath the pectineus muscle numerous branches of the obturator artery, vein, and nerve can now be visualized.

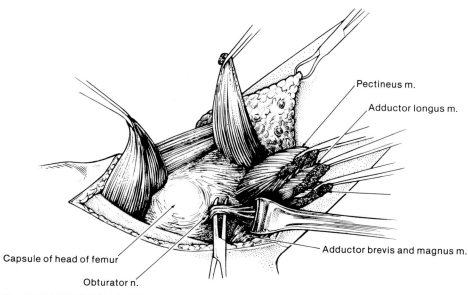

Pectineus m.

Adductor longus m.

Adductor brevis and magnus m.

Capsule of head of femur

Obturator n.

Figure 14–9. **TRANSECTION OF GRACILIS, ADDUCTOR LONGUS, BREVIS, AND MAGNUS MUSCLES FROM THEIR ORIGIN; DIVISION OF OBTURATOR VESSELS AND NERVE.** The remainder of the adductor muscles are transected at their origin on the symphysis pubis. These include the gracilis, adductor longus, adductor brevis, and adductor magnus muscles. Note that the obturator vessels and nerves usually bifurcate around the adductor brevis muscle. It is important that branches of the obturator artery be identified and secured during the dissection to prevent accidental rupture and retraction of the proximal ends up into the pelvis.

205

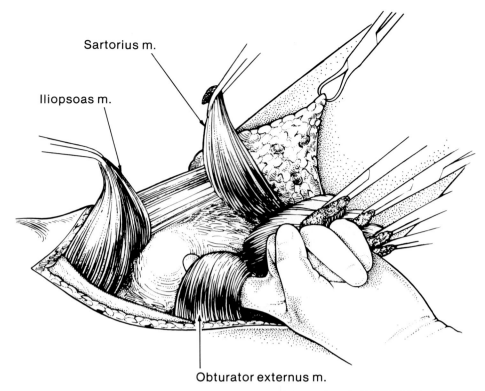

Figure 14–10. DIVISION OF OBTURATOR EXTERNUS MUSCLE AT ITS INSERTION. A finger is passed around the obturator externus muscle, and the muscle is isolated where it arises from the obturator foramen. Its tendon is severed at its insertion into the lesser trochanter with electrocautery.

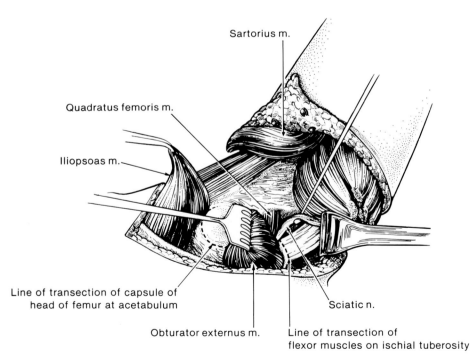

Figure 14–11. RELEASE OF THE FLEXOR MUSCLES FROM THE ISCHIAL TUBEROSITY. The extremity is hyperabducted to help localize the ischial tuberosity and to retract the cut ends of the adductor muscles. The flexor muscles, sciatic nerve, and quadratus femoris muscle are now identified. The large circumflex femoral vessels are nearby and should be avoided. The semimembranosus, semitendinosus, and long head of the biceps muscle are transected from their origin on the ischial tuberosity while preserving the quadratus femoris muscle and sciatic nerve.

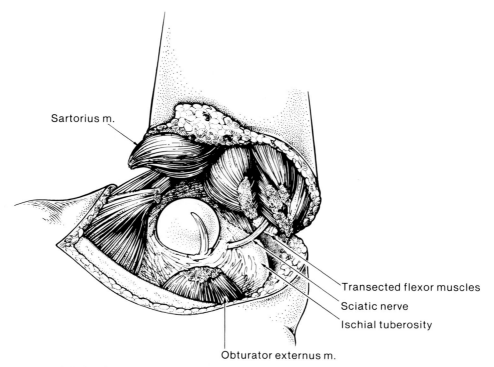

Sartorius m.

Transected flexor muscles

Sciatic nerve

Ischial tuberosity

Obturator externus m.

Figure 14–12. INCISION OF THE ANTERIOR PORTION OF THE HIP JOINT CAPSULE. At this point all the anterior and posterior muscle groups have been divided. The joint capsule overlying the head of the femur is incised, and the ligamentum teres is transected by electrocautery.

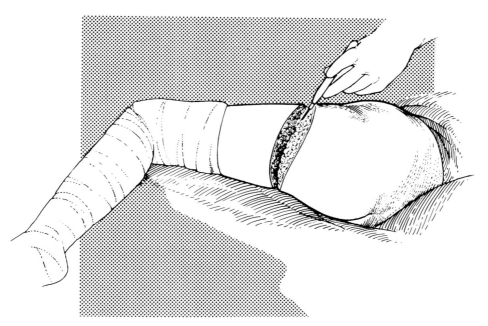

Figure 14–13. COMPLETION OF THE SKIN INCISION. The surgeon now moves from a position anterior to the patient to a posterior position. The patient's torso is tilted from posterolateral to anterolateral, and the skin incision is completed down through gluteal fascia.

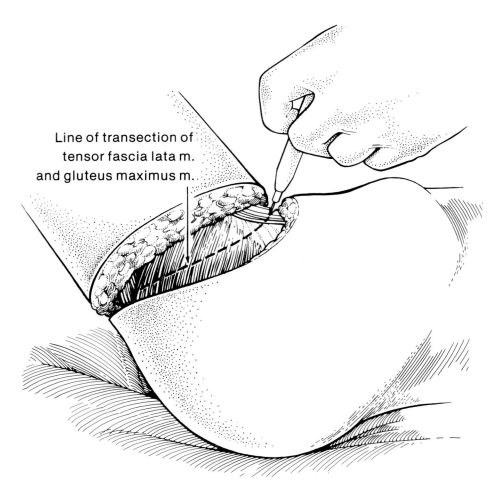

Line of transection of
tensor fascia lata m.
and gluteus maximus m.

Figure 14–14.   DIVISION OF TENSOR FASCIA LATA, GLUTEUS MAXIMUS, AND RECTUS FEMORIS
MUSCLES. The tensor fascia lata and gluteus maximus muscles are divided in the depths of the skin incision.
These are the only muscles not divided at either their origin or insertion in the procedure. Directly beneath these
muscles is the rectus femoris muscle, which is transected at its origin on the anterior inferior iliac spine by
electrocautery.

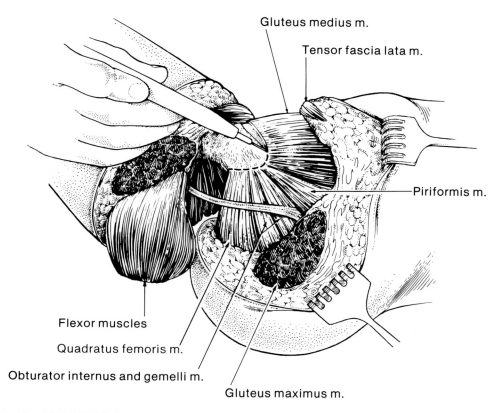

Gluteus medius m.

Tensor fascia lata m.

Piriformis m.

Flexor muscles

Quadratus femoris m.

Obturator internus and gemelli m.

Gluteus maximus m.

Figure 14–15. TRANSECTION OF THE MUSCLES INSERTING INTO GREATER TROCHANTER. After division of the gluteus maximus muscle the common tendon containing the multiple muscles inserting into the greater trochanter is exposed. This tendon receives contributions from the gluteus medius, gluteus minimus, piriformis, superior gemellus, obturator internus, inferior gemellus, and quadratus femoris muscles. These muscles are divided close to their insertions on the greater trochanter by electrocautery.

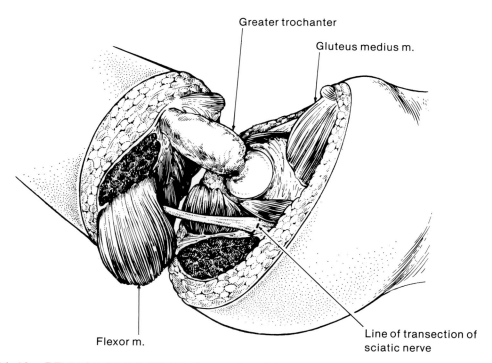

Greater trochanter

Gluteus medius m.

Flexor m.

Line of transection of sciatic nerve

Figure 14–16. RELEASE OF SPECIMEN. Transection of the hip joint capsule is completed by incising the posterior portion of the capsule. The sciatic nerve is dissected free of surrounding muscle, transected, and allowed to retract beneath the piriformis muscle.

209

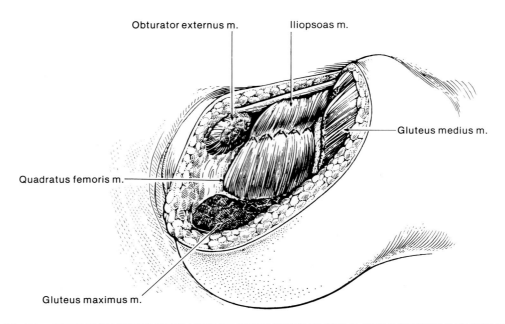

Figure 14–17. APPROXIMATION OF QUADRATUS FEMORIS MUSCLE AND ILIOPSOAS MUSCLE OVER THE JOINT CAPSULE. After the specimen is removed from the operative field, the area is copiously irrigated with saline solution, and all bleeding points are secured. The basic principle in closure is coverage of the protruding acetabulum with the muscles that have been preserved. The quadratus femoris muscle is secured to the iliopsoas muscle over the joint capsule with interrupted sutures. Often the lower portion of the iliopsoas can be used to fill the empty joint capsule.

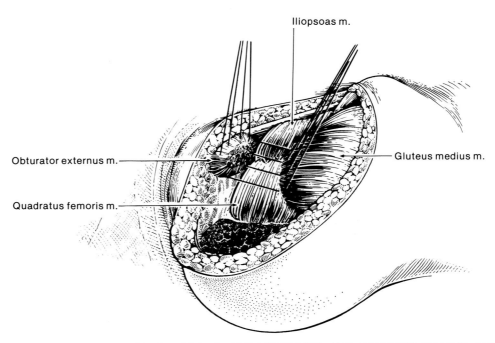

Figure 14–18. APPROXIMATION OF OBTURATOR EXTERNUS AND GLUTEUS MEDIUS OVER THE JOINT CAPSULE. To help provide soft tissue coverage of bony prominences, the obturator externus and gluteus medius muscles are sutured together over the acetabulum.

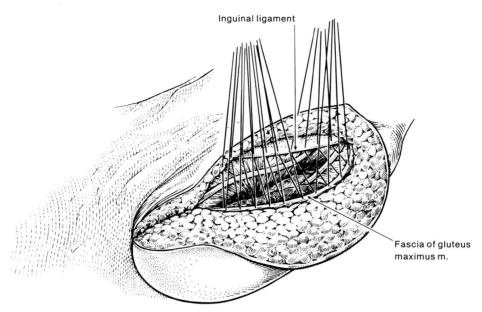

Figure 14–19.   APPROXIMATION OF GLUTEAL FASCIA TO THE INGUINAL LIGAMENT AND PUBIC RAMUS. The gluteal fascia is elevated and secured to the inguinal ligament and pubic ramus. In doing this, it becomes apparent that the posterior myocutaneous flap is much longer than the anterior fascia; therefore, multiple stitches are placed that bisect the fascial edge and uniformly gather the gluteal fascia as it is secured to the inguinal ligament. Sutures are individually placed and then tied. Prior to closure suction catheters are placed beneath the gluteal fascia.

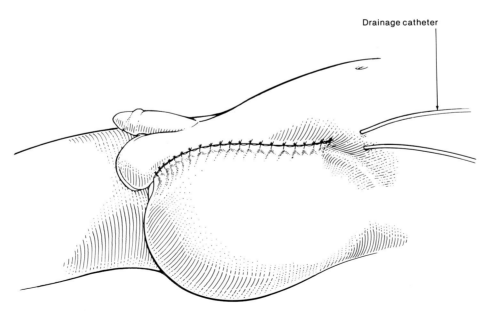

Figure 14–20.   SKIN CLOSURE. The skin is closed with interrupted sutures, Again care is taken to make sure that there is equal distribution of the excess tissue of the posterior flap. Not infrequently, additional suction catheters must be used to obliterate space within the subcutaneous tissue when the buttock flap is thick. Patency of the suction catheters must be maintained until drainage is diminished. Ambulation may proceed if the patient's hemodynamic status permits on the first postoperative day.

211

DISCUSSION

The hip disarticulation procedure as performed here is technically demanding. Considerable knowledge of the musculature around the hip and accurate dissection are required to preserve the iliopsoas, obturator externus, and quadratus femoris muscles. These muscles, used to cover the protruding acetabulum, provide a generous stump capable of bearing weight over extended time periods (Fig. 14–21).

Hip disarticulation is a well-tolerated procedure. Virtually none of the many problems seen after hemipelvectomy occur following this procedure. Wound infection may occur, but is much less frequent. Phantom limb pain is often noted, but is less severe than after hemipelvectomy.

One problem more frequently encountered in female patients concerns the discrepancy of the thick buttock subcutaneous tissue compared with that of the abdominal wall. When the incision is closed, considerable tension on the abdominal wall skin may result. Preservation of a small flap of skin extending

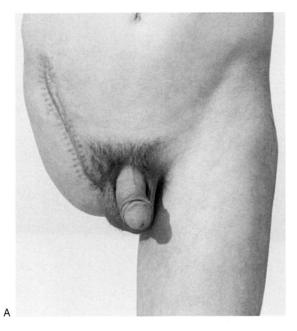

A

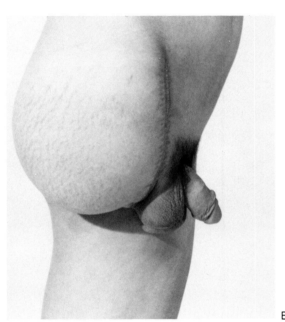

B

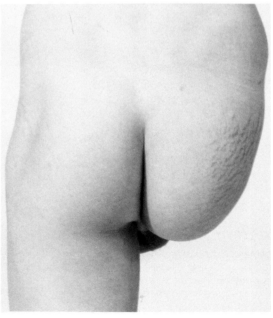

C

Figure 14–21. (A) Anterior, (B) lateral, and (C) posterior views of the stump constructed in a hip disarticulation procedure. Note the prominent stump; bone protuberances are covered with muscle so that prolonged weightbearing is well tolerated.

over the inguinal ligament provides a simple solution to this problem.

REFERENCES

1. Kirk NT: *Amputations.* Hagerstown, WF Pryor, 1943.

2. Boyd HB: Anatomic disarticulation of the hip. *Surg Gynecol Obstet* 1947;84:346.

3. Slocum DB: *An Atlas of Amputation.* St Louis, CV Mosby, 1949.

4. Bickel WH, Koch M: Amputations about the shoulder and about the hips, in Cooper P (ed): *The Craft of Surgery.* Boston, Little, Brown & Co, 1971.

15

Sacrectomy

CONSTANTINE P. KARAKOUSIS,
M.D., Ph.D.

OVERVIEW

Sacrectomy is used for the removal of pelvic tumors with sacral attachments or chordoma. It may be a satisfying dissection with clear margins or a difficult procedure with positive margins on nerve roots and considerable residual disability because of loss of nerve supply to anal and urethral sphincters. The tumors that involve the sacrum above the inferior border of the sacroiliac joints may require dissection or sacrifice of the S-3, S-2, or even S-1 nerve roots. Tumors with an anterior component are approached through a combined abdominolateral approach in a lateral position or sequential abdominosacral positions. Tumors with a large posterior component are approached with the patient prone. Tumors may require en bloc resection of the rectum or anal canal plus rectum. Following division of the origin of the gluteus maximus muscle from the sacral edge, the pudendal nerve must be spared, because it courses posterior to the ischial spine and then on the surface of obturator internus in the ischiorectal fossa. The dural sac ends at the S2-3 junction. If the dura is entered, it must be meticulously repaired to prevent a CSF leak. The fused sacral laminae are transected proximally with fine rongeurs. Sacral nerve roots are displaced laterally and the dura superiorly. The fused sacral bodies anteriorly may be divided with an osteotome. Closure is over generous closed suction drainage.

INTRODUCTION

Sacral tumors may present a difficult problem to the surgeon who desires to obtain a clear margin of excision. Frequently, tumors in this anatomic location are of low grade biologically and therefore unlikely to result in metastatic disease. Yet they may be locally persistent. The problem of local control may be made worse by tumor spill resulting from biopsy or incomplete excision by an inexperienced surgeon. Often it may be wise to remove a sacral tumor mass intact without previous biopsy in order to prevent tumor spillage into the resection site, particularly if the resection is not considered likely to result in denervation of the sphincters (Fig. 15–1).

INDICATIONS

Resections of the sacrum have been performed for several medical conditions. A limited resection of the distal sacrum (S-4 and S-5 vertebrae) along with the coccyx has been used in providing exposure, through a posterior approach, of the distal rectum for a resection of a villous adenoma or a low anastomosis above the dentate line following a low anterior resection. In the latter situation a combined abdominosacral approach may be used. With the patient in a right lateral position, the abdomen is opened and the resection of the appropriate portion of sigmoid and rectum performed. Simultaneously, through a transverse incision over the lower sacrum, the distal por-

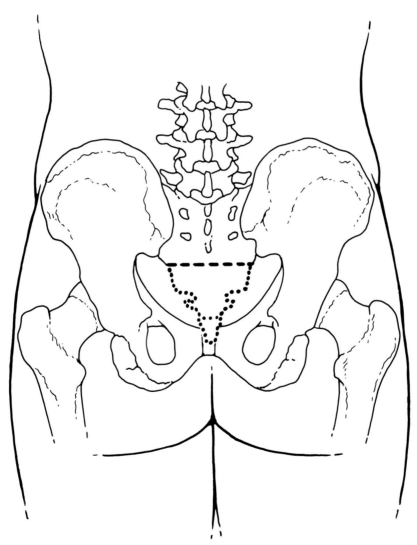

Figure 15–1. The sacrum and the attached tumor mass are removed at the level of the S2-S3 nerve root. The osteotomy is usually just below the sacroiliac joints.

tion of this bone and coccyx are removed, providing the necessary exposure for a very low anastomosis.[1] For extensive local recurrence involving the sacrum for colorectal carcinoma, a supine position has been advocated for an anterior transabdominal dissection initially, followed by the placement of the patient in a prone position[2] or a lateral position with the left side down[3] for completion of dissection and removal of the sacrum. This plan, although it requires repositioning of the patient and does not permit the guidance in posterior dissection afforded by a simul-taneously open abdominal incision, may be the preferable one if extensive, difficult dissection is anticipated anteriorly.

A primary tumor often involving the sacrum is chordoma.[4,5] Secondary involvement of the sacrum by direct spread is often due to a locally recurrent carcinoma of the rectum.[6,7]

Meticulous bowel preparation is advisable preoperatively along with perioperative antibiotics. The technique of resection is outlined below.

PROCEDURE

Position and Incision

Resection of the sacrum may be performed in three different positions depending on the clinical situation. These are a partial lateral position, true lateral position, or prone position. After the indications for the use of the first two positions are presented, the sacrectomy procedure will be demonstrated in the prone position.

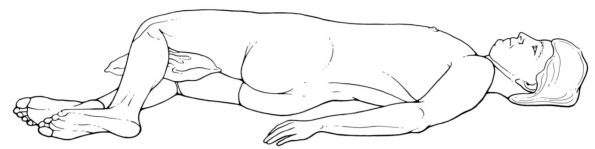

Figure 15–2. COMBINED ABDOMINOLATERAL SACRAL POSITION. A combined abdominolateral sacral position is preferred when it is known or highly suspected that the rectum is involved or when previous surgery in this area is expected to have caused dense adhesions between the rectum and the anterior surface of the sacrum. In most of these cases, the patient is placed in a lateral position with the left side up, because this makes the mobilization of the rectosigmoid easier. The anterior wall of the abdomen, the left flank, and the sacral area are prepped and draped as one continuous field, leaving exposed the iliac crest. The drapes are fixed to the desired position after their placement with skin clips. Posteriorly the entire sacrum is exposed, including the tip of the coccyx while anteriorly the midline is exposed from above the umbilicus to the pubic symphysis.

If, on the bases of the rectal and/or endoscopic examination, it is known that the rectum is involved, it is usually wise to start with the abdominal portion of the operation. As an abdominal incision, one may use an oblique incision extending from the left costal margin to the pubic symphysis, a left paramedian, or a midline incision extending from just above the umbilicus to the symphysis pubis. The midline incision is preferable and can easily be done with some rotation of the table. Not only is the opening and closure more rapid, but also it does not interfere with the construction of the end sigmoid colostomy, which is often needed.

Following entry into the peritoneal cavity, abdominal exploration is carried out to rule out the presence of metastatic disease.

The "white" lines are then incised along the descending and sigmoid colon in order to allow their mobilization. The left ureter is identified and traced down to its insertion to the bladder. The incision in the peritoneum is continued in the rectovesical or rectouterine area and then to the right of the rectosigmoid. Careful blunt and sharp dissection is now carried out in the presacral space, separating only that portion of rectosigmoid from the upper sacrum that can be dissected off with minimal effort. Obviously, one should be careful to avoid entering into tumor as the bowel is separated off the anterior sacral surface. On the other hand, it is important, when possible, to free the anterior surface of the first two sacral vertebrae, since their complete resection involves considerable difficulty. The lateral aspects of the rectum are dissected free further down, and the anterior surface is exposed by separating it from the bladder or uterus and upper vagina, to the extent possible through the abdominal approach.

As soon as the decision is made that the rectosigmoid should be resected en bloc with the sacrum, the bowel mesentery may be divided at the appropriate level. As is true generally of any bowel resection, the peritoneum should be incised first in a radial fashion on either side of the mesentery at the desired level. The adipose tissue is also incised, and the mesenteric arterial and venous branches are exposed. It then becomes obvious how these branches should be divided so that pulsatile blood flow will be present at the end colostomy. The bowel itself is then divided at the midsigmoid portion or distal descending colon as indicated. The distal end is dropped into the pelvis while the proximal end is brought out as an end colostomy.

It is best not to close the abdominal incision at this point lest further dissection be required transabdominally as the sacral resection proceeds. Careful technique should be used to avoid contamination of the incision. The incision over the sacrum is now performed. Flaps, consisting of skin and subcutaneous fat, are developed to the sacral margin, the fibers of gluteus maximus are divided along the sacral edge, and then the sacrotuberous and sacrospinous ligaments are divided. Following division of the anococcygeal raphe, gentle, blunt finger dissection is performed for a short distance on the anterior surface of the sacrum. If *preservation of the anal canal* is to be attempted, the rectum is divided above the dentate line and then dissection is carried out on the anterior surface of the bowel until the level of the transabdominal dissection is reached. Occasionally, in completing the dissection and providing guidance for its safe performance, the simultaneous presence of an operator on the abdominal side is very helpful.

When no part of the rectum can be saved, and an abdominal perineal resection en bloc with the resection of the sacrum has to be performed, the midline incision over the sacrum is extended inferiorly around and at an appropriate distance from the anal verge. The plane anteriorly between the lower rectum and the prostate or vagina is developed and continued on the sides of the rectum until the level of transabdominal dissection is reached. In this situation no attempt is made to expose the lower anterior surface of the sacrum.

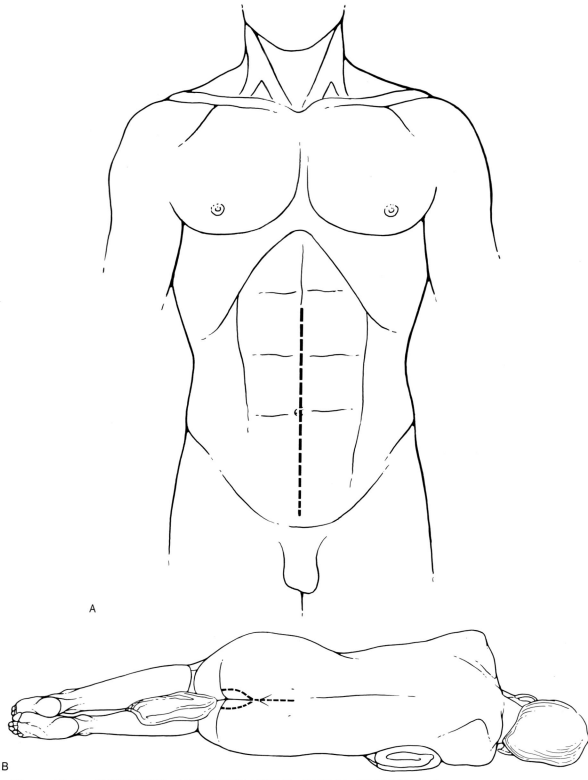

A

B

Figure 15–3. SEQUENTIAL ABDOMINOLATERAL SACRAL POSITION. Infrequently, wide abdominal dissection may be needed to completely mobilize the intra-abdominal portion of the specimen. If there is extensive visceral tumor involvement or pelvic adhesions, a full midline abdominal incision in a supine position is required (**A**). After all attachments to the sacral tumor specimen have been divided, the specimen is packed into the pelvis and the abdomen closed. The patient is turned to a full lateral position (**B**). Usually the left side is up, but this may be revised depending on the soft tissue component of the tumor lateral to the sacrum. Visualization is best on the superior margin of the sacrum as the patient is placed in a lateral position.

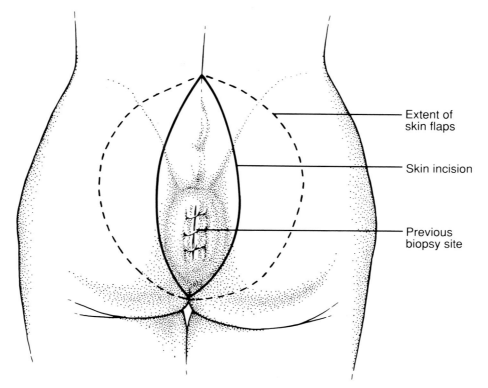

Extent of
skin flaps

Skin incision

Previous
biopsy site

Figure 15–4. PRONE POSITION. The prone position is utilized when the tumor mass remains posterior to the rectum and excision of the latter is not required to achieve a tumor-free margin of excision. In the case of a primary tumor of the sacrum, such as a chordoma, when, on rectal and endoscopic examination as well as radiologic evaluation by CT scan, it appears that the rectum is not involved and no prior surgery has been performed that would obliterate the plane between the rectum and the sacrum, it is best to start with the posterior approach. In a substantial portion of the patients this will suffice to complete the resection. If the tumor extends into the buttock(s) to a large extent or is recurrent with multiple deposits, wide exposure of the posterior surface may be needed, and then it is also best to place the patient in a prone position.

A longitudinal incision is performed through the midline. The two ends may curve leftward off the midline or toward the buttock with maximal involvement by tumor. In the presence of a previous biopsy, an elliptical incision is made. Curving the two ends of the incision provides greater length and exposure and makes initial development of the flaps easier, especially if tumor extends into the buttock, since the skin in the midline is tethered to the underlying fascia with dense fibrous tissue.

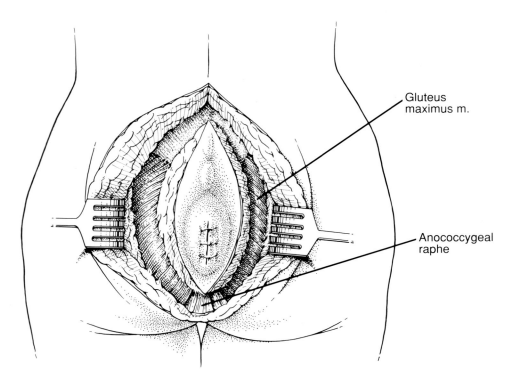

Figure 15–5.   CONSTRUCTION OF SKIN FLAPS. The incision is carried down to the deep fascia, and then flaps are raised to the palpable edges of the sacrum or beyond the soft tissue extent of the tumor. The incision stops distally just below the coccyx when it is known that the distal 4–5 cm of the rectum are uninvolved.

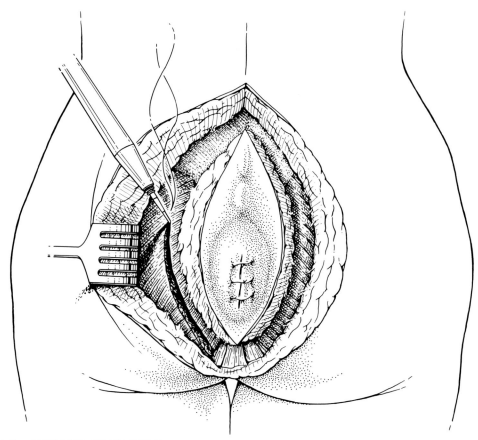

Figure 15–6. DIVISION OF GLUTEUS MAXIMUS MUSCLES WITH SPARING OF SCIATIC AND PUDEN-
DAL NERVES. The fibers of the gluteus maximus muscle are divided near their origin from the posterior sacral
surface. In the case of a tumor extending beyond the limits of the bone, obviously the dissection is guided by
the palpable extent of the tumor.

For large tumors it becomes necessary for a safe resection to expose the sciatic nerves bilaterally,
immediately distal to the greater sciatic notch. For such tumors it is also advisable to expose the pudendal
nerve, at least on one side, in the ischiorectal fossa. The anatomic landmark for its identification is the ischial
tuberosity. This is easily palpable and is exposed following division of the fibers of gluteus maximus coursing
over this bony prominence. The sacrotuberous ligament is divided just medial to the tuberosity, exposing the
ischiorectal fossa. The pudendal nerve is found on the lateral wall of this fossa on the surface of the obturator
internus muscle. This nerve can be traced proximally as it courses posterior to the sacrospinous ligament, and
should be retracted laterally as the latter is divided.

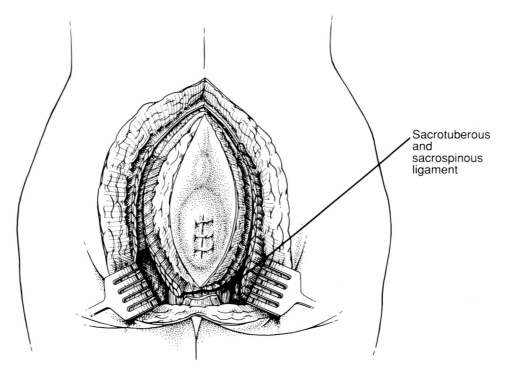

Figure 15–7. DIVISION OF THE ANOCOCCYGEAL RAPHE, SACROTUBEROUS AND SACROSPINOUS
LIGAMENTS. Division of the anococcygeal raphe allows one to enter the presacral space. The dissection
along either sacrococcygeal edge is carried out as guided by palpation of the edge of the tumor from the
outside and, upon occasion, by palpation of the tumor from within the rectum.

After division of the fibers of the gluteus maximus, the thick fibrous bands that constitute the sacrotuberous
and sacrospinous ligaments can be palpated. These are divided in order to gain free access to the ischiorectal
fossa. On the anterior surface of the sacrum, blunt finger dissection is used to separate sacrum from the
posterior rectum.

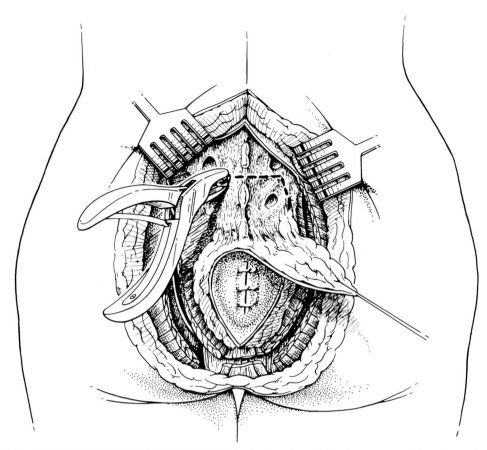

Figure 15–8. TRANSECTION OF THE SACRUM. So far the description has covered the dissection around the lower sacrum with preservation of the rectum. What remains is the dissection through the proximal portion of the bone to complete the resection. It is easier to identify and count the sacral foramina on the anterior surface when the latter is not obscured by tumor. On the basis of the preoperative radiologic studies, one should know the level at which the sacrum should be transected. The level of division of the sacrum is of critical importance. Division of this bone just below the lower border of S-3 vertebra is safe in preserving sphincteric function. Bilateral sacrifice of S-2, S-3, and S-4 nerve roots leads to urinary and fecal incontinence, and impotence for males. Patients about to undergo high sacral resection should be apprised of this risk, because the need for a clear margin of resection is obvious. The tumor, if not operated, is bound to interfere with these functions, and pain and further dissemination of the tumor will occur. Unilateral preservation of S-2, S-3 routes apparently suffices, and preservation of only one S-2 route leads to a weakened but present sphincter control.[8,9] There is some controversy, however, since some authors contend that unilateral preservation of S-2 root maintains perfect anorectal continence,[10] whereas others maintain that when both S-2 routes are preserved sphincter problems are mild and reversible.[11] Apparently early rehabilitative treatment for one year after surgery may restore normal bladder function.[12]

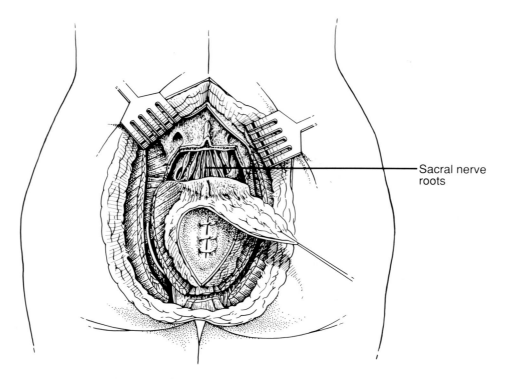

Sacral nerve roots

Figure 15–9. TRANSECTION OF PROXIMAL SACRUM. As one has completed the dissection on the sides of the sacrum, if it appears that one may go straight across the bone while maintaining some distance above the tumor to be resected, it is generally safe to do so. In other words, if one is able to divide the bone in a straight line, eg, with a Gigli saw, then one is well below the lower border of S-2 vertebra and generally below the S-3 vertebra. This is an anatomic point well illustrated previously by Sugarbaker.[3] The sacroiliac articulation does not allow dissection on the lateral surface of the sacrum, above S-3, unless one uses bone instruments. In order to divide the sacrum through S-2 or S-1 vertebrae, one has to reach at this level along either lateral side by using bone-cutting instruments and then divide the bone across the midline.

In the past, it was taught that division of the sacrum proximally should be carried out with an osteotome. However, this technique does not allow any discrimination of what one is dividing. Often it is a matter of 1–2 mm distance between this plane of division and proximal roots of the pudendal nerve. Furthermore, the subarachnoid space reaches the level of S-2 vertebra and may be entered when the bone is divided with an osteotome. The result can be a disturbing leak of CSF fluid in the wound, despite suturing of the dura, and potential infection resulting in meningitis.

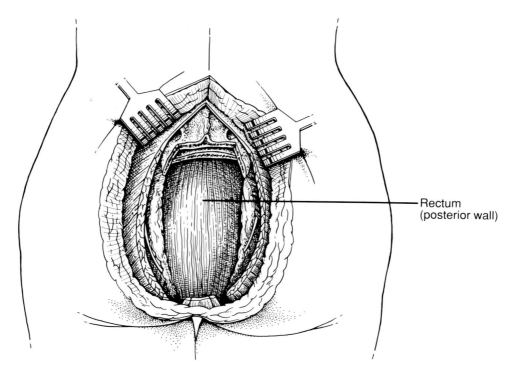

Rectum
(posterior wall)

Figure 15–10.   DISSECTING SACRAL NERVE ROOTS AT RESECTION SITE. A discriminating technique in dividing this bone proximally is the use of fine rongeurs with which the posterior sacral plate is divided at the desired level, and the sacral canal is entered. Nerve roots can then be displaced laterally and the dura superiorly. If one has dissected the pudendal nerve outside the sacrum, one can actually trace its continuity to the S-2 root, although the lower roots S-3 and S-4 may have to be sacrificed. The lower sacral roots may be seen as slender branches issuing from the tumor surface and entering the pudendal nerve at almost right angles. These nerve roots are divided close to the pudendal nerve. It might thus be possible, if the tumor permits, to salvage the S-2 and possibly the S-3 roots, unilaterally at least, and their continuation into the pudendal nerve. After the nerve roots have been isolated and preserved, one may then use an osteotome to divide the fused sacral bodies, anteriorly, at this level.

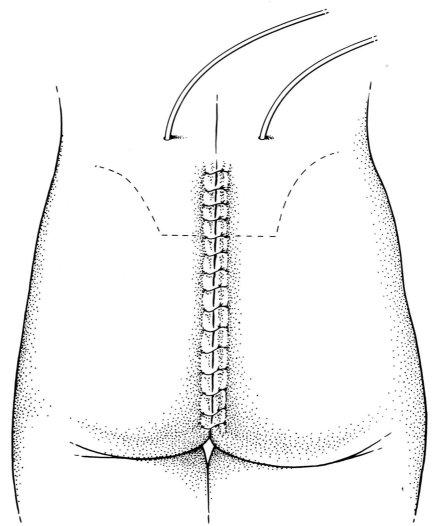

Figure 15–11.   CLOSURE. Following removal of the specimen, examination by the pathologist is requested. A frozen section may not be possible if the lesion is confined in the bone, but smears could be obtained from the proximal margins. For interosseous lesions clearly visible on preoperative films, some authors recommend a plain radiograph of the specimen before the incision is closed in order to assess the margin of resection. The wound is then irrigated, and a closed-system drainage with suction is used. The incision is closed in a routine fashion. These wounds have a high rate of wound infection, apparently due to proximity to the anus.

DISCUSSION

Resections of the sacrum are uncommonly performed, except in referral centers dealing with these problems. However, given a thorough knowledge of the anatomy of this area and a full consciousness of the principles of dissection, the operation can be performed safely and deliberately. Resections below the body of S-3 vertebra do not endanger continence of the anal and bladder functions (Fig. 15–12). Divisions of the bone immediately below or through S-2 vertebra or occasionally through S-1 are possible and can be done more safely in terms of avoiding nerve root injury or entrance in subarachnoid space by cutting first through the posterior sacral plate (the fused sacral laminae) with rongeurs. The sacral canal is thus entered, permitting in some patients the identification, dissection, and preservation of nerve roots that are not involved by the tumor (Fig. 15–13).

In two of our patients with high transection of the sacrum, the dural sac was entered. In the first as the bone was divided with an osteotome, a large amount of CSF fluid appeared in the wound, the dural sac was sutured after removal of the specimen, and the wound healed without complications, although the patient had sphincteric incontinence. She was required to self-catheterize her bladder three to four times daily, and, due to collection of feces in the

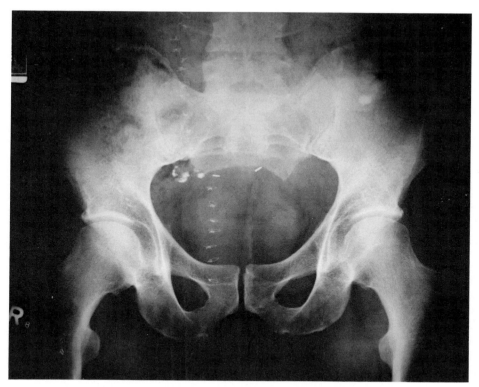

Figure 15–12.   Radiograph of patient following sacrectomy through S2-3.

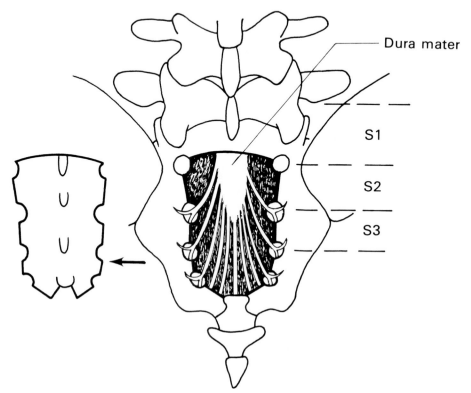

Figure 15–13.   Sacral nerve root distribution.

ampulla, she required frequent disimpaction. In the second patient with a chondrosarcoma reaching the level of S-1, the tumor was curetted at that level and treated with intraoperative radiation, but no evident CSF leak occurred intraoperatively. However, postoperatively he developed large collections of CSF fluid in the wound, thus requiring repeat aspirations, and developed meningitis, which required several weeks of antibiotic therapy before it resolved.

Tumors extending into S-1 vertebra present a special problem. These have been managed by transecting the bone through the middle of S-1. After opening the posterior sacral plate, one carefully dissects laterally whatever nerve roots can be preserved. Residual tumor into the proximal half of S-1 can be curetted out, and the area of potential microscopic residuum treated later with radiation. A dose of intraoperative radiation may also be given, when available, with the pelvic viscera appropriately shielded. The preliminary evidence from other centers also suggests that this may be helpful.[13]

Complete resection of the sacrum is seldom, if ever, practiced. There is a concern first for the removal of support for the spinal column that the sacrum provides. Experience, however, with hemicorporectomies, entailing division below the body of L-5, suggests that removal of the entire sacrum would not be likely to result in "collapse" of the spine, or some other catastrophic occurrence. However, the sciatic nerve comprises L-4–S-3 nerve roots. The lumbosacral trunk (L-4, L-5) courses over the sacral ala, and S-1, S-2, and S-3 roots issue through the upper three anterior sacral foramina. It is therefore clear that a radical resection of the entire sacrum would result, in addition to sphincteric incontinence, in considerable denervation of both lower extremities in the distribution of the sciatic nerves.

As in other anatomic areas, the cure rate following sacral resection depends on the adequacy of resection, the use of adjuvant modalities, and the biologic nature of the tumor. Local spill of tumor cells with biopsy or partial resection by an inexperienced surgeon may severely compromise the opportunity for a complete recovery.[14,15] This is very clear from experience with chordoma excision. For localized tumors, resection of the sacrum when involved can be performed safely if certain oncologic principles are followed. Often there is preservation of sphincteric control, and the result is cure or significant palliation.

REFERENCES

1. Localio SA, Eng K, Coppa GF: Abdominosacral resection for midrectal cancer. A fifteen-year experience. *Ann Surg* 1983;198:320–324.
2. Wanebo HJ, Marcove RC: Abdominal sacral resection of locally recurrent rectal cancer. *Ann Surg* 1981; 194:458–471.
3. Sugarbaker PH: Partial sacrectomy for en bloc excision of rectal cancer with posterior fixation. *Dis Colon Rec* 1982;25:708–711.
4. Karakousis CP, Park JJ, Fleminger R, et al: Chordomas: Diagnosis and management. *Am Surg* 1981; 47:497–501.
5. Azzarelli A, Quagliuolo V, Cerasoli S, et al: Chordoma: Natural history and treatment results in 33 cases. *J Surg Oncol* 1988;37:185–191.
6. Wanebo HJ, Whitehill R, Gaker D, et al: Composite pelvic resection. An approach to advanced pelvic cancer. *Arch Surg* 1987;122:1401–1406.
7. Wanebo JH, Gaker DL, Whitehill R, et al: Pelvic recurrence of rectal cancer. Options for curative resection. *Ann Surg* 1987;205:482–495.
8. Gunterberg B, Kewenter J, Peterson I, et al: Anorectal function after major resections of the sacrum with bilateral or unilateral sacrifice of sacral nerves. *Br J Surg* 1976;63:546–554.
9. Stener B, Gunterberg B: High amputation of the sacrum for extirpation of tumors: Principles and technique. *Spine* 1978;3:351–366.
10. Andreoli F, Balloni F, Bigiotti A, et al: Anorectal continence and bladder function. Effects of major sacral resection. *Dis Colon Rec* 1986;29:647–652.
11. Gennari L, Azzarelli A, Quagliuolo V: A posterior approach for the excision of sacral chordoma. *J Bone Joint Surg* 1987;69:565–568.
12. Torelli T, Campo B, Ordesi G, et al: Sacral chordoma and rehabilitative treatment of urinary disorders. *Tumori* 1988;74:475–478.
13. Hoekstra JH, Sindelar WF, Kinsella TJ: Surgery with intraoperative radiotherapy for sarcoma of the pelvis girdle: A pilot experience. *Int J Radiat Oncol Biol Phys* 1988;15:1013–1016.
14. Mindell ER: Current concepts review: Chordoma. *J Bone Joint Surg* 1981;63:501–505.
15. Kaiser TE, Pritchard DJ, Unni KK: Clinicopathologic study of sacrococcygeal chordoma. *Cancer* 1984;53: 2574–2578.

16

Above-Knee Amputation

PAUL H. SUGARBAKER, M.D.
MARTIN M. MALAWER, M.D.
ALAN R. BAKER, M.D.

OVERVIEW

Above-knee amputation is most often performed for advanced soft tissue sarcomas of the leg or osteosarcoma of the proximal tibia or fibula. Amputation is usually indicated because tumor involves the sciatic nerve or popliteal vessels. Osteosarcoma of the proximal tibia or fibula may require amputation if there is a posterior extension of the soft tissue tumor into the popliteal space. The amputation may be performed through the distal aspect of the femur (supracondylar), middle femur (diaphyseal), or just below the lesser trochanter. Muscles should be secured by myodesis over the end of the femur to allow purposeful motion of the stump. A rigid dressing and early ambulation are of great help in the rehabilitation process in most patients.

INTRODUCTION

Within the past two decades, limb-sparing procedures in combination with radiation therapy and chemotherapy have proved to be a safe and effective alternative to above-knee amputation for many patients with bony and soft tissue sarcoma. The regular use of infusional chemotherapy promises to reduce the requirement for limb ablation in an even greater percentage of patients. Also, for osteosarcoma limb-sparing surgery has been revolutionized by the development of new endoprosthetic devices. This technology and accompanying surgical technique allow for musculoskeletal reconstruction that combines a satisfactory cosmetic result with an excellent functional outcome.

Nevertheless, amputation continues to demand a definitive role in the management of lower-extremity bone and soft tissue sarcomas. Approximately 20% to 40% of all bone sarcomas of the distal femur are currently treated by amputation of the extremity along with the primary tumor. A lesser percentage of amputations are required with the soft tissue sarcomas of the thigh. Recurrence of high-grade cancer in the extremity following treatment of the primary tumor remains a common indication for above-knee amputation.

GENERAL INDICATIONS FOR ABOVE-KNEE AMPUTATION

Local recurrence of a high-grade primary tumor in the absence of evidence of disease spread to the lungs or other systemic sites demands a below-knee amputation. If a recurrent low-grade tumor can be removed and the function preserved, this is often acceptable.

Major vascular involvement, usually of the popliteal vessels or trifurcation, requires below-knee amputation in the majority of patients. The incidence of morbidity and the technical failures associated with limb-salvage surgery and reconstruction are significantly higher if a vascular graft is required.

Major nerve involvement may occur, usually in the popliteal space. In general, one nerve may be removed, but a two-nerve deficit results in a poorly functioning extremity. Worse than amputation is tissue left behind that has little or no function. If a useless extremity is maintained by the patient after sacrifice of major nerves, it can be compared to baggage that must be carried about but has no utility.

Extensive local *soft tissue contamination* may result from extensive hemorrhage into a large tumor mass often as a result of the biopsy. Also, a poorly planned and inappropriately located biopsy site can interfere with limb salvage surgery. Certainly local dissemination of tumor cells especially in an extensive hematoma increases the risk for local recurrence.

Pathologic fracture through a tumor in a weight-bearing bone results in a hematoma and the traumatic dissemination of tumor extensively into the soft tissues. Except under unusual circumstances this local tumor contamination makes limb-salvage surgery difficult.

Infection usually is the result of tumor ulceration through the skin, or it may be caused by wound infection at the biopsy site. It may negate attempts at local resection especially if prosthetic materials must be used in the limb-salvage effort. Also infection will markedly impair the ability of the oncologist to administer adequate preoperative or postoperative chemotherapy.

Skeletal immaturity is of great concern when irradiating or replacing the proximal tibia. Eighty percent of this bone's growth is from the proximal epiphysis. If the tibia has not reached its full length, prosthetic replacement will result in leg-length discrepancies. Also, high-dose radiation therapy will limit the growth of all other tissues (muscle, tendon) contained within the field. Contractures may be an additional problem that result from high-dose radiation therapy in the young patient. Irradiation across the knee joint carries a high incidence of late contracture.

In addition to the anatomic location of the tumor and the probable spread that has occurred prior to definitive therapy, the pathologic *grade of the malignancy* is extremely important in deciding the proper surgical procedures. It is unusual to perform an amputation with a grade I malignancy. Only if removal of the tumor causes severe functional impairment of the extremity should amputation be considered with a grade I sarcoma. In other patients, the malignancy may be of an advanced stage and makes systemic spread of disease a high probability. In this instance induction systemic or regional chemotherapy with or without local radiation therapy may be considered prior to definitive amputation at a later time. This "surgical procrastination" allows one a three- to four-month time interval with a repeat thorough search for metastatic disease prior to definitive amputation.

A common neoplastic indication for above-knee amputation is osteosarcoma of the distal femur in an adolescent patient for whom a limb-sparing procedure would not ensure local control (Fig. 16–1). Soft tissue sarcomas arising from the proximal leg and large lesions of the popliteal space are often considered not resectable with a reasonable margin. They

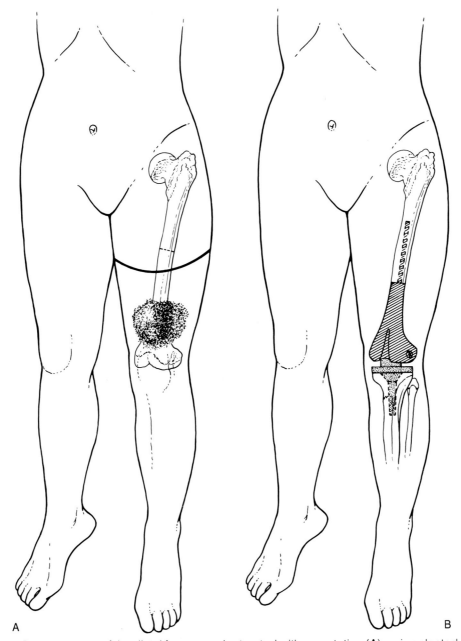

Figure 16–1. Osteosarcoma of the distal femur may be treated with amputation (**A**) or, in selected patients, a prosthetic replacement of the femur and reconstruction of the knee joint (**B**).

are usually best treated by above-knee amputation (Fig. 16–2).

CLINICAL CONSIDERATIONS

Timing of the surgical procedure is important. Physiological and psychological factors must be optimized. If the patient has received a recent course of chemotherapy, it is essential that leukocyte and platelet counts be permitted to return toward normal. Significant deficits in red blood cell mass should be corrected by preoperative transfusion. Also, recent chemotherapy may impair wound healing. Vascular insufficiency is rarely a complicating factor in these patients. The nausea and vomiting associated with an aggressive chemotherapy regimen may result in poor nutritional intake and weight loss. Because of potential healing difficulties, stump wound closure must be meticulous. Hematoma or seroma must be avoided by the adequate use of closed-suction drains. If possible, one should defer remov-

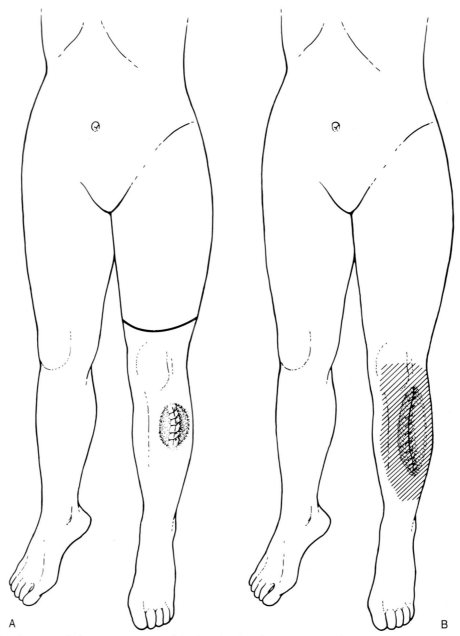

Figure 16–2. Large soft tissue sarcomas of the leg that involve neurovascular structures or bone are usually treated by amputation (**A**). Wide local excision plus radiation therapy is always the preferred option if local recurrence can be avoided (**B**).

ing skin sutures for approximately three weeks after operation. The stump may mold and mature slowly if the amputation required unusual dissection or skin flap construction.

REHABILITATION AND EMOTIONAL SUPPORT

Psychosocial support and rehabilitation are necessary prerequisites for above-knee amputation. The rehabilitation process should start at the time of the staging studies. The entire health care team must develop an honest relationship with the patient and family and include them in the early stages of the decision-making process. Building upon this basis, the patient will be better able to accept the above-knee amputation and set realistic goals for recovery. The patient should be told about the possible phantom limb sensations that might occur following surgery. They should be presented as normal sensations that are to be expected as a part of the recovery process. Generally the phantom limb problems with above-knee amputations are controlled by the passage of time and the judicious use of analgesics. It is not unusual for depression to be a part of the postoperative period. The judicious use of professional psychological intervention and pharmacologic treatment of depression may be of great help to the patient and family for a time.

LEVEL OF AMPUTATION

Sarcomas of the leg and tibia that require an amputation are treated by a standard above-knee procedure. The surgical planning, operative procedure, and management of these patients are similar to those used for amputation for other causes. In contrast, patients requiring an above-knee amputation for osteosarcoma of the distal femur or distal thigh soft tissue sarcoma must undergo thorough anatomic studies in order to determine the level of amputation. The level of tumor involvement of bone and of soft tissue must be evaluated. In general, the more proximal of the two levels of involvement (bone *v* soft tissue) determines the site of amputation. The type of flaps to be used must also be determined at this time.

RADIOLOGIC STUDIES

Computerized tomography is useful in determining the proximal extent of soft tissue sarcoma or the extraosseous extent of osteosarcoma of the femur. The level of bone transection should be at least 5 to 10 cm proximal to this point. Bone scintigraphy, combined with computerized tomography and MRI, will accurately predict proximal intraosseous extension. MRI provides an extremely accurate evaluation of intraosseous involvement of bone marrow by tumor.

The level of marrow involvement should be marked by the nuclear medicine physician the day prior to the surgical procedure. This ensures the surgeon that there will be no tumor visualized at the time of amputation thus avoiding tumor contamination of the operative field. This may occur upon transection of the femur at a site of bone marrow involvement by cancer. Often the level of amputation as determined by the preoperative studies is above the mid-femur. As a rule, any length of femur makes fitting of a prosthesis easier than if there were no residual femur. Even amputations at the subtrochanteric level are preferred to hip disarticulation; if 3 to 5 cm of bone distal to the lesser trochanter remain, the patient can be fitted with a prosthesis in the manner used for above-knee amputation.

To rule out systemic spread of cancer, a computerized tomogram of the chest and a bone scan should be performed.

ONCOLOGIC CONSIDERATIONS

It should be emphasized that an extremity involved by a cancer is never exsanguinated with a compressive tourniquet. However, a sterile Esmarch tourniquet is placed just proximal to the level of the tumor and distal to the planned incision in order to prevent tumor emboli or hematoma and edema fluid from previous manipulation from contaminating the operative field.

A more proximal tourniquet may be utilized if the stump is long enough. Following transection of the femur for a bony sarcoma, cytological examination and a frozen section of the proximal marrow canal must be performed to determine with certainty that no occult intraosseous extension has occurred. A frozen section of any questionable site tissue margins should be performed as indicated.

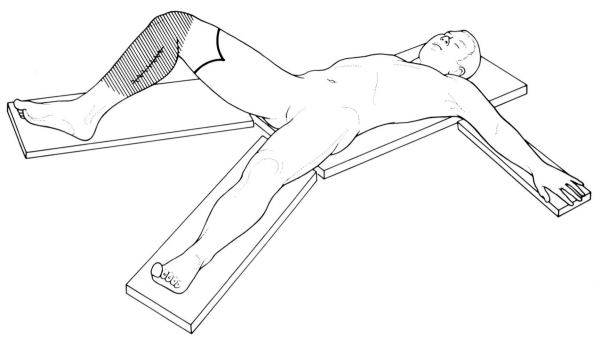

Figure 16–3.　POSITION.

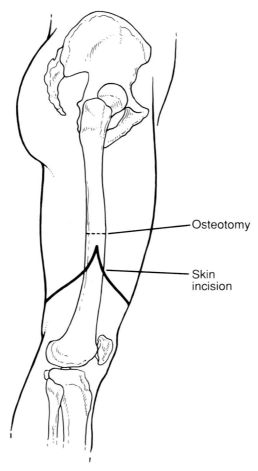

Osteotomy

Skin
incision

Figure 16–4. INCISION. The skin flaps are marked out with a pencil on the patient's skin. The main factors that determine the type of flaps are the extent of soft tissue tumor, areas of prior radiation, and previous scars. The greatest priority in performing the surgical procedure is to avoid local recurrence. No attempt is made to adhere to "standard flaps"; at this level a skin or muscle flap of almost any length will heal primarily in the young patient. Furthermore, it is not necessary to utilize equal flaps; long posterior, anterior, or medial flaps will heal. Often, the tumors that require amputation will have failed radiation therapy or regional chemotherapy. If this is so, the radiation therapy ports or skin distribution of the chemotherapy should be avoided if possible in fashioning the skin flaps.

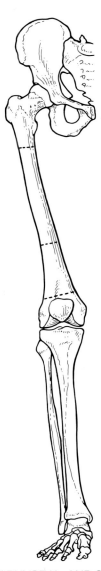

Figure 16–5.   OSTEOTOMY FOR HIGH, DIAPHYSEAL, AND SUPRACONDYLAR ABOVE-KNEE AMPUTA-TION. Above-knee amputation is preferable to hip disarticulation even though the osteotomy is only a few cm below the greater trochanter. With the hip joint intact, movement of a prosthesis is greatly facilitated. Also even a remnant of proximal femur allows the prosthetist a deeper cup in the prosthetic device in which to secure the stump. The higher above-knee amputations are generally used for osteosarcoma of the distal femur. Low above-knee amputations are used for sarcoma of the leg, especially those that involve the popliteal fossa or arterial trifurcation.

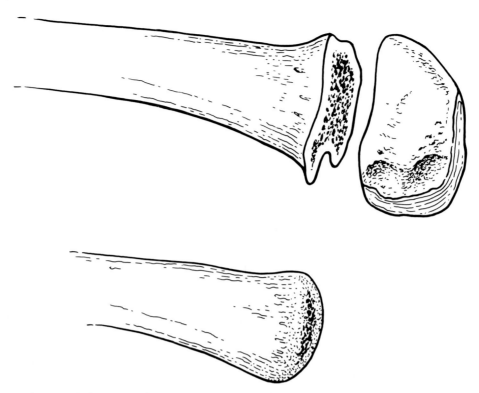

Figure 16–6.   SHAPING OF THE DISTAL FEMUR WITH A SUPRACONDYLAR AMPUTATION.

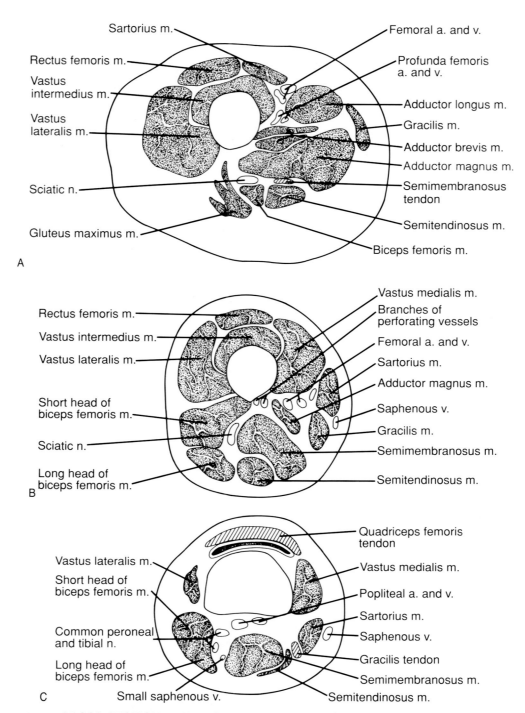

Figure 16–7.   CROSS-SECTIONAL ANATOMY FOR A HIGH ABOVE-KNEE AMPUTATION (**A**), DIAPHYSEAL AMPUTATION (**B**), AND SUPRACONDYLAR AMPUTATION (**C**).

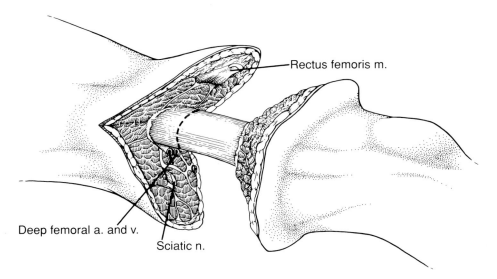

Rectus femoris m.

Deep femoral a. and v.

Sciatic n.

Figure 16–8. TRANSECTION OF MUSCLE AND BONE. One moves through the skin, superficial fascia, and subcutaneous tissue vertical to the skin edges. Then the muscle flaps are beveled in their transection down to bone. The CO_2 laser or electrocautery is used to transect muscle. Large vessels are dissected, ligated in continuity, and transected in a bloodless fashion. The large vessels should be suture-ligated. Nerves are treated with great respect. The nerve should be gently pulled down from its muscular bed for approximately 2 cm. It is doubly ligated with a nonabsorbable monofilament suture, and then it is transected with a knife and allowed to retract back into the muscle mass. The area is generously infiltrated with local long-lasting anesthetic.

Electrocautery is used to score the periosteum. The bone is transected with a saw or a Gigli saw without traumatizing the soft tissue. The distal femur is contoured to remove sharp edges.

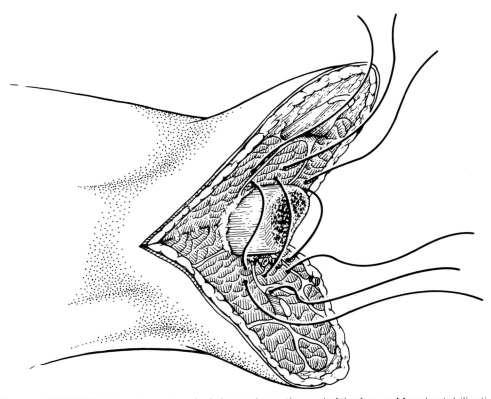

Figure 16–9. MYODESIS. A two-layer myodesis is used over the end of the femur. Muscle stabilization of the femur is essential if muscular strength of the limb is to be retained. The quadriceps and/or hamstring muscles are myodesed to each other in covering the bony end of the femur. This is especially important if there is a short proximal femoral stump that has a strong tendency to go into flexion. Hip flexor muscles are routinely stronger than the extensor muscle; thus, the hamstrings should be cut longer than the quadriceps and attached to one another. The myodesis should be made with the hamstring muscles somewhat tighter than the quadriceps and secured over the end of the femur. In addition, the adductors should be tendodesed to the muscles over the end of the femur. A well-balanced extremity requires strong adductors.

239

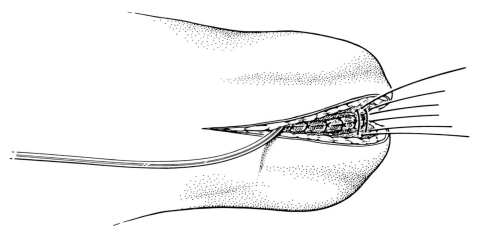

Figure 16–10.   CLOSURE OF SUPERFICIAL FASCIA.

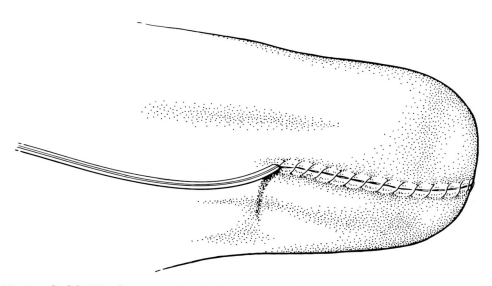

Figure 16–11.   CLOSURE. Closed-suction drains are brought out the medial and lateral aspects of the incision. It is important not to stitch these catheters to the skin, for they will be removed from inside the rigid dressing.

It is important to place all sutures by halving the incision, especially if unusual skin flaps have been utilized. It is important to avoid a large fold of skin. This can be done by dividing with individual sutures the superficial fascia and skin equally with each stitch. This will result in small pleats in the longer skin flap rather than unsightly skin folds.

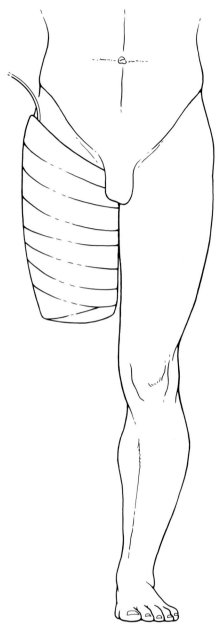

Figure 16–12. APPLICATION OF THE RIGID DRESSING. As soon as the surgery is completed, a rigid dressing is applied. A stump sock is placed over the stump. Usually no felt pads are required beneath the above-knee rigid dressing. The cast should be continued up to the groin and held in place with a belt. Preoperative or early postoperative chemotherapy is not a contraindication to a rigid dressing and early ambulation. With early ambulation, patients tend to have less pain and experience less psychological difficulties. They invariably mobilize earlier than those who are furnished with a standard soft dressing. Patients with short stumps are fitted with a pelvic band that decreases the possibility of hip flexion contractures.

PAIN CONTROL

Pain occurs more frequently in the young patient following a transmedullary amputation than in the dysvascular patient. If pain had been present preoperatively, it may increase and be particularly difficult to control. Large doses of narcotics may be necessary, and patient-controlled analgesia devices have been well utilized. Intraoperative epidural morphine has also been used with satisfactory effects. One should make sure that the surgery is performed under deep narcosis so that the patient has no recollections of the amputative procedure. Especially bothersome may be inadequate anesthesia when large nerves are being transected or the femur is being divided. In some patients with high amputations, small catheters are positioned parallel to the distal portion of transected nerves. A continuous infusion of local anesthetic has been successful in minimizing stump pain postoperatively.[1] Some clinicians suggest that good pain control in the early postoperative period may help avert chronic phantom limb pain problems later in the patient's recovery.

REFERENCE

1. Malawer MM: Infusion of nerves for post-operative relief of stump pain, to be published.

17

Distal Femoral Resection for Sarcomas of Bone

MARTIN M. MALAWER, M.D.

OVERVIEW

Patients with osteosarcoma of the distal femur have traditionally been treated with a high above-knee amputation. With earlier diagnosis and induction chemotherapy the soft tissue component of the cancer can usually be resected with tumor-free margins. Careful preoperative evaluation and strict adherence to established criteria for resection of bone cancers are required to keep local recurrences at a minimum. Prosthetic reconstruction of the distal femur is an option that must be evaluated in all of these patients. Results with the modular segmental replacement system (MSRS) described here can provide limb salvage in a large population of patients. The functional results are excellent and patient satisfaction is high.

INTRODUCTION

Many recent studies have demonstrated a low risk of local recurrence (<5%) following limb-sparing surgery of osteosarcomas.[1–5] Similarly, the continuous disease-free survival rates in patients who have undergone resection are the same or better than those of patients undergoing amputation (presumably due to selection criteria). Eckardt et al, from UCLA, reported their experience with stage IIB osteosarcoma for the period 1972–1984. Seventy-eight of 116 patients (67%) were treated by a limb-sparing procedure, with a local recurrence rate of 8%.[6] Simon et al compared results of limb-sparing procedures with amputation in 277 patients with osteosarcoma of the distal femur; there was no difference between the two groups in rate of metastasis or local recurrence.[7]

As a result of these and other studies, limb-sparing surgery is now considered the preferred treatment for carefully selected patients with osteosarcomas and other high-grade sarcomas involving the distal femur. Amputations are reserved principally for patients whose primary tumor is unresectable. The most common factors necessitating an amputation are significant contamination of the tumor site resulting from a poor biopsy, fracture, or extreme neurovascular involvement.[8] The size and extent of the tumor are important only to the degree that they affect these three factors and influence the amount of soft tissue required to be resected and thus the resultant functional outcome. Even tumors with large extraosseous components can be resected in conjunction with most of the musculature of the distal thigh. If there is insignificant quadriceps remaining to power a prosthesis, hamstrings transfers can be performed or a primary arthrodesis implanted. Muscle power is then not necessary since the "knee" will not bend.

PREOPERATIVE EVALUATION AND STAGING STUDIES

Staging studies should be performed before biopsy if the plain radiograph suggests a malignant tumor.[9] Preoperative studies allow the surgeon to conceptualize the local anatomy and thereby appreciate the volume (en bloc) of tissue to be resected and the extent of surgical reconstruction that will be needed. All patients should be considered candidates for limb-sparing procedures unless a surgical oncologist familiar with these procedures feels that a nonamputative option has little chance of success.

Bone Scans

Bone scintigraphy is useful in determining intraosseous extension of tumor. In general, the area of uptake accurately corresponds to tumor extent.

Computed Tomography (CT)

CT allows accurate determination of intraosseous and extraosseous extension of skeletal tumors. CT accurately depicts the transverse relationship of the tumor, enabling the surgeon to detect which portion of the quadriceps muscle is involved and the relationship of the tumor to the popliteal vessels.

Magnetic Resonance Imaging (MRI)

MRI allows detailed evaluation of tumor involvement and extent within the marrow of the medullary canal. It also provides details of soft tissue extension. Of all preoperative studies, MRI is generally the most affected by a prior biopsy or manipulation of the tumor.

Angiography

Biplane angiography is essential in determining the relationship of the tumor to the popliteal vessels.[10,11] The angiogram serves as a road map for the surgeon during the operative procedure, thus permitting safe exposure of the popliteal vessels. Two views, anterior posterior and lateral, are required to evaluate the relationship of the vessels to the tumor and the potential plane of resection and to detect any anatomic distortions or anomalies. The increasing preoperative use of intra-arterial chemotherapy has made angiography almost routine. The decrease in vascularity of osteosarcomas following neoadjuvant chemotherapy correlates well with tumor necrosis.[12]

A careful evaluation of all data from the preceding studies allows extremely accurate preoperative determination of tumor extent and permits the operating surgeon to form an accurate three-dimensional image of the amount of bone and soft tissue to be resected.

Biopsy

If a resection is to be performed, it is crucial that the location of the biopsy be in line with the anticipated incision for the definitive procedure. Extreme care should be taken *before* biopsy not to contaminate potential tissue planes or flaps that would compromise the management of the lesion. To minimize contamination, a needle biopsy of soft tissue masses or of extraosseous components should be attempted prior to an incisional biopsy whenever possible. Radiographs should be obtained to document the position of the trocar. Needle biopsy usually provides an adequate specimen for diagnosis. If it proves to be inadequate, a small incisional biopsy is performed. Care should be taken to avoid contamination of the knee joint, sartorial canal, popliteal space, and rectus femoris muscle. A medial biopsy is preferred if an option exists.

Regardless of the biopsy technique utilized, tumor cells will contaminate all tissue planes and compartments traversed. All biopsy sites must therefore be removed en bloc when the tumor is resected.

CONTRAINDICATIONS FOR LIMB-SPARING SURGERY

The contraindications of limb-sparing surgery are as follows[3–5,9]:

1. *Major neurovascular involvement*—specifically the popliteal vessels.
2. *Pathologic fractures.* A fracture through a bone affected by a tumor spreads tumor cells via the hematoma beyond accurately determined limits. The risk of local recurrence increases following a pathologic fracture, making resection inadvisable.
3. *Inappropriate biopsy sites.* An inappropriate or poorly planned biopsy jeopardizes local tumor control by contaminating normal tissue planes and compartments.
4. *Infection.* Implantation of a metallic device (or allograft) in an infected area is contraindicated. Sepsis jeopardizes the effectiveness of adjuvant chemotherapy.
5. *Immature skeletal age.* In the lower extremity the predicted leg-length discrepancy (when the patient has achieved adult stature) should not be greater than 6 to 8 cm. Upper-extremity reconstruction is independent of skeletal maturity. An expandable prosthesis or a rotation plasty can be utilized in the young child.[13,14]
6. *Extensive muscle involvement.* Enough muscle must remain to reconstruct a functional extremity.

SURGICAL GUIDELINES

The surgical guidelines and technique of limb-sparing surgery utilized by the author are summarized as follows[9]:

1. The major neurovascular bundle (popliteal vessels) must be free of tumor.
2. The resection of the affected bone should leave a wide margin and a normal muscle cuff in all directions.
3. All previous biopsy sites and all potentially contaminated tissues should be removed en bloc.
4. To avoid intraosseous tumor extension, bone should be resected 5–6 cm beyond abnormal uptake, as determined by preoperative studies.
5. The adjacent joint and joint capsule should be resected.
6. Adequate motor reconstruction must be accomplished by regional muscle transfers. The type of transfer depends on functional requirements.
7. Adequate soft tissue coverage is needed to decrease the risk of skin flap necrosis and secondary infection.

Description of the Modular Segmental Replacement System

The modular segmental replacement system (MSRS) was developed to meet the unique needs of patients who require reconstruction of large segmental defects for tumors.[15,16] Most clinical experience has been with distal femoral replacements. This system is designed to

1. Reconstruct large segmental defects of the knee, shoulder, or hip.
2. Reconstruct osteoarticular defects of varying sizes.
3. Decrease the time required to obtain a "custom" implant. The prosthesis is immediately available and assembled intraoperatively.
4. Allow for variation in both planned and unsuspected necessary intraoperative changes.
5. Strengthen the implant by extracortical fixation.

The system consists of articular components, body segments, and stem sections. It also includes a set of trial components. The articular components utilize a male/female Morse taper locking mechanism. The components are assembled during surgery by impacting them together. The impaction causes the male/female tapers to produce a cold-weld-type lock.

The body segments are available in 40–120-mm lengths in 20-mm increments. This component features a male/female taper for attaching proximal and distal components. The body sections have an overall diameter of 28 mm.

The stem sections have a 40-mm replacement length with a tapered 127-mm stem that is available in 11-, 13-, and 15-mm diameters; their respective seat diameters are 24, 28, and 32 mm, which allows close matching of host bone. The body of the stem segment has an area that is porous-coated. The porous coating offers the option for bone graft and extracortical fixation. The stem segments are designed to be cemented into the medullary canal.

The condylar section has a 65-mm replacement length and is available in left or right. The condyle has a built-in 6° offset, so when a stem or body unit is attached the condyle is made to utilize standard or custom rotating hinge knee components.

TRIAL COMPONENTS

The implant systems are complemented with a complete set of *trial components*. The trial components are replicas of their corresponding implant; however, they have nonlocking trunnions. The articulating trials are satin-finished so that they can easily be distinguished from the prosthesis. The body sections have several large holes drilled through the major diameter to distinguish them from the implant. The stem sections do not have porous coating, and the stem diameters are 2 mm oversize to account for a cement mantle. All trial articulating components are made of cast Vitallium, and all body segments are made of machined stainless steel.

INTRAMEDULLARY REAMERS

Intramedullary facing reamers correspond to the diameter of the proximal stem. The reamers are used to plane the seat area of bone for the prosthesis. The cutting flutes recreate in bone the radius at the stem/seat junction. The reamers are available in 11-, 13-, and 15-mm diameters, with corresponding seat diameters for the femoral system.

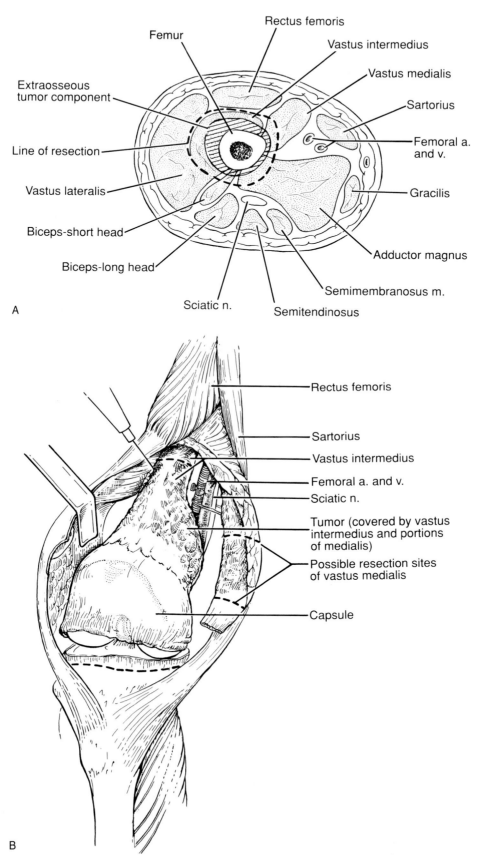

A

B

Figure 17–1(A,B). ANATOMICAL LOCATION OF MALIGNANCY. Adequate en bloc resection includes 15–20 cm of the distal femur and proximal tibia and portions of the adjacent quadriceps. An intra-articular resection is usually performed. The surgical planes of resection are shown.

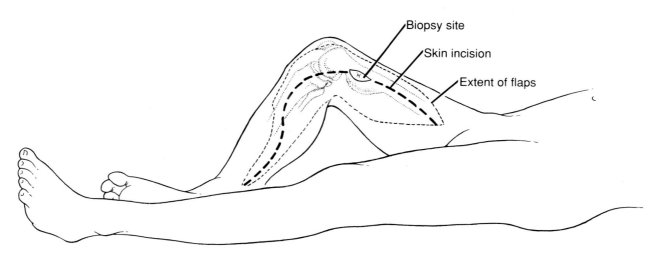

Figure 17–2. SURGICAL APPROACH AND INCISION. The patient is placed supine on the operating table. A sandbag is placed under the ipsilateral buttock to facilitate taking a bone graft. The entire extremity, including the groin and pelvis, is prepped and draped. The groin should always be included to allow for the rare instance in which exposure of the common femoral vessels is required. The pelvis (used for bone graft) is draped separately.

A long medial incision begins in the mid-thigh, crosses the knee joint along the medial parapatellar area and distal to the tibial tubercle, and then passes gently posterior to the inferior border of the pes muscles. The biopsy site is included, with a 3-cm margin in all directions.

This approach allows an extensile exposure of the distal one-third to one-half of the femur and knee joint and identification of the important muscle intervals. It allows simple and safe exploration of the sartorial canal, the superficial femoral vessels, and the popliteal space. It permits distal extension of the incision to develop a medial gastrocnemius muscle transposition for prosthetic coverage. Fasciocutaneous (*not* subcutaneous) flaps are developed.

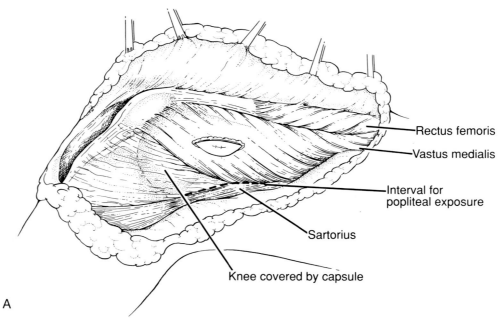

A

Figure 17–3A. POPLITEAL EXPLORATION. Resectability is determined by initial exploration of the popliteal space and vessels. The popliteal space is approached by detaching or retracting the medial hamstrings. The sartorius is identified. The superior border is opened with the knee in a flexed position. This allows direct entry to the popliteal space. This permits exploration of the popliteal vessels and the sciatic nerve.

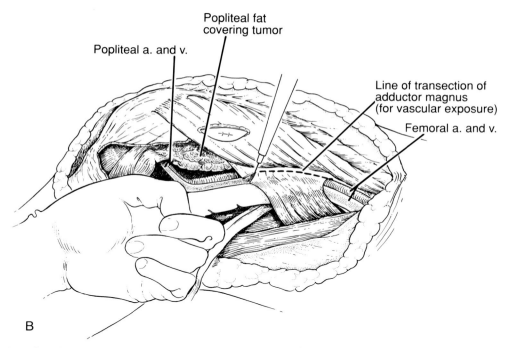

B

Figure 17–3B. SUPERFICIAL FEMORAL ARTERY EXPLORATION. The superficial femoral artery (SFA) is identified within the sartorial canal. If resection length is greater than 15 cm, the SFA must be mobilized from the adductors within Hunter's canal (as shown). If this is not done, the artery can be inadvertently damaged due to its proximity to the canal and its contents as the SFA passes anteriorly to posteriorly. The adductor magnus tendon is released at the foramen to facilitate retraction of the SFA.

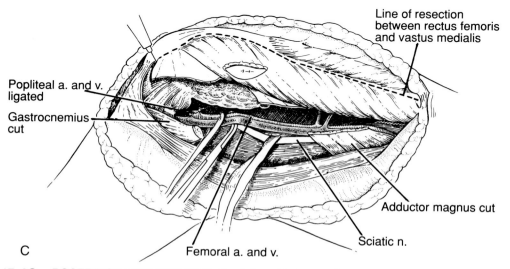

C

Figure 17–3C. POSTERIOR EXPLORATION. The interval between the popliteal vessels and the posterior femur is then developed and explored. The popliteal artery is mobilized, and all the geniculate vessels are ligated and transected. If the vessels are free of tumor, resection proceeds.

249

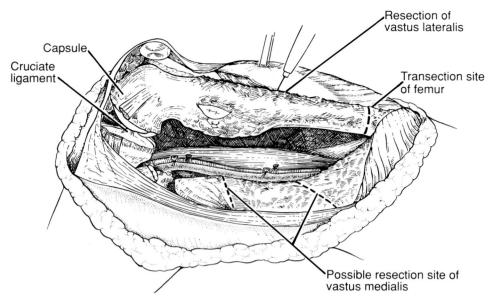

Figure 17–4. DISTAL FEMORAL RESECTION. The interval between the rectus femoris and vastus medialis muscle is identified and opened, exposing the underlying v. intermedius muscle. The v. intermedius must remain intact around the femoral shaft and the extraosseous tumor component. If there is a medial extraosseous component, a cuff of normal muscle must remain as a covering around it. If necessary, the entire portion of the v. medialis muscle can be removed en bloc with the tumor, at their insertion under direct vision. The entire capsular insertion onto the tibia may be partially or completely released. (The stability of the prosthesis is *not* dependent on the capsule.) The majority of the soft tissue detachments of the distal femur structures should now be performed prior to osteotomy. The remaining muscle attachments to the distal femur, which must be severed, include the medial and lateral intermuscular septa, the short head of the biceps, and both medial and lateral heads of the gastrocnemius muscles.

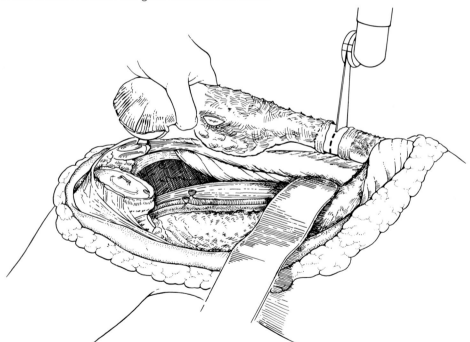

Figure 17–5. PROXIMAL FEMORAL OSTEOTOMY. The length of the resection is measured from the medial joint line to the correct area on the femur and then marked. All remaining soft tissue at the level of transection is cleared. The osteotomy is performed after the posterior and medial structures have been protected and retracted; special care is taken to protect the SFA. A frozen section of the bone marrow from the proximal end is performed.

Following the osteotomy, it is helpful to pull the distal end of the femur forward in order to expose the remaining soft tissue attachments, usually remaining fibers of the short head of the biceps, intermuscular septums, and capsular structures. The distal femur is then passed off the operative field.

CAUTION: It is *extremely* important not to distract the extremity following the resection; one assistant must be assigned to monitor this. The end of the proximal femoral osteotomy should be kept well padded to avoid injuring the popliteal/SFA vessels. The length of the resected specimen should be checked and measured again following resection.

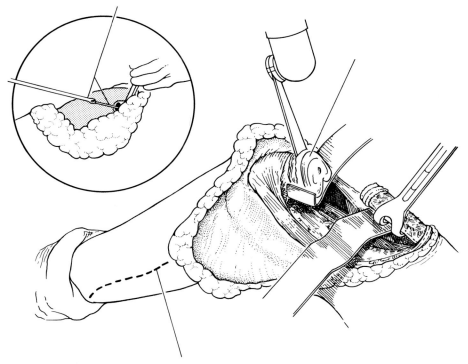

Figure 17–6. TIBIAL OSTEOTOMY AND PREPARATION OF THE FEMUR. The tibial osteotomy is performed in the same manner as the standard knee joint replacement. Approximately 1 cm of bone is removed. The cut should be perpendicular to the long axis of the tibia. Do *not* discard this bone; it can be utilized for bone graft for the extracortical fixation of the distal femoral component.

A flexible guide wire is inserted into the femoral canal. Flexible reamers are utilized to widen the canal to the appropriate diameter. To permit an adequate cement mantle, the canal should be reamed to 2 mm larger than the selected stem of the prosthesis. (Note: The three femoral stem widths are 11, 13, and 15 mm.)

A stem/seat rasp is used to plane the osteotomy site so as to ensure *direct contact* and accurate seating of the prosthesis upon the cortices. The rasp is also designed to expand the diameter of the shaft to allow the increased radius of curvature of the stem/prosthesis junction to fit accurately into the canal.

The chosen trial femoral component is inserted to ensure ease of insertion. (Note: The trials are 2 mm oversized.) If there is any difficulty, one must ream an additional 1 mm. It is *extremely important* to verify the close apposition of the *seat* of the femoral trial to the cortex. If necessary, a high-speed burr is used to adjust or trim the osteotomy site.

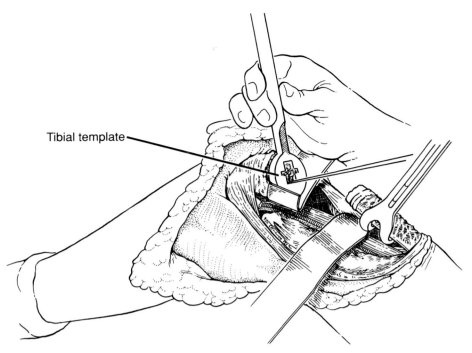

Figure 17–7. PREPARATION OF THE PROXIMAL TIBIAL CANAL. The tibial canal is located with a curette. The canal is reamed to the appropriate size, as determined by the preoperative evaluation of the width of the proximal diaphyseal canal. (The stem diameters of the tibial-bearing plug component are 8, 11, 16, and 21 mm; the tibial trial components are *not* oversized.) The canal is reamed 2 mm larger than the chosen stem diameter to permit an adequate cement mantle. All trial components, with their respective sizes, are marked as trials. The standard tibial template from the Kinematic II (Howmedica, Inc, Rutherford, NJ) rotating hinge is used to outline the rectangular cut for the box portion of the tibial-bearing plug component. The *trial* tibial-bearing plug component is then impacted with a mallet. The seating of the component must be checked carefully. If necessary, the fit can be adjusted with a small curette and/or high-speed burr.

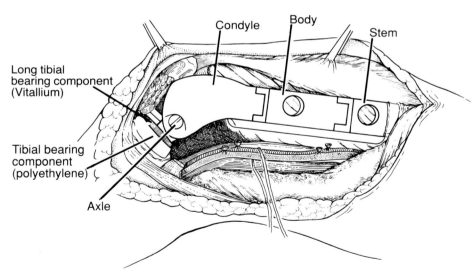

Figure 17–8. TRIAL REDUCTION WITH TEMPLATES. The purpose of the trial reduction is to determine the ease of insertion of the femoral and tibial components prior to cementing and to determine whether the length of the prosthesis is appropriate.

If the prosthesis is too long, too much tension will be placed upon the neurovascular structures when the knee is extended. In addition, the extensor mechanism will be tight, causing loss of flexion and difficulty in closing the soft tissues. To determine the appropriate length, one must extend the knee and monitor the distal pulse with the trial prosthesis in place. A sterile Doppler can be used to evaluate the posterior tibial and dorsalis pedis pulses.

Insert the trial tibial-bearing component into the tibia and impact it with a mallet. Insert the femoral stem segment into the femur. Align the femoral stem segment using the linea aspera as a guide (see Fig 17–11). Construct an imaginary perpendicular line that passes directly anterior, originating from the linea aspera. The horizontal axis of the prosthesis should be perpendicular to this line. Construct the trial femoral prosthesis by joining the femoral stem segment with the trial femoral body segment and condylar segment.

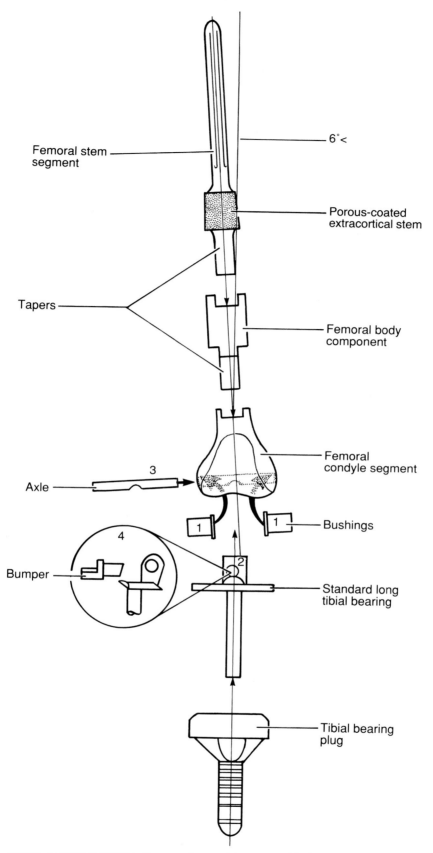

Figure 17–9. TRIAL ARTICULATION. Four parts must be assembled to articulate the femoral and tibial components: standard long tibial bearing (Vitallium), an axle, two bushings, and a bumper. They are assembled as pictured in Figure 17–10. Once the prosthesis is articulated, hold the femoral components in one hand to prevent rotation, and extend the legs fully. Palpate the femoral vessels to determine the status of the pulse or evaluate the pulses at the ankle with a sterile Doppler. If the pulse is diminished, flex the knee to determine if it increases. This will indicate the need for either modifying the length of the prosthesis or for removing additional bone from the distal femur. Test the range of motion of the knee with the patella relocated. A full range of motion should be obtained. Note whether the capsular mechanism can be easily closed. These factors, taken together, will determine the adequacy of the length of the resection.

253

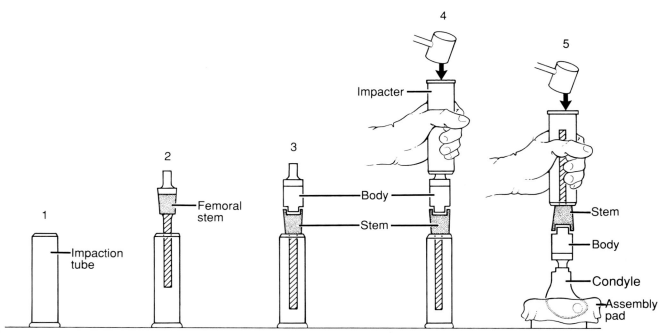

Figure 17–10.   PREPARATION, IMPLANTATION, AND ASSEMBLY OF PROSTHESIS. The femoral prosthesis consists of three components: the femoral stem segment, femoral body component, and femoral condyle segment. There are two femoral condyle components, right and left. Check the correct side and the lengths of all components *before* assembly. The three instruments necessary for the assembly/impaction are the impaction tube, impactor, and assembly pad. Before joining any of the tapers, make sure the male and female components are completely dry. The femoral body component and femoral stem segment are assembled first. The femoral stem segment is placed into the impaction tube (1,2) and the femoral body component is mated with it (3). The impaction tool is placed over the taper of the femoral body component (4) and impacted with a swift blow of the heavy mallet.

The femoral condyle component is then placed onto the distal end of the femoral body component (5). The entire prosthesis is then removed from the impaction tube and placed with the femoral condyles against the assembly pad. The impaction tool is placed over the stem against the base of the prosthesis and impacted with a swift blow. Once the prosthesis is assembled, *do not* disengage the tapers.

To implant the tibial (bearing plug) component, a cement plug is inserted at the appropriate distance. A trial tibial (bearing plug) prosthesis (polyethylene component) is inserted to ascertain the plug is placed distal. The medullary canal is irrigated and dried. Two packs of PMMA are injected with a cement gun to fill the canal and coat the undersurface of the tibial prosthesis. The prosthesis is aligned with the tibial tubercle and impacted. Excess PMMA is removed.

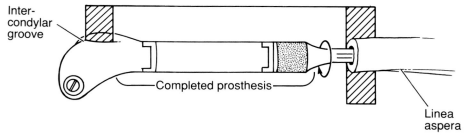

Figure 17–11.   IMPLANTATION AND ORIENTATION OF THE FEMORAL PROSTHESIS. The femoral canal is thoroughly irrigated. A cement plug is placed at the appropriate depth. This depth is checked by inserting the actual prosthesis and verifying complete seating. The femoral canal is again irrigated and dried. The soft tissues, especially those that are near the neurovascular structures, are protected and packed off with wet lap pads. Two packs of PMMA are mixed and injected into the canal to ensure complete filling of the canal. Some PMMA is then placed around the stem of the prosthesis.

The femoral prosthesis is oriented with the *linea aspera* as the guide. This is the only landmark. There is *no* guide for femoral alignment. The prosthesis is then impacted. Excess cement is removed from around the prosthesis. Care is taken to prevent cement from getting into the porous-coated section. The articulation of the actual prosthesis is identical to that of the trial structure.

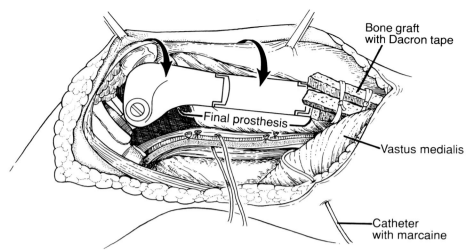

Bone graft
with Dacron tape

Final prosthesis

Vastus medialis

Catheter
with marcaine

Figure 17–12. BONE GRAFTING. This prosthesis offers the *option* of obtaining additional fixation by extracortical fixation. Bone graft is obtained from the ilium *after* the surgeons change gloves and gowns. Separate instruments must be utilized to avoid contamination of the donor site. Long iliac strips of corticocancellous grafts are placed along the porous-coated segment of the prosthesis, with overlapping of the distal 2–3 cm of the femur. The cortical surface of the femur can be roughened with a mechanical burr. The grafts are held in place with two or three Dacron tapes. Care must be taken *not* to place bone graft adjacent to the SFA.

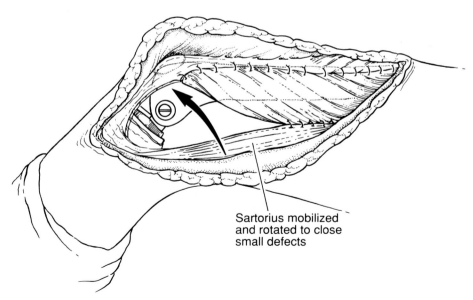

Sartorius mobilized
and rotated to close
small defects

Figure 17–13. CLOSURE OF SOFT TISSUE RECONSTRUCTION WITH MEDIAL GASTROCNEMIUS TRANSFER. It is essential to completely cover the prosthesis with soft tissue. The prosthesis should *not* be left in a subcutaneous position.

The remaining vastus medialis muscle is sutured to the rectus femoris. The sartorius muscle can be mobilized and rotated anteriorly for closure of a small remaining defect. A large defect requires a medial gastrocnemius transfer. Similarly, a lateral defect is closed with a lateral gastrocnemius transfer.[17]

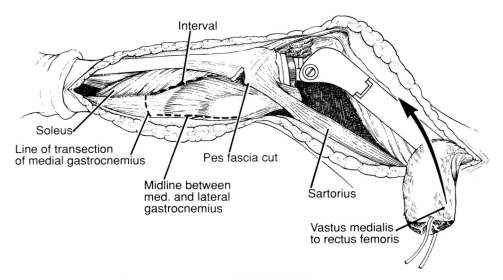

Figure 17–14. EXPOSURE OF THE MEDIAL GASTROCNEMIUS. To adequately expose the medial portion of the gastrocnemius muscle one must: 1. Increase the length of the incision distally to the level of the musculotendinous junction. 2. Create a posterior-based midline fasciocutaneous flap in order to expose the midline of the two gastrocnemius muscle bellies. 3. Expose and open the interval between the medial gastrocnemius muscle and soleus muscle by lifting the medial gastrocnemius muscle by finger dissection. Stop at the midline.

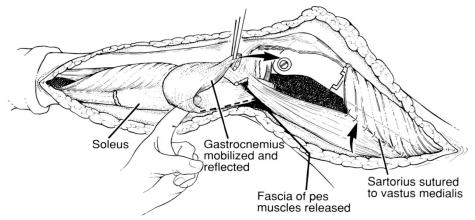

Figure 17–15. FASCIA OF PES MUSCLES RELEASED. Detach the medial portion of the musculotendinous junction and separate the two muscle bellies along the midline.

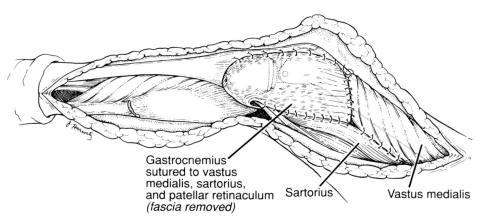

Figure 17–16. ROTATION OF THE MUSCULAR FLAP. Rotate the flap anteriorly over the prosthesis. Occasionally, the fascia of the pes musculature must be released to increase the arc of rotation. Remove the thick anterior and posterior fascia of the medial gastrocnemius in order to spread the muscle over a larger area.

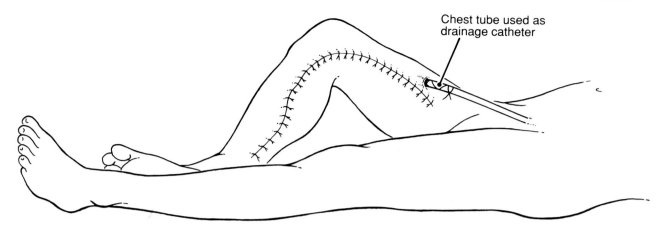

Figure 17–17. WOUND CLOSURE. A 28-gauge chest tube attached to Pleurovac suction (20 cm of water) is used. The pulses are checked following wound closure and prior to removing the patient from the table. A knee immobilizer is used.

POSTOPERATIVE MANAGEMENT

1. The extremity is kept elevated for three to five days until the wound is checked. This prevents postoperative edema, a risk to wound healing.
2. Continuous suction is required for three to five days to avoid fluid collection. This operative procedure involves a large dead space. A 28-gauge chest tube to 20 cm of suction is used.
3. Routine perioperative antibiotics are continued until drainage tubes are removed, usually within three to five days.
4. Isometric exercises are started the first postoperative day. Knee motion is not generally permitted until the wound is examined and there is adequate muscle control.
5. Muscle control is essential to prevent rotation of the prosthesis in the early postoperative period. This is a unique consideration associated with this procedure. A knee immobilizer or posterior splint is required.

DISCUSSION

The distal femur is the most common site for osteosarcoma.[18] Limb-sparing surgery is now considered the preferred treatment for the majority of patients with osteosarcoma as well as those with other high-grade sarcomas (malignant fibrous histiocytoma, fibrosarcoma, and malignant giant cell tumors).[2,3,14,19–21] Almost all low-grade sarcomas of the distal femur (especially parosteal osteosarcoma and chondrosarcoma) can be treated safely with a limb-sparing resection.

Careful preoperative planning and patient selection are crucial to a successful outcome. All patients with high-grade bone sarcomas of the distal femur should be evaluated by CT, MRI, bone scintigraphy, and biplane angiography (see indications) *before* a limb-sparing resection is undertaken. Similarly, all patients should be evaluated for a limb-sparing option *prior* to preceding with an amputation. Today, it appears that preoperative (neoadjuvant) chemotherapy has changed our indications for patient selection.[2,3,20,22,23] In a recent study, approximately three-fourths of patients considered unresectable were converted to limb-sparing procedures following induction chemotherapy utilizing two cycles of intra-arterial *cis*-platinum and continuous intravenous adriamycin.[15]

This chapter describes prosthetic replacement as the method of reconstruction of a large tumor defect. We assume a prosthesis such as that described here may have to be revised. The use of improved cement techniques, extracortical fixation, and newer metals (titanium) will, it is hoped, increase the longevity of the prosthesis. Osteoarticular allografts are favored by some surgeons.[8,16] In general, they are not recommended for patients with high-grade sarcomas requiring adjuvant chemotherapy due to the increased risk of infection. Alternatively, arthrodesis (fusion) is a reliable procedure that may last the life of the patient.[24,25] The major drawback of an arthrodesis is a stiff knee.

There are several considerations that we have found to be important in decreasing the complications of limb-sparing procedures:

1. A single medial incision allows adequate exposure for most lesions.
2. A wide exposure is necessary in order to avoid

inadvertent tumor contamination. Large fasciocutaneous flaps are required.

3. Adequate soft-tissue reconstruction is *mandatory* in order to avoid wound breakdown. A medial (occasionally, lateral) gastrocnemius transfer is required to cover the prosthesis. This has greatly decreased the problems associated with flap necrosis.[9]

4. Adequate and prolonged tube drainage of the resection site to decrease secondary wound problems is essential. We recommend the use of a 28-gauge chest tube for three to five days, along with continuous extremity elevation, to avoid flap edema and secondary necrosis.

The modular segmental replacement system, as described here, is a new design that incorporates the advantages of several different features of prosthetic design, with the goal of increasing longevity of the prosthesis.[10] The Kinematic rotating hinge component is one of the most effective means of decreasing stress on the stem and of ensuring stability.[26] It has been in use since 1981. In general, the stem is the most vulnerable site of potential prosthesis loosening and failure. Mechanical stability is required, since all soft-tissue attachments to the knee are usually removed in order to adequately resect the tumor. The hinge component provides stability, and the rotary component permits a large amount of rotation. In comparison with a straight hinge or earlier knee designs, there is significantly less stress on the bone/cement interface.

The MSRS mates this design with a modular system that permits *immediate* availability of different sizes of a prosthesis without the customary wait of six to ten weeks. In addition, the extracortical porous coating may provide additional bony fixation with the prosthesis. This may further decrease the stress on the stem and permit more physiologic cortical transmission of forces.

REFERENCES

1. Campanacci M, Bacci G, Bertoni F, et al: The treatment of osteosarcoma of the extremities: Twenty years' experience at the Instituto Orthopedico Rizzoli. *Cancer* 1981;48:1569–1581.
2. Eilber F, Morton DL, Eckardt J, et al: Limb salvage for skeletal and soft tissue sarcomas: Multidisciplinary preoperative therapy. *Cancer* 1984;53:2579–2584.
3. Eilber FR, Eckhardt J, Morton DL: Advances in the treatment of sarcomas of the extremity. Current status of limb salvage. *Cancer* 1984;54:2695–2701.
4. Kotz R, Winkler K, Salzer-Kuntchik M, et al: Surgical margins influencing oncological results in osteosarcoma, in Yamamuro T (ed): *New Developments for Limb Salvage in Musculoskeletal Tumors.* Tokyo, Springer-Verlag, 1989, pp 83–91.
5. Morton DL, Eilber FR, Townsend CM Jr, et al: Limb salvage from a multidisciplinary treatment approach for skeletal and soft tissue sarcomas of the extremity. *Ann Surg* 1976;184:268.
6. Eckardt JJ, Eilber FR, Grant TG, et al: The UCLA experience in the management of stage IIB osteosarcoma: 1972–1983, in *Limb Salvage in Musculoskeletal Oncology.* New York, Churchill Livingstone, 1987, pp 314–326.
7. Simon MA, Aschliman MA, Thomas N, et al: Limb-salvage treatment versus amputation for osteosarcoma of the distal end of the femur. *J Bone Joint Surg Am* 1986;68:1331–1337.
8. Malawer M, Priebat D, Buch R, et al: The impact of preoperative intraarterial chemotherapy on the choice of surgical procedure for high grade bone sarcomas. *Clin Orthop,* to be published.
9. Malawer MM, Link M, Donaldson S: Bone sarcomas, in DeVita VT Jr, Helman S, Rosenberg SA (eds): *Principles and Practice of Oncology,* ed 3. Philadelphia, JB Lippincott, 1989, chap 41.
10. Malawer M, McHale KA: Limb-sparing surgery for high-grade malignant tumors of the proximal tibia: Surgical technique and a method of extensor mechanism reconstruction. *Clin Orthop* 1989;239:231–248.
11. Hudson TM, Hass G, Enneking WF, et al: Angiography in the management of musculoskeletal tumors. *Surg, Gynecol Obstet* 1975;141:11–21.
12. Chuang VP, Wallace S, Benjamin RS, et al: The therapy of osteosarcoma by intra-arterial cis platinum and limb preservation. *Cardiovasc Intervent Radiol* 1981;4:229–235.
13. Kotz R, Salzer M: Rotation-plasty for childhood osteosarcoma of the distal part of the femur. *J Bone Joint Surg* 1982;64A:959.
14. Salzer M, Knahr K, Kotz R, et al: Treatment of osteosarcoma of the distal femur by rotation-plasty. *Arch Orthop Traum Surg* 1981;99:131.
15. Malawer M, Canfield D, Meller I: Porous-coated segmental prosthesis for large tumor defects. A prosthesis based upon immediate fixation (PMMA) and extracortical bone fixation, in Yamamuro T (ed): *International Symposium on Limb-Salvage in Musculoskeletal Oncology.* New York, Springer-Verlag, 1988, pp 247–255.
16. Malawer M, Meller I: Extracortical fixation of large segmental prostheses and description of a modular segmental replacement system (MSRS), in *Fifth International Symposium of Limb-Sparing Surgery.* St Malo, France, Sept 1989.
17. Malawer MM, Price WM. Gastrocnemius transposition flap in conjunction with limb-sparing surgery for primary sarcomas around the knee. *Plast Reconstruc Surg* 1984;73:741–749.
18. Dahlin DC: *Bone Tumors: General Aspects and Data on 6,221 Cases,* ed 3. Springfield, Ill, Charles C Thomas, 1978.
19. Kotz R: Possibilities of limb-preserving therapy for bone tumors today. *J Cancer Res Clin Oncol* 1983;106(Suppl):68–76.
20. Marcove RC, Rosen G: En bloc resection for osteogenic sarcoma. *Cancer* 1980;45:3040.
21. Rosen G, Marcove RD, Caparros B, et al: Primary osteogenic sarcoma. The rationale for preoperative

chemotherapy and delayed surgery. *Cancer* 1979;43: 2163–2177.

22. Huvos AG, Rosen G, Marcove RC: Primary osteogenic sarcoma. Pathologic aspects in 20 patients after treatment with chemotherapy, en bloc resection, and prosthetic bone replacement. *Arch Pathol Lab Med* 1977;101:14.

23. Winkler K, Beron G, Kotz R, et al: Neoadjuvant chemotherapy for osteogenic sarcoma: Results of a cooperative German/Austrian study. *J Clin Oncol* 1984;2:617.

24. Campanacci M, Costa P: Total resection of distal femur or proximal tibia for bone tumours. Autogenous bone grafts and arthrodesis in twenty-six cases. *J Bone Joint Surg* 1979;61B:455.

25. Enneking WF, Shirley PD: Resection-arthrodesis for malignant and potentially malignant lesions about the knee using an intramedullary rod and local bone graft. *J Bone Joint Surg Am* 1977;59:223–235.

26. Eckardt JJ, Eilber FR, Mirra JM: Kinematic rotating hinge knee-distal femoral replacement, in Enneking WF (ed): *Limb Salvage in Musculoskeletal Oncology.* New York, Churchill Livingstone, 1987, pp 392–399.

18

Below-Knee Amputation

PAUL H. SUGARBAKER, M.D.
MARTIN M. MALAWER, M.D.
ALAN R. BAKER, M.D.

OVERVIEW

Below-knee amputation is usually performed for high-grade soft tissue sarcomas of the ankle or foot. Extensive infiltration of tendons and ligaments in this area may preclude an adequate wide excision. Rarely, an osteosarcoma of the distal tibia, fibula, or ankle bones may occur and require below-knee amputation. Skin flaps for oncologic procedures are rarely standard; most heal without difficulty. Muscle and fascia should be secured by myodesis over the end of the bones. A rigid dressing and early ambulation are of great help in the rehabilitation process in most patients.

INTRODUCTION

Below-knee amputation is usually performed for malignant tumors of the ankle and foot. Fortunately, within the last two decades wide excision of the tumor in combination with radiation therapy and chemotherapy have proven to be safe and effective alternatives to amputation for patients with soft tissue tumors. Nevertheless, amputation remains a clear-cut and definitive requirement in the management of most bone and cartilage tumors and an appreciable proportion of the soft tissue sarcomas located at the ankle or in the foot (Fig. 18–1). The need to perform below-knee amputation stems from the fact that many soft tissue sarcomas infiltrate in and around the musculoskeletal structures of the foot and ankle. In these circumstances, procedures that entail a wide excision may lead to a functionless foot and ankle. Also, unless the procedure achieves clear margins of resection it will be associated with an unacceptably high rate of local recurrence.[1,2]

A major responsibility of the oncologist is to determine which patients are best served by an amputation and which patients may benefit from a limb-salvage procedure. Such decisions, especially with ankle and foot sarcomas, must be made on a case-by-case basis. All patients should be considered and evaluated for limb salvage surgery, and the decision to proceed with amputation should be made only after this option has been ruled out. Guidelines are

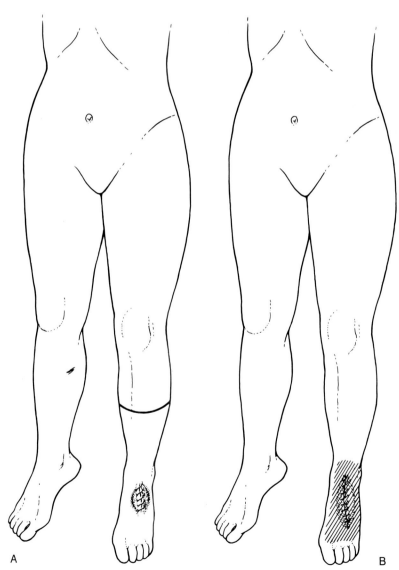

Figure 18–1.   Amputation remains the treatment option of choice in many cartilage and bone sarcomas of the ankle and foot (**A**). Most soft tissue sarcomas in this region are treated by wide local excision plus radiation therapy (**B**).

based on (1) the stage and grade of the malignancy and (2) its anatomic location.

GENERAL INDICATIONS FOR BELOW-KNEE AMPUTATIONS

Amputations in this area, as in other portions of the extremities, are performed for high-grade sarcomas that do not have a limb-salvage option, for *recurrent high-grade cancers* previously treated by a limb-sparing approach, and for recurrent low-grade tumors that lack a local excision option. Rarely will amputation be performed as the initial procedure in patients with a low-grade tumor. Rather, in those sarcomas that are unlikely to result in systemic disease, one or even several local failures are tolerated as long as local treatment options remain and function is acceptable.

The most common indication for amputation in ankle and foot sarcomas is *extensive infiltration* in the longitudinal structures that occupy this option of the anatomy. Frequently, negative margins of excision cannot be attained without extensive removal of tendons, muscles, nerves, and other tissues that provide function for the lower extremity. Yet, major vascular or nerve involvement is rarely an indication for below-knee amputation, because at this distal point on the extremity, vascular and nerve structures are widely separated by bony structure.

Not uncommonly extensive local soft tissue contamination may occur due to prior surgery, to *hematoma* developing within a biopsy site, or even from a *poorly planned biopsy. Pathologic fracture* in this area will usually result in a hematoma that spreads tumor cells widely around the ankle or foot. This will make a conservative procedure unable to achieve tumor-free margins.

Infection, usually of the tumor itself or of the biopsy site, may negate an attempt at local resection. Local infection will always seriously jeopardize the use of prosthetic materials. It may also interfere with preoperative regional chemotherapy or postoperative systemic chemotherapy.

Skeletal immaturity caused by radiation therapy is unlikely to result in a limb-length discrepancy with ankle or foot irradiation. Rather the problems with high-dose radiation therapy comes from the need to treat the heavily traumatized skin on the plantar surface of the foot or the skin around the ankle.

Ankle and foot sarcomas present a particular problem for limb-sparing surgery. Because of anatomic constraints, tumor size, and the difficulty of achieving a complication-free recovery, functional results following major resections in and around the foot

and ankle are often poorer than the below-knee amputation itself. In addition a special consideration related to wide excision and radiation therapy for the sarcomas of the foot concerns the difficulty in delivering and tolerating large doses of radiation therapy especially in the weight-bearing tissues. In contrast to the questionable long-term results with limb salvage surgery for ankle or foot sarcomas, the results with below-knee amputation are almost universally good.

CLINICAL CONSIDERATIONS FOR BELOW-KNEE AMPUTATIONS

The timing for the surgical procedure is important. Both physiological and psychological factors must be optimized. If the patient has received preoperative chemotherapy, it is essential that the quantity of leukocytes and platelets be permitted to return toward normal. Significant deficits in red blood cell mass should be corrected by preoperative transfusion. Although vascular insufficiency is rarely a complicating factor of below-knee amputation in this patient population, suboptimal wound healing may be a problem in patients who have received high-dose regional or systemic chemotherapy. Also, associated poor nutrition from nausea and vomiting induced by preoperative chemotherapy may further compound the wound-healing problem. Because of potential wound-healing difficulties, stump closure must be meticulously performed. Hematoma and seroma must be avoided by the use of adequate closed-suction drainage. One should defer removal of skin sutures for as long as possible. If unusual skin flaps or muscle resection occurred with the amputation, the stump may require additional time to mold and mature.

REHABILITATION AND EMOTIONAL SUPPORT

The cancer patient faces unique psychological problems. Not only is there a threat in the loss of a body part but also a threat to life itself. Rehabilitation of a patient undergoing a major amputation, especially a cancer patient, begins at the time of the staging studies. The entire health care team must develop an honest relationship with the patient and include him or her in the early stages of all decision making. Building upon this, the patient will be better able to accept the amputation and set realistic rehabilitation goals. All patients undergoing an amputation will experience some phantom sensation. This is minimal in patients with below-knee amputation. However, it should be discussed with the patient prior to surgery. The patient needs to understand that this is an expected phenomenon, that it can be treated with analgesics, and that it will subside in its severity over time. The patients who report severe pain are often those who find it most difficult to adapt to surgery and to the malignant process. It is important to distinguish between stump pain, which is more common in this amputation, and phantom pain, which is relatively uncommon.

Although successful rehabilitation depends to a great extent on the patient's attitude, the physiatrist can help tremendously in these efforts. A *positive attitude* toward functional recovery augmented by early or immediate postoperative ambulation and prosthesis use help patients move rapidly toward their goals. The prosthesis must often be readjusted several times before stump stability is achieved. A positive approach is amplified by contact with other patients who have successfully met some of the rehabilitative challenges. This can provide an immeasurable psychological boost to the patient. The surgical or orthopedic oncologist, rehabilitation therapists, and others involved in the postoperative care must coordinate their efforts carefully, realizing the possibility of conflicting demands on the patient's time and a different interpretation of the same clinical information presented to the patient. The entire team must not only be supportive but must also be positive about the complete rehabilitation that can be achieved following a below-knee amputation.

LEVEL OF BELOW-KNEE AMPUTATION

The longer the stump is, the better the functional result. A minimum of 5 cm is required for good function and prosthesis fitting. The fibula should always be cut shorter than the remaining tibia. The fibula head should not be removed even if this bone must be greatly shortened.

Below-knee amputation for sarcomas for the distal tibia is done at a higher level than the standard below-knee amputation and often requires modified flaps. Neoplasms in the foot and ankle, usually soft

tissue sarcomas, may be managed with the standard below-knee procedure. Below-knee amputation in young patients or adults without ischemia heal well. These patients are ideal candidates for an immediate fit prosthesis.

RADIOLOGIC STUDIES

The level for below-knee amputation in patients with osteosarcoma of the leg and distal tibia must be carefully determined. Evidence of tumor contamination of muscle or fascia and proximal extent of the intramedullary tumor must be carefully evaluated. Computerized tomography and MRI are used to determine soft tissue extension. Bone scintigraphy combined with MRI is useful in determining intraosseous extension of tumor. Prior to surgery, the nuclear medicine physician should mark the level of osseous involvement on the skin. The skin flaps utilized may often be atypical. Here, as with other amputations, the highest priority in performing the surgery is to eliminate the possibility of local recurrence. Tumors that show by radiologic studies that they are below the level of the musculotendinous junction of the gastrocnemius can generally be treated by a high below-knee amputation. In a child, almost any level of below-knee amputation is acceptable. With growth a functional stump will be obtained. Seventy percent of the growth of the tibia is from the proximal epiphysis.

ONCOLOGIC CONSIDERATIONS

A double-tourniquet technique is recommended to prevent contamination of the operative site from the tumor. A tourniquet is placed just above the tumor, but the blood is not evacuated from the extremity. A second tourniquet is placed above the knee and provides absolute hemostasis while the amputation is being performed. A cryostat section and touch prep of the marrow from the medullary canal is performed for osteosarcomas. For soft tissue sarcoma, the margins of resection should be examined by the pathologist before the amputation is completed.

PROCEDURE

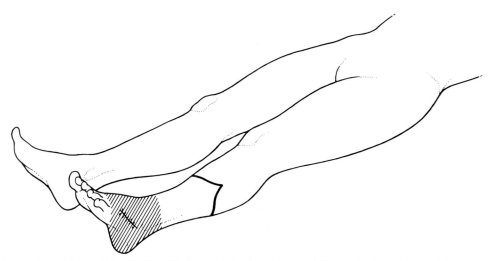

Figure 18–2.   **POSITION AND INCISION.** The skin incision is carefully marked out to provide well-vascularized and nonirradiated skin for coverage of the stump. A long posterior flap is less frequently used in amputations for cancer in order to maximize the margins of resection. Anterior, lateral, or the standard long posterior flap may be used. In the patient shown, nearly equal anterior and posterior flaps were utilized.

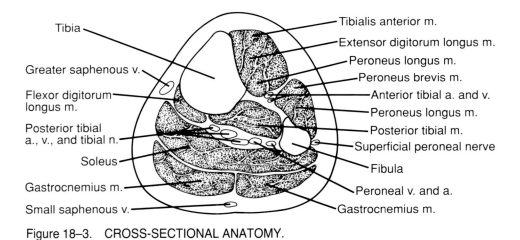

Tibia

Greater saphenous v.

Flexor digitorum longus m.

Posterior tibial a., v., and tibial n.

Soleus

Gastrocnemius m.

Small saphenous v.

Tibialis anterior m.

Extensor digitorum longus m.

Peroneus longus m.

Peroneus brevis m.

Anterior tibial a. and v.

Peroneus longus m.

Posterior tibial m.

Superficial peroneal nerve

Fibula

Peroneal v. and a.

Gastrocnemius m.

Figure 18–3.   CROSS-SECTIONAL ANATOMY.

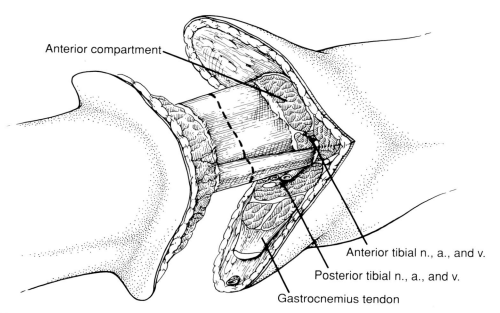

Anterior compartment

Anterior tibial n., a., and v.

Posterior tibial n., a., and v.

Gastrocnemius tendon

Figure 18–4. SOFT TISSUE DISSECTION AND BONE TRANSECTION. The skin, superficial fascia, and subcutaneous tissue are cut perpendicular to the skin surface. The muscles are transected with electrocautery or the CO_2 laser. Major vascular structures are ligated in continuity and then divided. Large vessels should be suture-ligated. Nerves are meticulously transected. They are gently pulled approximately 2 cm out of their surrounding muscle mass. They are double-ligated with a monofilament nonabsorbable suture. They are then infiltrated with a long-acting anesthetic agent prior to being meticulously transected with a knife. They are allowed to retract into the muscle mass.

The large muscles in the posterior compartment are tapered so that they can be secured over the cut ends of the bone.

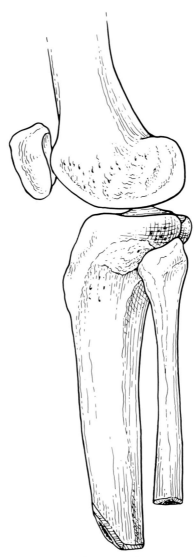

Figure 18–5.   OSTEOTOMY OF THE TIBIA AND FIBULA. The longer the stump, the better is the functional result. A minimum of 5 cm of tibia is required for good function and prosthesis fitting. An exception is the child. The tibia will continue to grow from its proximal epiphysis in the child. The fibula should always be cut shorter than the remaining tibia. The tibial edge is beveled as indicated.

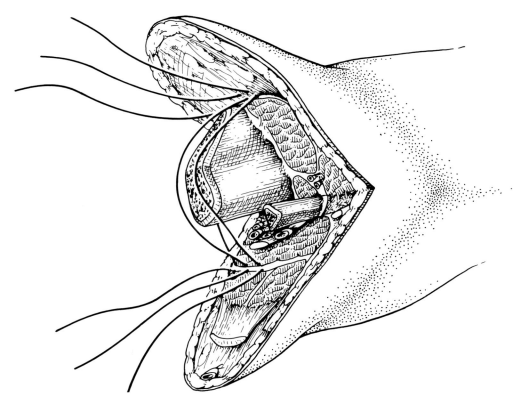

Figure 18–6.   MYODESIS AND TENODESIS OVER DISTAL TIBIA AND FIBULA. The muscle is closed in two layers over the distal tibia and fibula.

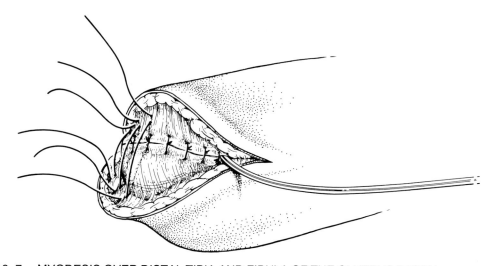

Figure 18–7.   MYODESIS OVER DISTAL TIBIA AND FIBULA OF THE GLUTEUS FASCIA.

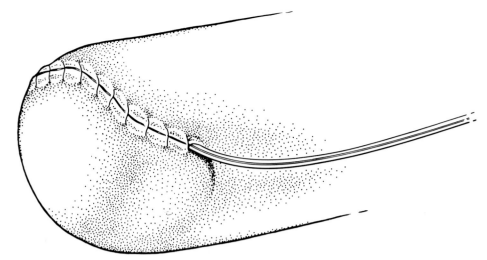

Figure 18–8.   CLOSURE OF SUPERFICIAL FASCIA AND SKIN OVER SUCTION DRAINS. It is important that the superficial fascia be closed by repeatedly dividing with the sutures the extent of the incision. This will ensure that there are no skinfolds after the closure is completed. Extensive posterior flaps can be smoothly approximated to smaller anterior flaps with uniform pleating of the posterior skin flap.

Closed-suction drains are placed on the medial and lateral aspects of the incision. These should not be sutured in place because they will be removed from beneath the rigid dressing in the first postoperative week.

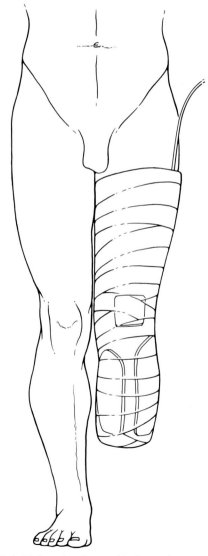

Figure 18–9.   RIGID DRESSING. A rigid dressing is used in the early postoperative period. A pylon is applied, and early ambulation is begun in most patients. Felt pads are placed longitudinally along the tibia in order to prevent skin ischemia where there is only skin over bone.

REFERENCES

1. Rosenberg SA, Kent H, Costa J, et al: Prospective randomized evaluation of the role of limb-sparing surgery, radiation therapy, and adjuvant chemoimmunotherapy in the treatment of adult soft-tissue sarcomas. *Surgery* 1978;84:62–69.

2. Rosenberg SA, Tepper J, Glastein E, et al: Prospective randomized evaluation of adjuvant chemotherapy in adults with soft tissue sarcomas of the extremities. *Cancer* 1983;52:424–434.

19

Limb-Sparing Surgery for Malignant Tumors of the Proximal Tibia

MARTIN M. MALAWER, M.D.

OVERVIEW

Resection of the proximal tibia is a limb-sparing option for low-grade bony sarcomas and carefully selected high-grade sarcomas (eg, osteosarcoma) arising from the proximal tibia. In the past, several unique surgical and technical problems prevented successful limb-sparing surgery for tumors at this site. These included anatomic constraints, a difficult surgical approach, inadequate soft tissue coverage, vascular complications, and the need to reconstruct the patellar/extensor mechanism. Most surgeons have traditionally recommended above-knee amputation for these lesions. The limb-sparing technique illustrated here allows a safe approach to the dissection of popliteal vessels and resection plus replacement of the proximal one half to two thirds of the tibia. Preoperative evaluation of tumor extent requires a detailed understanding of the anatomy and careful evaluation by computerized axial tomography, magnetic resonance imaging, bone scintigraphy, and biplane angiography. The major contraindications to this procedure are a pathologic fracture, neurovascular involvement, and/or contamination from a poorly positioned biopsy. One half to two thirds of the tibia is removed, along with a portion of all muscles inserting on the tibia and the entire popliteus muscle, in combination with an extra-articular resection of the proximal tibiofibular joint. The peroneal nerve is preserved. A primary arthrodesis, prosthetic replacement, or allograft replacement is performed following resection. One key to success of this procedure is the use of a gastrocnemius muscle transfer to obtain reliable soft tissue coverage that helps prevent skin flap necrosis and secondary infections, and provides for extensor mechanism reconstruction. Most patients with low-grade sarcomas and approximately one half of all those with high-grade sarcomas of the proximal tibia can be treated by a limb-sparing resection.

INTRODUCTION

The proximal tibia is the second most common site for primary bony sarcomas.[1] Despite advances in limb-sparing techniques, this anatomic site remains a difficult area in which to perform a safe limb-sparing resection that preserves function. This is due to several unique surgical problems and the difficulty of reconstruction. There have been only a few reports of limb-sparing resections for high-grade bony sarcomas of the proximal tibia.[2–6] Most surgeons still recommend above-knee amputations. This contrasts markedly to the good results, widespread acceptance, and varied techniques for limb-sparing resections of bony sarcomas of the distal femur, the most common site for primary bony sarcomas.[3,7–9] Most proximal tibia resections reported to date have been for giant cell tumors and low-grade sarcomas, especially chondrosarcomas.[5,10–12]

The difficulty in performing a successful resection for a high-grade sarcoma of the tibia arises from surgical problems related to the local anatomy rather than to any inherent properties of the tumor. In fact, persons with osteosarcomas of the proximal tibia have a higher survival rate than those with tumors of the distal femur.[13–15] The surgical and technical problems include intimate anatomic relationships, a difficult surgical approach, inadequate soft tissue coverage, and possible vascular complications. In addition, unique to an arthroplasty of the proximal tibia is the need to reconstruct the patellar tendon (extensor mechanism). Finally, one must deal with a second adjacent joint, the proximal tibiofibular joint. These difficulties have often led to a high rate of early postoperative complications, foremost among which is failure of reconstruction. These difficulties resulted in a poor functional outcome.

This chapter describes a technique developed over a ten-year time span that permits safe and easy access to the popliteal vessels, resection and replacement of a large segment of the tibia and knee joints, a method of patellar/extensor mechanism reconstruction and soft-tissue coverage that utilizes a transferred gastrocnemius muscle. The unique anatomic considerations are emphasized as well as the staging studies that are necessary to determine resectability.[6,16–18]

INDICATIONS

Indications for proximal tibia resections include low-grade bony sarcomas (usually chondrosarcomas), recurrent aggressive benign tumors (especially giant cell tumors), and carefully selected high-grade sarcomas.[4,5,11,12] The most common high-grade bony sarcoma is osteosarcoma; malignant fibrous histiocytoma and fibrosarcoma are less common.[6,16] Round cell sarcomas (eg, Ewing's sarcoma of bone) are usually not treated by resection but by a combination of radiation and chemotherapy. Selection of patients for resection is based on a complete and careful evaluation of the local tumor extent, placement of any previous biopsy sites, and the patient's functional demands. Careful preoperative assessment must evaluate the length of bone resection (usually not more than one half to two thirds of the tibia) that would be required; the degree of soft tissue, capsular, and patellar tendon involvement; and the tumor-free status of the popliteal trifurcation. Absolute contraindications to resection include a pathologic fracture, extensive contamination from a poorly positioned biopsy, tumor penetration through the skin, and local sepsis. Relative contraindications include a large posterior extraosseous component or immature skeletal age. Recently, expandable prostheses have been used in younger patients in the hope of avoiding an amputation because of leg-length discrepancy.

STAGING STUDIES

Detailed radiographic analysis is necessary before surgery in order to determine the local tumor extent. The following studies are required:

Bone scintigraphy is done to rule out skip lesions and to determine the extent of local intraosseous tumor. The site of resection is 5–6 cm distal to the area of abnormality. For resections, a minimum of one third of the remaining distal tibia must appear normal.

Computerized axial tomography (CAT) is useful to determine intraosseous as well as extraosseous extension of the primary tumor. Attention is paid to the possibility of posterior extension and tibiofibular joint and intra-articular knee involvement. *MRI* is most helpful in determining intraosseous extent, skip lesions, and soft tissue extension.

Biplane angiography is essential and is used for local arterial evaluation, especially if CAT has revealed posterior soft tissue extension. The anterior-posterior view is used to evaluate the popliteal trifurcation; of particular relevance is the presence or absence of the posterior tibial artery, which may be the sole blood supply to the leg after resection. The lateral view is required to evaluate the interval between the tibia and the neurovascular bundle (Fig. 19–1). The popliteus muscle often separates a posterior tumor mass from the vessels.[2,19] This is seen as a clear interval on the lateral angiogram and is an indication that an adequate resection margin exists.

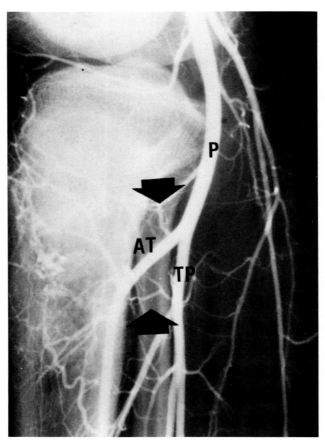

Figure 19–1.   Angiogram showing lateral view of the popliteal artery. The space between tumor in the head of the tibia and the popliteal trifurcation is best appreciated by this study. The popliteal artery (P), tibioperoneal trunk (TP), and anterior tibial (AT) arteries are all visualized. It is essential that the soft tissue posterior to the tumor mass (between arrows) be free of cancer along the popliteal artery and tibioperoneal trunk. The popliteus muscle covers the bone in this interval and usually protects the vessels from tumor invasion.

Biopsy

Extreme caution must be taken to minimize contamination when the biopsy is performed. The biopsy site must be placed along the line of the definitive incision, ie, the anteromedial aspect of the tibia. It is important to avoid contamination of the anterior muscles, the peroneal nerve, the patella tendon, and the knee joint. A small core biopsy of the extraosseous tumor component is optimal. There is no need to open the cortex unless no extraosseous component is easily accessible. If the cortex must be opened, a tourniquet is used to decrease local contamination, and the cortical window is plugged with a small amount of polymethyl methacrylate (PMMA).

PROCEDURE

The limb-sparing procedure has three phases: (1) resection of the tumor, (2) skeletal reconstruction (arthrodesis or prosthetic replacement), and (3) muscle transfer and soft tissue reconstruction using the medial gastrocnemius muscle.

Resection of the Tumor

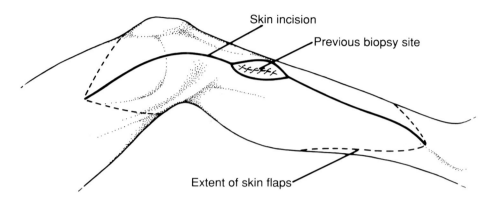

Figure 19–2. INCISION. A single anteromedial incision is made, beginning proximally at the distal one third of the femur and continuing to the distal one third of the tibia. The approach includes excision of biopsy sites with at least a 2-cm margin. Medial and lateral flaps of skin and subcutaneous tissue are developed. Uninvolved flaps are raised with the underlying fascia to decrease flap ischemia.

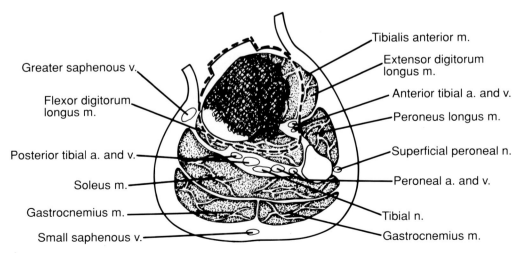

Figure 19–3. CROSS-SECTION OF THE LEG THROUGH THE PROXIMAL TIBIA SHOWING THE PLANES OF DISSECTION.

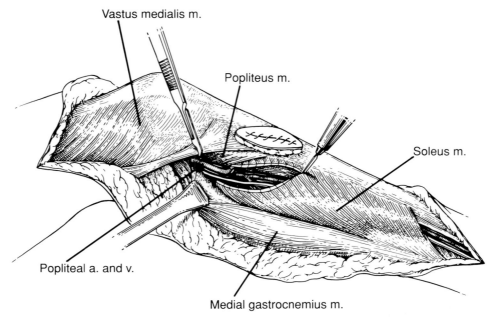

Vastus medialis m.

Popliteus m.

Soleus m.

Popliteal a. and v.

Medial gastrocnemius m.

Figure 19–4. EXPLORATION OF POPLITEAL ARTERY TRIFURCATION. Careful exploration of the popliteal fossa is needed to determine resectability. The medial flap is continued posteriorly, and the medial hamstrings are released at 2–3 cm proximal to their insertion to expose the popliteal fossa. The popliteal vessels are identified, and the trifurcation is initially explored through the medial approach. The medial gastrocnemius is partially mobilized, and the soleus muscle is split to expose the neurovascular structures. Care is taken to preserve the medial sural artery, which is the main pedicle to the medial gastrocnemius muscle. If the interval between the posterior aspect of the tibia and the tibioperoneal trunk (separated by popliteus muscle) is free of tumor, resection can proceed.

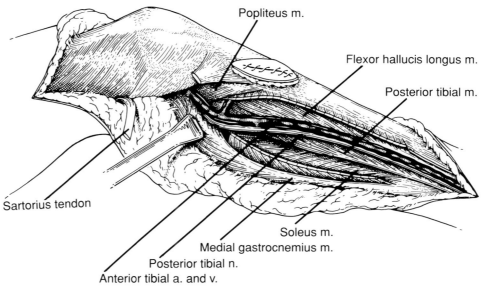

Popliteus m.

Flexor hallucis longus m.

Posterior tibial m.

Sartorius tendon

Soleus m.

Medial gastrocnemius m.

Posterior tibial n.

Anterior tibial a. and v.

Figure 19–5. DISSECTION AND EXPOSURE OF THE NEUROVASCULAR BUNDLE. Identification and mobilization of the major vessels are often difficult because the tumor has distorted the normal anatomy. Care should be taken to identify all major vascular branches to any ligation. The anterior tibial artery, which is the first takeoff of the popliteal artery, is located at the inferior border of the popliteus muscle. As it passes directly anterior through the interosseous membrane, this artery ties down the entire neurovascular bundle.

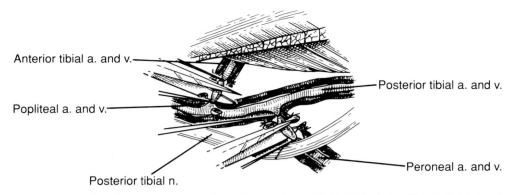

Anterior tibial a. and v.

Popliteal a. and v.

Posterior tibial a. and v.

Peroneal a. and v.

Posterior tibial n.

Figure 19–6. LIGATION OF THE ANTERIOR TIBIAL AND PERONEAL ARTERY AND VEIN. Applying posterior traction proximal to the popliteal artery permits visualization of the takeoff of the anterior tibial artery and its accompanying veins. The anterior tibial vessels are individually ligated, allowing the entire neurovascular bundle to fall away from the posterior aspect of the tibia and/or tumor. If the mass is large, the peroneal artery must occasionally also be ligated.

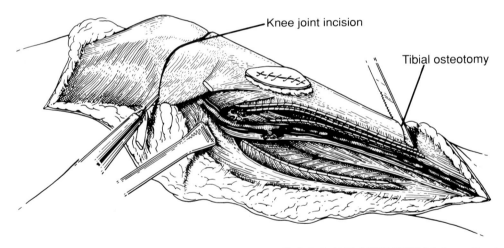

Knee joint incision

Tibial osteotomy

Figure 19–7. KNEE JOINT EXPLORATION, CAPSULAR INCISION, AND OSTEOTOMY. A small arthrotomy is performed. The meniscus and cruciate ligament are carefully evaluated. If there is no evidence of hemarthrosis (indicating tumor contamination) or direct tumor extension, an intra-articular resection is performed. The patellar tendon is sectioned 1–2 cm proximal to the tibial tubercle, and the entire capsule of the knee is detached circumferentially by electrocautery 1–2 cm from the tibial insertion. The posterior capsule is dissected carefully under direct vision after the popliteal vessels have been mobilized by ligation of the inferior geniculate vessels. The cruciate ligaments are sectioned close to the femoral attachments, and frozen sections of the proximal stumps are obtained. The capsular excision is done to the distal tibial osteotomy.

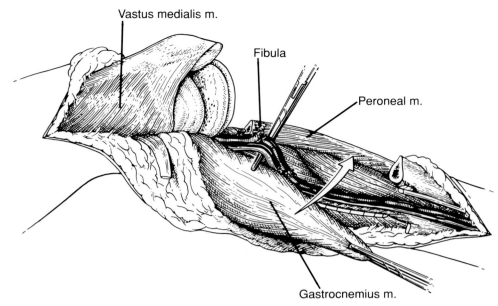

Vastus medialis m.

Fibula

Peroneal m.

Gastrocnemius m.

Figure 19–8. EXPOSURE OF THE PERONEAL NERVE AND RESECTION OF THE TIBIOFIBULAR JOINT.
A portion of the anterior tibialis muscle is routinely removed along with the tibia. The remaining anterior
compartment muscles are preserved. Care must be taken to protect the branches of the peroneal nerve that
enervate the anterior muscles. Posteriorly, a portion of the soleus origin and the entire popliteus muscle are left
on the tibia.

The peroneal nerve is identified proximal to the fibular head and below the fascia of the biceps tendon. The
biceps is transected 2 cm proximal from insertion. The peroneal nerve is freed from the proximal fibula, and the
fibula is osteomized approximately 6–8 cm from its head. An extra-articular resection of the proximal tibiofibular
joint is routinely performed. A sleeve of muscle is left on the joint in order to avoid inadvertent contamination by
tumor. Again it should be emphasized that care should be taken not to place tension on the peroneal nerve.

Finally, to release the specimen, the tibia is osteomized 5–6 cm distal to the lesion, as determined by bone
scintigraphy, MRI, and CAT. The intermuscular septum is released under direct vision. An intra-articular
resection of the knee joint is then completed. (From Malawer and McHale.[17] Reprinted with permission.)

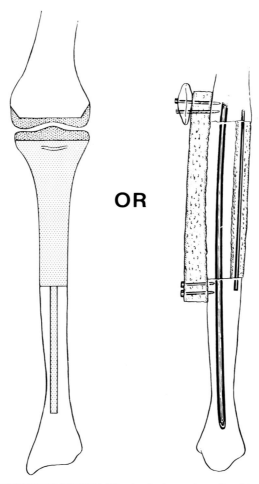

OR

Figure 19–9. **SKELETAL RECONSTRUCTION.** The technique described by Enneking et al[4,5] is used for arthrodesis. Cancellous bone from the femoral condyles is used as graft around all host/graft junctions. The ipsilateral fibula is used for reconstruction.

To complete the arthroplasty the bone ends are reamed with flexible reamers and prepared for a custom-made prosthesis. The components are then cemented into place. (From Malawer and McHale.[17] Reprinted with permission.)

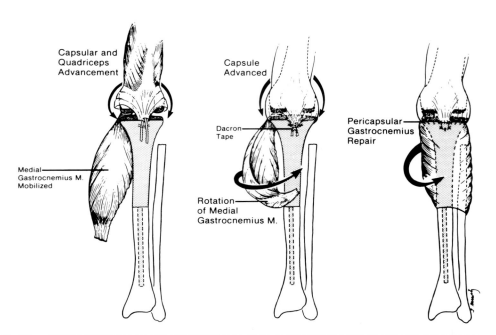

Figure 19–10.   SOFT TISSUE RECONSTRUCTION AND GASTROCNEMIUS TRANSPOSITION. Irrespective of the type of skeletal reconstruction, a medial gastrocnemius transposition flap (GTF) is used in all cases to provide adequate soft tissue coverage.[20] The medial sural artery was carefully preserved to the medial gastrocnemius muscle. The muscle graft is spread out, rotated anteriorly over the defect, and sutured to the border of the anterior muscles, forming a complete soft tissue envelope around the prosthesis. Dacron tapes sewn into the patellar tendon are tied to a highly polished loop on the prosthetic tibia.

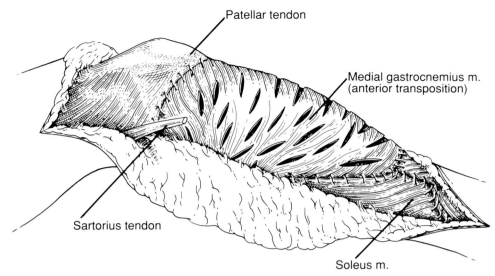

Figure 19–11. MUSCULAR CLOSURE. The patellar tendon and anterior capsule are advanced and sutured to the transferred GTF with nonabsorbable sutures. The proper tension on the quadriceps mechanism is determined by bending the knee through a 30°–40° range of motion. The medial hamstrings are reattached to the transferred medial gastrocnemius muscle. If possible, the soft tissue posterior to the prosthesis or arthrodesis should be closed to avoid direct contact of the neurovascular bundle with metal or allograft. At the level of the knee joint, the origins of the gastrocnemius heads are approximated; more distally, fibers of the posterior tibialis muscle and/or soleus are approximated.

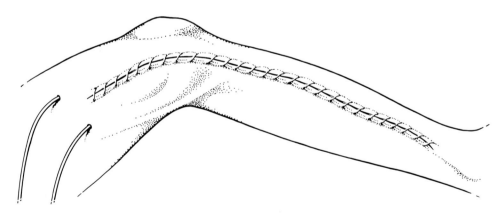

Figure 19–12. CLOSURE OF SUPERFICIAL FASCIA AND SKIN.

POSTOPERATIVE MANAGEMENT

Large closed-suction drains are utilized to prevent hematoma. The extremity is elevated five to ten days to prevent edema of the flaps. If the flaps develop areas of ischemia, they are allowed to demarcate and are excised at about ten days after surgery, and the underlying muscle is covered with a split-thickness skin graft. Patients with knee fusions are placed in a long-leg cast until there is radiographic evidence of bone healing, usually within three to four months. The patients are then fitted for a long-leg brace, which is worn for approximately a year. Patients with arthroplasty are immobilized for three weeks in a long-leg cast to permit healing of the extensor mechanism to the gastrocnemius transfer. A long-leg brace with the knee restricted to 0°–30° is then fitted. Rehabilitation emphasizes extensor strength rather than flexion. Knee flexion is increased only after full active extension has been obtained.

DISCUSSION

In general, patients with proximal tibial osteosarcoma have an overall higher survival rate than those with femoral tumors, probably because the former are smaller and are generally detected earlier.[13–15] Fortunately, most proximal tibial sarcomas tend to be smaller and have less of an extraosseous component than such lesions have in other locations. Posterior extension and vascular involvement are rare; when extension does occur, the popliteus muscle often acts as a barrier to involvement of the popliteal and tibioperoneal arteries.[19]

Since 1978, 11 of 21 patients presenting with sarcomas of the proximal tibia at our institution have undergone limb-sparing resection. The remainder underwent an above-knee amputation, the majority of which were performed prior to 1980. The technique and surgical approach described here are reliable and have decreased the previously high complication rates. They permit a choice of reconstructive procedures (ie, an arthrodesis or a prosthetic or allograft replacement). Contraindications to resection have generally included sepsis or local contamination, significant posterior tumor extension, and/or the absence of a posterior tibial artery. We believe that patients with tibial sarcomas should be considered as potential candidates for limb-sparing procedures and should undergo appropriate staging studies to determine resectability before amputation is performed.

Accurate radiographic studies are required for patient selection. Biplane radiography and angiography in conjunction with CAT, MRI, and bone scintigraphy accurately depict local tumor extent. Angiography is particularly helpful in this anatomic location, where anomalies and vascular distortion make dissection difficult. Because the tibiofibular joint is at high risk for microscopic capsular involvement, we routinely perform an extra-articular resection and do not rely upon imaging studies for that determination.

The location and technique of the biopsy are major determinants of outcome of a limb-sparing resection, especially in this location. This point cannot be overemphasized. It is essential to avoid contamination of the anterolateral muscles, peroneal nerve, popliteal space, and knee joint. To minimize contamination, we recommend a small core biopsy of the medial flare of the tibia that is in line with the definitive incision.

The technique of quadriceps reconstruction as described here has proven to be a reliable method of soft tissue coverage and reconstruction of the extensor/patellar mechanism.[6,16,21] Reconstructing

this mechanism has heretofore been one of the major barriers to a successful outcome of an arthroplasty. Several techniques of extensor mechanism reconstruction have been attempted, including direct suture to the prosthesis or allograft and osteotomy of the fibula with attachment to the lateral collateral ligament.[22] The muscle transfer technique described in this chapter uses muscle-to-muscle attachment to provide two important functions: it covers the prosthesis, which reduces the possibility of secondary infections, and provides a means for reconstruction of the extensor mechanism.

Following proximal tibial resections, intensive rehabilitation of the quadriceps is necessary. The postoperative rehabilitation following an arthroplasty of the proximal tibia is almost the opposite from that following a distal femoral arthroplasty. The aim is to avoid an extensor lag; thus, the patient is placed in a cast for three weeks to permit healing of the extensor mechanism to the transferred gastrocnemius. Immediate postoperative motion must be avoided. Active flexion exercises do not begin until extension is obtained.

REFERENCES

1. Dahlin DC: *Bone Tumors: General Aspects and Data on 6,221 Cases*, ed 3, Springfield, Ill, Charles C Thomas, 1978.
2. Campanacci M, Costa P: Total resection of distal femur or proximal tibia for bone tumors. *J Bone Joint Surg* 1979;61B:445–463.
3. Eilber FR: Limb salvage for high grade sarcomas: UCLA experience. Presented at the NIH Consensus Development Conference, Limb-Sparing Treatment, Adult Soft-Tissue and Osteogenic Sarcomas, Bethesda, Maryland, Dec 3–5, 1984.
4. Enneking WF, Eady IL, Burchardt H: Autogenous cortical bone grafts in the reconstruction of segmental skeletal defects: *J Bone Joint Surg* 1980;62A:1039–1058.
5. Enneking WF, Shirley PD: Resection arthrodesis for malignant and potentially malignant lesions about the knee using intramedullary rod and local bone grafts: *J Bone Joint Surg* 59A:223–236.
6. Malawer MM, McHale KC: Limb-sparing surgery for high-grade malignant tumors of the proximal tibia, abstract. Fourth International Symposium on Limb Salvage in Musculoskeletal Oncology, Kyoto, Japan, Oct 28–31, 1987.
7. Eckhardt JJ, Eilber FR, Grant TT, et al: Management of stage IIB osteogenic sarcoma: Experience at the University of California, Los Angeles. *Cancer Treat Symp* 1985;3:117–130.
8. NIH Consensus Development Conference on Limb-Sparing Treatment of Adult Soft-Tissue Sarcomas and Osteosarcomas. *Cancer Treat Symp* 3:1985.
9. Sim FH, Chao EYS: Prosthetic replacement of the knee and a large segment of the femur or tibia. *J Bone Joint Surg* 1979;61A:887–891.

10. Blouth W, Schuchardt E: Resection arthrodesis in bone tumors located near the knee joint (German). *Zeitschrift Orthop* 1976;114:931–935.
11. Dunham WK, Calhoun JC: Resection arthrodesis of the knee for sarcoma. Preliminary results. *Orthopedics* 1984;7:1810–1818.
12. Jenson JS: Resection arthroplasty of the proximal tibia. *Acta Orthop Scand* 1983;54:126–130.
13. Ivins JC, Taylor WF, Golenzer H: A multi-institutional cooperative study of osteosarcoma: Partial report with emphasis on survival after limb salvage, abstracts. Fourth International Symposium on Limb Salvage in Musculoskeletal Oncology, Kyoto, Japan, Oct 28–31, 1987.
14. Larson SE, Lorentzon R, Wedron H, et al: The prognosis in osteosarcoma. *Inter Orthop* 1981;5:305–310.
15. Lockshin MD, Higgins TT: Prognosis in osteogenic sarcoma. *Clin Orthop* 1968;58:85–101.
16. Malawer MM: The use of the gastrocnemius transposition flap with limb-sparing surgery for knee sarcomas: Indications and technique. Presented at the Second International Workshop on the Design and Application of Tumor Prostheses for Bone and Joint Reconstruction, Vienna, Sept 5–8, 1983.
17. Malawer MM, McHale KC: Limb-sparing surgery for high-grade tumors of the proximal tibia: Surgical technique and a method of extensor mechanism reconstruction. *Clin Orthop Rel Res* 1989;239:231–248.
18. Malawer MM, Link M, Donaldson S: Sarcomas of bone, in DeVita VT, Helman S, Rosenberg SA (eds): *Cancer: Principles and Practice of Oncology*, ed 3. Philadelphia, JB Lippincott, 1989, chap 41.
19. Hudson TM, Springfield DS, Schiebler M: Popliteus muscle as a barrier of tumor spread: Computer tomography and angiography. *J Comput Assist Tomogr* 1985;8:498–501.
20. Malawer MM, Price WM: Gastrocnemius transposition flap in conjunction with limb-sparing surgery for primary bone sarcoma around the knee. *Plas Reconstr Surg* 1984;73:741–750.
21. Malawer MM, Abelson HT, Suit HD: Bone sarcomas, in DeVita VT (ed): *Cancer: Principles and Practice of Oncology*. Philadelphia, JB Lippincott, 1984, chap 37.
22. Kotz R: Possibilities and limitations of limb-preserving therapy for bone tumors today. *J Cancer Res Clin Oncol* 1983;106:68–76.

20

Adductor Muscle Group Excision

PAUL H. SUGARBAKER, M.D.

OVERVIEW

The adductor muscle group excision is performed for malignant tumors that are confined to the medial compartment of the thigh. A longitudinal incision is used to include the previous biopsy site. After dissecting the superficial femoral artery and vein free, the saphenous vein and inguinal lymphatics are preserved if they are not directly involved by cancer. The profunda femoris artery and vein are ligated with an attempt to spare the medial circumflex femoral artery. The adductor muscles are severed from their origin on the pelvic bone, but the external oblique muscle and quadratus femoris muscle, which may be inadvertently traumatized, are spared. After Hunter's canal is opened, the tendinous insertion of the adductor muscles are severed. The subcutaneous tissue and skin are meticulously closed over generous suction drainage.

INTRODUCTION

A successful treatment plan for extremity soft tissue sarcoma must employ sound management principles based on natural history of this disease.[1-5] As a group, soft tissue sarcomas progress locally by extension along fascial planes. In addition, they are known to perforate the surrounding connective tissue (called a "pseudocapsule") and develop microfoci of disease well beyond the grossly apparent tumor mass. This pattern of growth necessitates treatment of the entire anatomic structure from which the primary tumor originates. For example, involvement of a single muscle group requires a tumor-destructive treatment, but not necessarily surgical removal of the involved muscles, from origin to insertion; to ensure adequate margins, at least one intact anatomic plane surrounding the tumor mass must be treated.

For patients with soft tissue sarcoma of the medial thigh, these principles of management have been maintained to varying degrees by three different treatment plans. The standard of treatment by which all other modalities must be evaluated is radical amputation of the thigh and hemipelvis. Often reserved for patients with advanced disease, this approach has produced five-year survival rates of 40%.[6-8] Local recurrences as low as 2% may be obtained with adequate resection performed above the joint proximal to the tumor. Another strictly surgical approach for selected soft tissue sarcomas of the medial thigh is a muscle group excision.[9] Enneking and co-workers have reported local recurrence rates of 25% and distant metastases in 50% of selected patients treated with this type of surgery.

More recently, a multimodality approach to extremity sarcomas has been advocated.[10] In this approach, a wide local surgical excision of the primary tumor is followed by high-dose large-field radiation therapy. Suit and his co-workers[11] treated 57 patients by using only local excision and radical radiotherapy, with results comparable to radical surgery alone. Other work has supported the usefulness of radiation as an adjunct to surgical therapy.[12-15]

The adductor muscle group excision may be used without postoperative radiation therapy in selected sarcomas of the medial thigh. If tumor is contained by the muscles excised from origin to insertion, few failures of local control are expected. However, postoperative irradiation is recommended if the margins of excision are not completely adequate, if tumor spillage occurs during dissection, or if hematoma occurring with the biopsy is found beyond the excised specimen.

A review of the experience with adductor muscle group excision for soft tissue sarcoma at the National Cancer Institute showed high postoperative morbidity.[16] Prolonged suction catheter drainage in several patients led to infection, a protracted hospital convalescence, and a significant delay in the initiation of adjunctive radiation therapy.

If the combination of prolonged drainage and infection occurred, it resulted in an extended hospital convalescence. The clinical review revealed a strong association between lymph node dissection and a complicated postoperative course. As shown in Table 20–1, in the patients with uncomplicated postoperative courses, none had nodal dissections. In contrast, seven of eight patients with complicated postoperative course had lymph node dissections. Indication for removal of inguinal lymph nodes was generally their proximity to the primary sarcoma; in no instance did the tumor involve these nodes. Chi-square analysis showed the association of lymph node dissection and a complicated postoperative course to be significant ($P \le .01$). Lymphatic return from the extremity will be disrupted by the dissection. The only indication for removal of the inguinal nodes is their direct involvement by tumor.

Table 20–1. Postoperative Complications without and with Inguinal Node Dissection*

STATUS	INGUINAL LYMPH NODES SPARED	INGUINAL LYMPH NODES REMOVED
No complications	4	0
Complications†	1	7

*From Mentzer SJ, Sugarbaker PH.[16]
†Prolonged suction drainage and wound infection.
Chi-square analysis: $P < .01$.

PROCEDURE

As a result of these studies, we recommend that the surgical technique of an adductor muscle group excision proceed as shown in the following illustrations. In the revised procedure, the lymphatic drainage of the lower extremity is spared as completely as possible while the best principles of sarcoma surgery are maintained.

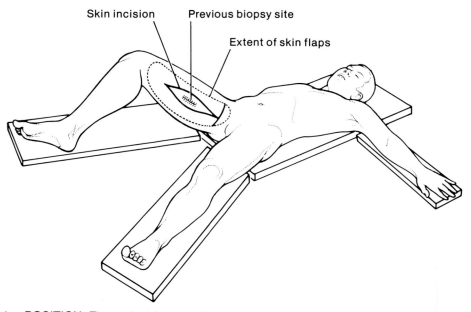

Figure 20–1. POSITION. The patient is placed on an exenteration table. The incision must be generous, extending from the pubic tubercle to the area of the medial epicondyle of the tibia. If a previous biopsy site is present, this must be widely excised and included in the operative specimen. A T of the incision along the superior and inferior pubic rami may be needed if the tumor is large or in the upper portion of the adductor muscles. Skin flaps are raised laterally to the sartorius and medially to the flexor muscles. The extent of these flaps is shown by dashed lines. The knee is slightly flexed and partially abducted during the dissection.

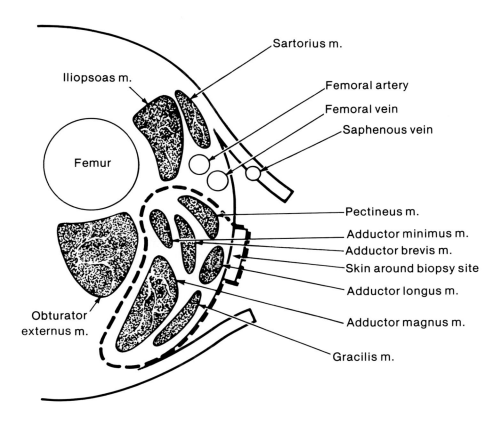

Figure 20–2. CROSS SECTION OF THE FEMORAL TRIANGLE. The femoral triangle overlies the pectineus and other adductor muscles. Unless special care is taken to preserve the lymphatic structures and saphenous vein within the femoral triangle, a majority of the lymphatic return from the extremity will be disrupted by the dissection. The only indication for removal of the inguinal nodes is their direct involvement by tumor.

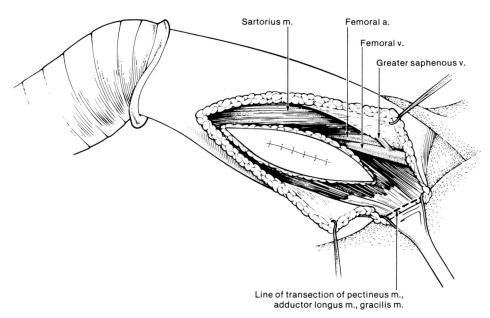

Figure 20–3. CONSTRUCTION OF THE SKIN FLAPS. Proximally the superior skin flap is dissected free of the superior pubic ramus. Its lateral extent is to the iliopsoas muscle, the femoral vein, and the sartorius muscle. The inferior skin flap is dissected back to the flexor muscles.

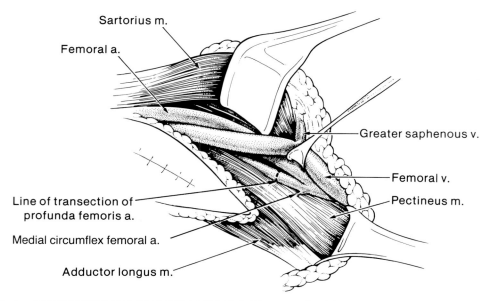

Figure 20–4. DISSECTION OF FEMORAL VESSELS. The superficial femoral artery is dissected free of the adductor muscles from the superior pubic ramus to the area of Hunter's canal. If the margin of resection around the tumor is close to these vessels, they should be dissected clean. If the margin is more adequate, some loose areolar tissue and the lymphatic channels on the vessels should be preserved. The profunda femoris vessels are ligated and divided below the origin of the medial circumflex femoral vessels.

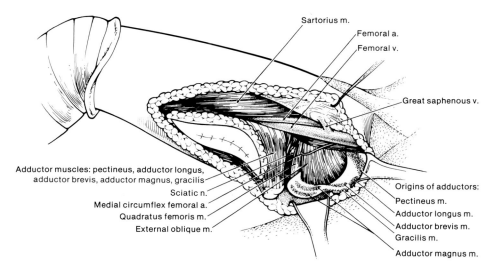

Figure 20–5. RELEASE OF ADDUCTOR MUSCLES FROM PUBIC RAMI. The dissection proceeds from superior to inferior. Superiorly, starting with the pectineus, the adductor muscles are released from their origins on the pubic rami. Care is taken to preserve the obturator externus muscle, which with the pelvic bones forms the proximal limits of the dissection. The origins of the flexor muscles and the quadratus femoris muscle are left intact on the ischial tuberosity.

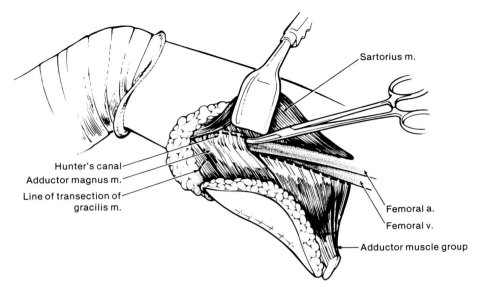

Figure 20–6. DIVISION OF THE INSERTIONS OF THE ADDUCTOR MUSCLES. The insertions of the adductor muscles are transected from the shaft of the femur. The insertions of the adductor magnus and the gracilis are divided at Hunter's canal as they cross over the superficial femoral artery.

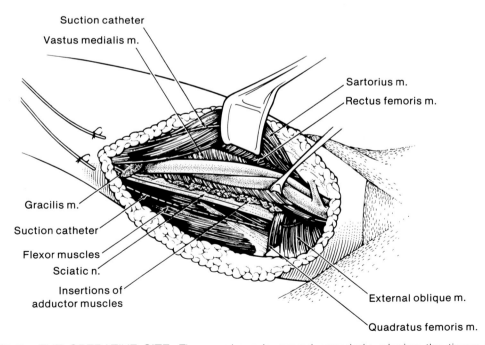

Figure 20–7. THE OPERATIVE SITE. The specimen is moved superiorly, placing the tissue between adductor muscles and flexor muscles under tension. By sharp and blunt dissection the adductor muscle group is released from the flexor muscles and sciatic nerve. When this is completed, the specimen may be removed. It is carefully marked and then oriented for the pathologist so that the margins of excision can be assessed histopathologically. The operative site is copiously irrigated, and any bleeding points are secured. The margins of the dissection are marked by metal clips.

287

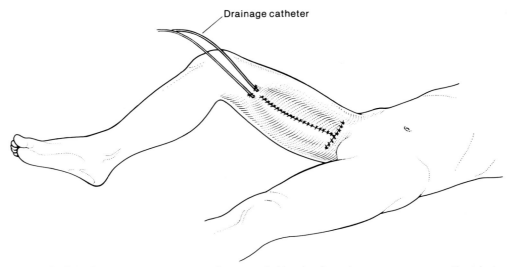

Figure 20–8. CLOSURE. The subcutaneous tissue and skin are closed over generous suction drainage.

DISCUSSION

Excision of regional lymph nodes is not indicated in an adductor muscle group excision unless there is direct involvement by tumor. Their excision does little or nothing to improve the probability for long-term survival, but it does substantially increase the morbidity of the procedure. Reviews of the incidence of sarcoma metastases show that regional lymph node involvement with tumor occurs infrequently.[17–27] Occasionally, patients with rhabdomyosarcoma or synovial cell sarcoma will metastasize to regional lymph nodes; however, nodal disease occurs in only about 20% of these patients.[27,28] In the majority of histologic subtypes, lymph node metastases occur much less frequently. The overall frequency of nodal disease is approximately 8% to 10%.

In general, lymph node metastases are a very poor prognostic sign. An ultimate fatal course of the patient's disease is unlikely to be affected by lymph node dissection (Table 20–1).

An exception to this observation may be the occurrence of primary nodal disease in childhood rhabdomyosarcomas. Suit and associates,[26] Mauer and associates,[22] and Lawrence and associates report that 17% to 25% of children with rhabdomyosarcoma have isolated lymph node disease. The implication of these observations on survival is not yet clear.[29]

Undertaking the treatment of an extremity sarcoma involves consultation with the radiation therapist prior to surgery. The radiation ports that are planned for the tumor must be known so that the incision and dissection do not extend beyond the field. For example, with sarcoma of the adductor muscle group that is to receive postoperative radiation therapy, the lowest part of the dissection should be kept above the knee, so the knee joint does not need to be included in the irradiation field. This means that insertions of the gracilis and adductor magnus muscles below the knee joint must be excluded from the dissection. Also, if there is a complete muscle bundle between tumor and margin of resection, postoperative radiation therapy may be needed. In any case, always mark the extent of the dissection with metal clips for radiation therapy treatment planning.

The initial biopsy incision must be planned with the subsequent definitive surgery in mind. Although a transverse incision across the inner thigh heals nicely, it makes an adductor muscle group incision much more difficult. An incisional rather than excisional biopsy is almost always indicated when soft tissue sarcoma is entertained as a diagnosis.

During completion of a limb-sparing approach to extremity soft tissue sarcoma, the tissue planes through which an amputation would be performed should not be contaminated by tumor. Also, the skin flaps that would be created in an amputation should be spared from the irradiation field if at all possible.

REFERENCES

1. Bowden L: The principles and methods of surgical management of soft part tumors, in *Proceedings of the Sixth National Cancer Conference*. Philadelphia, JB Lippincott 1968, pp 771–774.
2. Bowden L, Booher RJ: The principles and techniques

of resection of soft parts for sarcoma. *Surgery* 1958;44:963–977.

3. Das Gupta TK, Ghosh BC: Principles of diagnosis and management of soft tissue sarcomas. *Surg Annu* 1973;7:115–136.

4. Fortner JG: Operative management of soft tissue sarcomas, in Najarian JS, Delaney JP (eds): *Advances in Cancer Surgery*, New York, Stratton Intercontinental Med Book, 1976, pp 393–399.

5. Liberman Z, Ackerman LV: Principles in management of soft tissue sarcomas. *Surgery* 1964;35:350–365.

6. Douglas HO, Razack M, Holyoke ED: Hemipelvectomy. *Arch Surg* 1975;110:82–85.

7. Higinbotham NL, Marcove RC, Casson P: Hemipelvectomy: A clinical study of 100 cases with five year follow-up on 60 patients. *Surgery* 1966;59:706–708.

8. Miller TR: Hemipelvectomy in lower extremity tumors. *Orthop Clin N Am* 1977;8:903–919.

9. Simon MA, Enneking WF: The management of soft-tissue sarcomas of the extremities. *J Bone Joint Surg* 1976;58:319–327.

10. Suit HD, Russell WO, Martin RG: Sarcoma of soft tissue: Clinical and histopathologic parameters and response to treatment. *Cancer* 1975;35:1478.

11. Suit HD, Russell WO: Radiation therapy of soft tissue sarcomas. *Cancer* 1975;36:759–764.

12. McNeer GP, Cantin J, Chu F, et al: Effectiveness of radiation therapy in the management of sarcoma of the soft somatic tissues. *Cancer* 1968;22:391–397.

13. Rosenberg SA, Kent H, Costa J, et al: Prospective randomized evaluation of the role of limbsparing surgery, radiation therapy, and adjuvant chemoimmunotherapy in the treatment of adult soft-tissue sarcomas. *Surgery* 1978;84:62–68.

14. Spittle MF, Newton KA, MacKenzie DH: Liposarcoma. A review of 60 cases. *Br J Cancer* 1971;24:696–704.

15. Windeyer B, Dische S, Mansfield CM: The place of radiotherapy in the management of fibrosarcoma of the soft tissues. *Clin Radiol* 1966;17:32–40.

16. Mentzer SJ, Sugarbaker PH: Surgical considerations in the treatment of sarcomas of the adductor muscle group. *Surgery* 1982;91:662–668.

17. Cardman NL, Soule EH, Kelly PJ: Synovial sarcoma. An analysis of 134 tumors. *Cancer* 1965;18:613–627.

21

Quadriceps Muscle Group Excision

PAUL H. SUGARBAKER, M.D.

OVERVIEW

A quadriceps muscle group excision may be selected for definitive treatment of intra-compartmental soft tissue sarcomas within this muscle group. After making a skin incision from anterior superior iliac spine to patella, skin flaps are dissected superficial to the fascia lata to the flexor muscles laterally and to the gracilis muscle medially. The superficial femoral artery is dissected free of the quadriceps muscles over the entire thigh. The origins of the sartorius, tensor fascia lata, and rectus femoris are transected from their origins on the pelvis, and the vastus lateralis, vastus medialis, and vastus intermedius are transected from their origins on the femur. To free the specimen, the quadriceps femoris tendon is divided just proximal to its attachment to the patella. The gracilis muscle medially and the short head of the biceps muscle laterally are transected at their insertions and secured to the patella. The subcutaneous tissue and skin are closed over generous suction drainage. An ankle/foot orthosis is used postoperatively to provide relatively unrestricted ambulation.

Soft tissue sarcoma of an extremity has been successfully treated by amputation,[1,2] muscle group excision,[3,4] or wide local excision plus high-dose radiation therapy.[5,6] All three of these treatment modalities provide an acceptable incidence of local control in properly selected patients because a wide margin of normal tissue surrounding the primary sarcoma is treated. If normal tissue planes surrounding the primary tumor are not achieved, inadequate margins of resection will result and an extremely high local recurrence rate will occur. Ultimate survival following a local recurrence is reported to be poor, because the occurrence of systemic disease in many patients will have a cause and effect relationship to locally recurrent tumor.

Enneking and co-workers have suggested that two factors operate to determine the success or failure of muscle group excision as a treatment modality.[7] First, low-grade lesions can be definitively treated with a lesser margin of excision, and maintenance of a low local recurrence rate can be maintained. That is, the margin of excision required for local control (narrow *v* radical margin of excision) is dictated in part by the biologic aggressiveness of the primary tumor.

Secondly, the necessary margin of excision that can be achieved surgically while sparing the extremity depends on the anatomic location of the primary tumor.[7] Intracompartmental tumors arise within a muscle group and do not involve bone or essential neurovascular structures that border on the muscle group. These lesions are ideally suited for a muscle group excision. Tumors confined to the adductor muscle group or quadriceps muscle group and not involving femur or superficial femoral artery are the most frequent examples of tumors treatable by muscle group excision.

An extracompartmental lesion arises de novo between muscle groups or, as a result of surgically induced tumor contamination, involves more than a single muscle group. Also, lesions that involve a bone or essential neurovascular structure are categorized as extracompartmental tumors. These tumors should not be treated by muscle group excision.

This chapter presents a surgical technique for muscle group excision of soft tissue sarcomas contained within the quadriceps muscle. The rationale for an ankle/knee orthosis that maintains 5° of plantar flexion of the ankle is discussed. The procedure has been associated with a minimal amount of morbidity postoperatively and with good mobility.

INDICATIONS

Quadriceps muscle group excision is indicated for intracompartmental soft tissue sarcomas that arise within the quadriceps mechanism. By physical examination, patients selected to undergo this procedure should have a tumor that is freely mobile over the femur and confined to the extensor compartment. Occasionally a low-grade (grade I or II) tumor may be excised adequately by removing some but not all portions of this muscle group. However, higher-grade tumors need removal of the entire muscle mass for adequate margins of resection. A bone scan should indicate no involvement of patella, femur, or anterior superior iliac spine. A computerized tomogram of the thigh is helpful to rule out involvement of the other muscular compartments, but does not predict accurately involvement of bones or neurovascular structures, because normal muscle compressed by tumor usually cannot be distinguished from tumor itself. A femoral arteriogram must show some normal tissue between the superficial femoral artery and the tumor mass detected by tumor blush. Involvement of the superficial femoral artery by tumor is the most common reason for recommending amputation after attempting quadriceps muscle group excision.

PROCEDURE

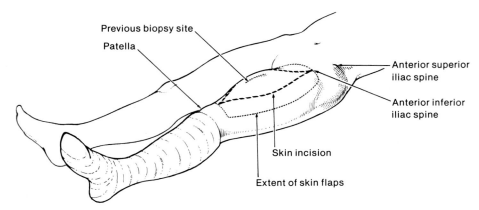

Figure 21–1. INCISION. The incision extends longitudinally from the anterior inferior iliac spine to the patella. It should be elliptical in configuration and widely encompass the biopsy site. If physical examination or tomography shows that the tumor encroaches on the patella, this bone and its tendon should also be excised. If this clinical situation arises, the incision should be continued over the knee to the tibial tubercle.

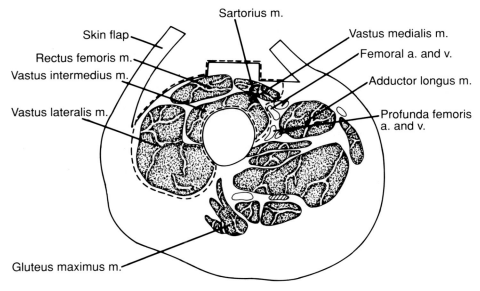

Figure 21–2. CROSS-SECTIONAL ANATOMY.

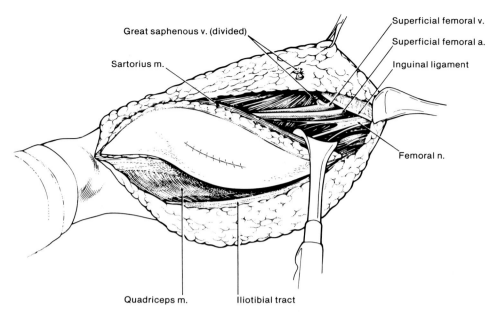

Figure 21–3.   SKIN FLAPS. Flaps composed of skin and subcutaneous tissue are made just superficial to the fascia lata. They extend to the adductor muscle group medially and to the greater trochanter and flexor muscles laterally. The saphenous vein is divided as it enters the fossa ovalis. The inguinal ligament and the femoral triangle are uncovered, exposing the common femoral artery and vein and the femoral nerve.

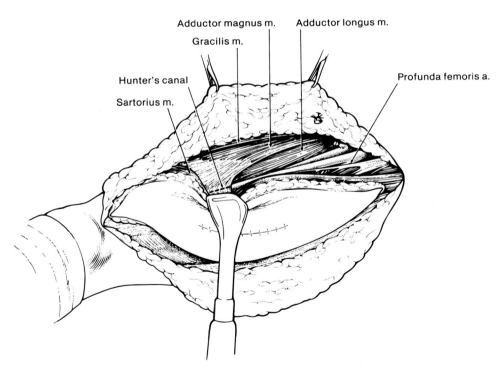

Figure 21–4.   DISSECTION OF THE SUPERFICIAL FEMORAL VESSLES. Lateral traction is placed on the quadriceps muscle group so that muscular branches coming from the superficial femoral artery and vein into the quadriceps muscle are exposed. Working from cranial to caudal, these vessels are clamped, divided, and ligated; included are the profunda femoris artery and vein. In the area of Hunter's canal when strong lateral traction is placed on the sartorius muscle, muscular insertions from the adductor magnus muscle coursing over the superficial femoral artery are identified. These muscle fibers should be divided as they cross the superficial femoral artery.

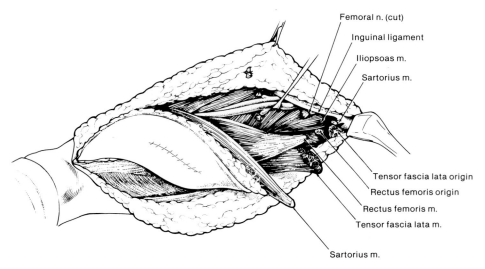

Femoral n. (cut)

Inguinal ligament

Iliopsoas m.

Sartorius m.

Tensor fascia lata origin

Rectus femoris origin

Rectus femoris m.

Tensor fascia lata m.

Sartorius m.

Figure 21–5.   TRANSECTION OF MUSCLE ORIGINS ON THE PELVIS. A plane beneath the tensor fascia lata muscle and above the gluteus medius and minimus is identified. By electrocautery the tensor fascia lata muscle is released from its origin on the wing of the ilium. Then the origin of the sartorius muscle on the anterior superior iliac spine is identified and divided. The origin of the rectus femoris muscle on the anterior inferior iliac spine is likewise identified and divided through its tendinous portion.

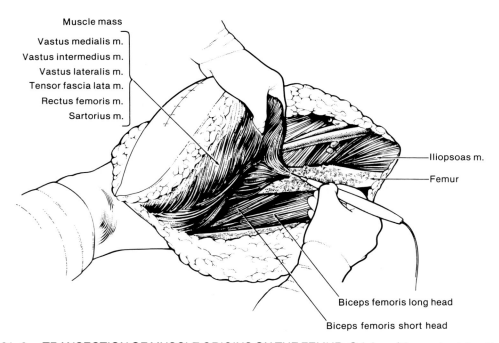

Muscle mass

Vastus medialis m.

Vastus intermedius m.

Vastus lateralis m.

Tensor fascia lata m.

Rectus femoris m.

Sartorius m.

Iliopsoas m.

Femur

Biceps femoris long head

Biceps femoris short head

Figure 21–6.   TRANSECTION OF MUSCLE ORIGINS ON THE FEMUR. Origins of the vastus lateralis, vastus intermedius, and vastus medialis on the femur are transected from bone by using electrocautery. Strong upward traction on the muscle group facilitates this dissection.

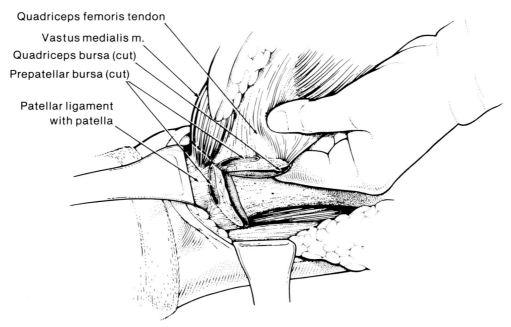

Quadriceps femoris tendon

Vastus medialis m.

Quadriceps bursa (cut)

Prepatellar bursa (cut)

Patellar ligament
with patella

Figure 21–7.   TRANSECTION OF THE MUSCLE INSERTIONS OF THE QUADRICEPS MUSCLE. Using strong upward and medial traction on the specimen, insertions of the vastus lateralis, vastus medialis, and rectus femoris into the patellar tendon are divided on the patella bone. One cannot avoid transecting both the prepatellar and quadriceps (postpatellar) bursae. The insertion of the vastus medialis into the medial collateral ligament is likewise divided, and the specimen is then free. The dissection site is copiously irrigated, and any bleeding points are secured with ligatures or electrocautery.

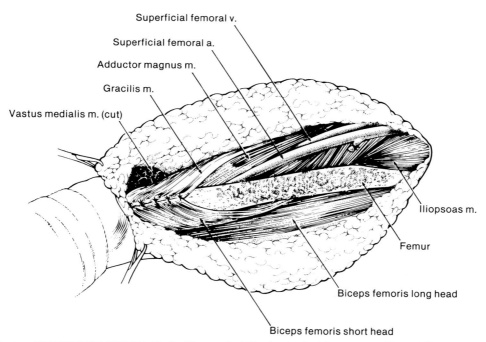

Superficial femoral v.

Superficial femoral a.

Adductor magnus m.

Gracilis m.

Vastus medialis m. (cut)

Iliopsoas m.

Femur

Biceps femoris long head

Biceps femoris short head

Figure 21–8.   RECONSTRUCTION. To facilitate rehabilitation by helping to provide stability to the knee, the gracilis muscle medially and the short head of the biceps muscle laterally are transected at their insertions on the medial and lateral collateral ligaments. This transection should be as far distal on the muscle as possible so that a tendinous portion of the muscle is retained on the muscle belly. Then, using heavy nonabsorbable sutures, these two muscles are transplanted onto the patellar tendon. The prepatellar and quadriceps bursae are closed within these sutures. The muscles are approximately in the midline so that they cover the distal one third of the femur.

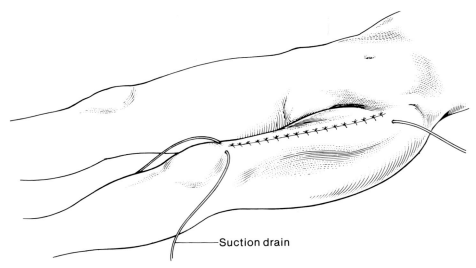

Suction drain

Figure 21–9. CLOSURE. Suction catheters are placed beneath the skin flaps and the subcutaneous tissue is approximated with interrupted absorbable sutures. The skin is closed. No immobilization using plaster is required and the incision is merely covered with povidone-iodine ointment and a loose dry sterile dressing. The patient may begin ambulation when the suction catheters have been removed and edema of the leg has resolved. Because lymphatics along the superficial femoral artery and within the buttock remain intact, prolonged swelling is not usually a problem. Also, because muscles have been removed from origin to insertion, serous drainage from transected muscle bundles does not occur in large amounts. The patient is ambulated initially with crutches and a touchdown gait.

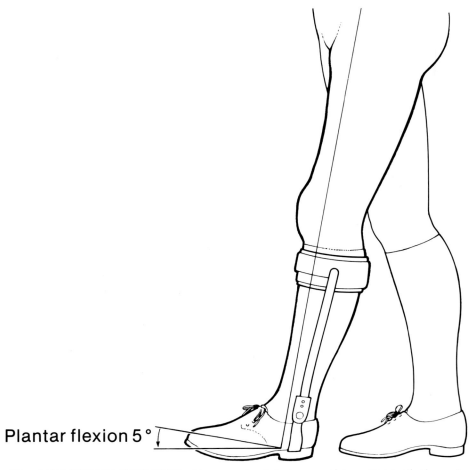

Plantar flexion 5°

Figure 21–10. ANKLE/FOOT ORTHOSIS. At approximately two weeks postoperatively a dual channel aluminum ankle/foot orthosis (AFO) is provided which blocks out dorsiflexion and permits 5 or more degrees of plantar flexion. This prevents flexion of the knee on contact of the foot with the floor. Patients continue to use a cane held in their contralateral hand.[8,9]

DISCUSSION

Quadriceps muscle group excision is a definite treatment alternative for selected soft tissue sarcomas involving this anatomic site. Enneking and co-workers[7] emphasize that a decision to use this treatment modality depends almost exclusively on the anatomic location of the primary tumor. An intracompartmental tumor located near the center of the muscle mass that can be removed en bloc with a generous margin of muscle and fascia on femur, superficial femoral artery, and the neighboring adductor and flexor muscle groups is ideal for this surgical approach. If adequate margins are achieved radiation therapy is not required postoperatively, and yet local recurrence rates of 5% or less are to be expected.

If radiation therapy can be avoided, the morbidity and sexual dysfunction seen with high-dose, wide-field irradiation therapy of the thigh (especially the upper thigh) does not occur. This side effect is a very real concern to the young male or female who wishes to remain fertile. The amount of x-ray scatter from wide-field irradiation of the thigh makes further childbearing impossible or unadvisable.

Some tumors have no other good treatment option short of quadriceps muscle group excision except amputation. Large tumors that intimately involve the patellar tendon cannot be treated successfully by wide local excision plus wide-field irradiation therapy. To achieve negative margins of resection these tumors demand sacrifice of the patellar tendon. Reliable, long-term continuity between the upper quadriceps muscles and the patella is nearly impossible to achieve using a prosthetic device or other anatomic structure. Irradiation therapy up to 6,000 rads used in the postoperative period will almost invariably result in breakdown of a tendon reconstruction with the passage of time. Functional results are better if the muscle is sacrificed along with the patellar tendon as in the quadriceps muscle group excision and x-ray therapy is not employed. Also, severe stiffness of the knee will result if high-dose radiation therapy is delivered to the entire knee joint as would be required in the multimodality approach.

The rehabilitation potential with quadriceps muscle group excision (as with adductor muscle group excision) is excellent. The number of patients that can learn to stabilize the knee through use of the transplanted gracilis and short head of the biceps

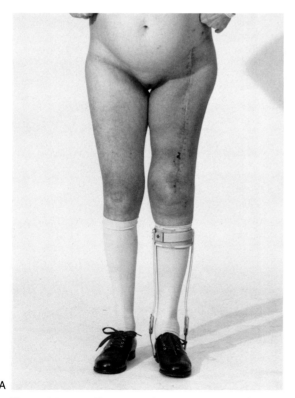
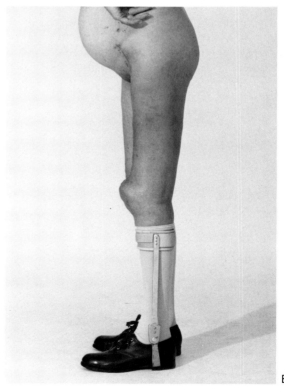

A   B

Figure 21–11. Postoperative appearance of a patient under quadriceps muscle group excision for a myxoid liposarcoma, **(A)** anterior view and **(B)** lateral view. The patella appears prominent because of some residual fluid within the knee joint. The patient walks with a nearly normal gait using an ankle/foot orthosis.

muscles is unknown; long-term follow-up on a large number of patients is as yet unavailable. Transplantation of these muscles from both the medial and lateral muscle groups over the top of the femur not only allows the patient to fix the patella and thus keep the knee from collapsing with weight bearing, but also brings some soft tissue over the femur in an area that may be frequently traumatized with normal daily activity.

Even if transplanted muscles cannot be developed to sufficient strength (at least the "good" range) to stabilize the knee, orthotics can be used to provide the patient with excellent mobility. The AFO shown in Figure 21–10 allows for functional and safe ambulation. As the patient gains experience, crutches are not required, but a cane is usually retained to help with balance (not weight bearing) on irregular terrain.

The orthotic device used to provide ambulation after quadriceps muscle group excision is lightweight and generally not found to be cumbersome. When dorsiflexion is blocked out by an anterior stop in the AFO, and at least 5 degrees of plantar flexion is allowed, an extension moment is created at the knee on weight bearing. In doing so, the ground reactive force lies ahead of the knee axis. The thigh–knee–ankle line (TKA) forces the knee into extension and prevents flexion as the foot makes contact with the floor. As the trunk moves forward even more weight is distributed posteriorly at the knee, and only as the extremity becomes non-weight-bearing is flexion allowed to occur.[8,9] Episodes of knee instability are liable to occur if patients forget to wear their AFO (for example, when getting up from bed at night). Patients need to be cautioned against any ambulation without the AFO (Fig. 21–11).

REFERENCES

1. Douglass HO, Razack M. Holyoke ED: Hemipelvectomy. *Arch Surg* 1976;110:82–85.
2. Higinbotham NL, Marcove RC, Casson P: Hemipelvectomy: A clinical study of 100 cases with five year follow-up on 60 patients. *Surgery* 1966;59:706–708.
3. Fortner JG: Operative management of soft tissue sarcomas, in Najarian JS, Delaney JP (eds): *Advances in Cancer Surgery*. New York, Stratton Intercontinental Med Book, 1976, pp 393–399.
4. Simon MA, Enneking WF: The management of soft-tissue sarcomas of the extremities. *J Bone Joint Surg* 1976;58:319–327.
5. Rosenberg SA, Kent H, Costa J, et al: Prospective randomized evaluation of the role of limb-sparing surgery, radiation therapy, and adjuvant chemoimmunotherapy in the treatment of adult soft-tissue sarcomas. *Surgery* 1978;48:62–68.
6. Suit HD, Russell WO: Radiation therapy of soft tissue sarcomas. *Cancer* 1975;36:759–764.
7. Enneking WF, Spanier SS, Malawer MM: The effects of the anatomic setting on the results of surgical procedures for soft parts sarcoma of the thigh. *Cancer* 1981;47:1005–1022.
8. Perry J, Hislop HJ (eds): *Principles of Lower-Extremity Bracing*. Washington, DC, American Physical Therapy Association, 1976, pp 70–80.
9. Lehmann JF: Biomechanics of ankle–foot orthoses: Prescription and design. *Arch Phys Med Rehabil* 1979; 60:200–207.

22

Resection of the Posterior Compartment of the Thigh

PAUL H. SUGARBAKER, M.D.

OVERVIEW

Soft tissue sarcoma of the posterior thigh may be completely surrounded by the hamstring muscles. This allows for a dissection of tumor with clear margins of excision by removal of the hamstring muscles from their origins on the ischial tuberosity to insertions at the medial and lateral femoral condyles. If all margins are clear on histopathologic examination, no postoperative radiation therapy is required. Rather, this muscle group excision is interpreted as the definitive ablative procedure, similar to an amputation. If tissues at the margin of excision are directly adjacent to tumor, postoperative radiation therapy must be employed. The structure most commonly contaminated by tumor is the sciatic nerve. The sciatic nerve may be sacrificed with a compromised but satisfactory functional result. After their origins are excised from the ischial tuberosity, muscles are reflected inferiorly off of the sciatic nerve. The insertion of the long head of the biceps is transected laterally and the semitendinosus and semimembranosus are divided through their tendinous portion medially. The superficial fascia and skin are meticulously closed over generous suction drainage.

INDICATIONS

Patients with malignant tumors optimally treated by posterior muscle group excision are not frequently encountered. The best candidates for this procedure are patients with low-grade malignancies so that little normal tissue margin is required surrounding the tumor mass. For grade II or greater soft tissue sarcomas, the tumor mass must be quite small and completely confined to the posterior compartment. If the size of the tumor or its anatomic location suggests that postoperative radiation therapy is required, then a wide local excision rather than a complete dissection of the posterior compartment should be performed.

If tumor penetration of the muscle group at its deep margin is observed during the dissection, it is possible that the sciatic nerve should be sacrificed. The sciatic nerve will almost always need to be removed along with the muscle group if the tumor is of neural origin. The sciatic nerve can be removed with satisfactory function of the leg. If the sciatic nerve is involved and there is contamination of the periosteum of the posterior femur, then hemipelvectomy should be recommended. In general, if an amputation is required, the best results are with anterior flap hemipelvectomy.

PROCEDURE

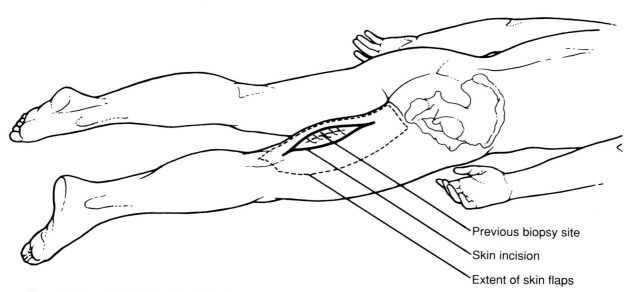

Figure 22–1. **INCISION AND SKIN FLAPS.** The patient is placed in the prone position. An ellipse of skin is outlined so that there is a 2-cm margin of skin around the old biopsy site. The extent of the skin flaps are dissected, care being taken to taper the flaps, as one encounters the lateral margins of the dissection. It is helpful to mark on the skin the extent of the dissection of the skin flaps so that one does not inadvertently exceed this during the dissection. The medial extent of the dissection is the gracilis muscle, and the lateral extent is the iliotibial tract.

Previous biopsy site

Skin incision

Extent of skin flaps

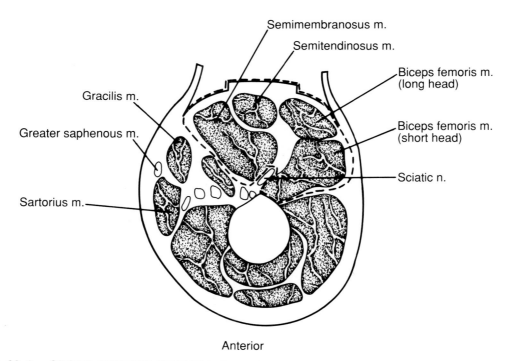

Semimembranosus m.

Semitendinosus m.

Biceps femoris m. (long head)

Biceps femoris m. (short head)

Sciatic n.

Gracilis m.

Greater saphenous m.

Sartorius m.

Anterior

Figure 22–2. **CROSS SECTION OF THE MID-THIGH.** The near proximity of the sciatic nerve to large sarcomas within the posterior compartment is clearly indicated by this diagram.

301

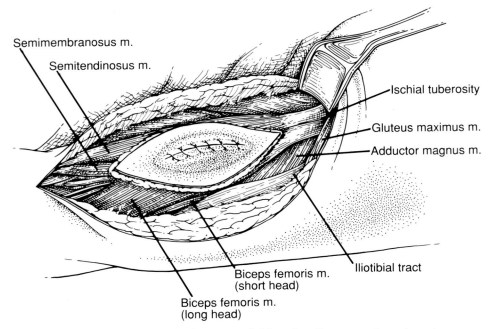

Figure 22–3. **CREATION OF SKIN FLAPS.** The medial (semitendinosus and semimembranosus muscles) and lateral (biceps femoris long head and short head) muscle bundles are exposed.

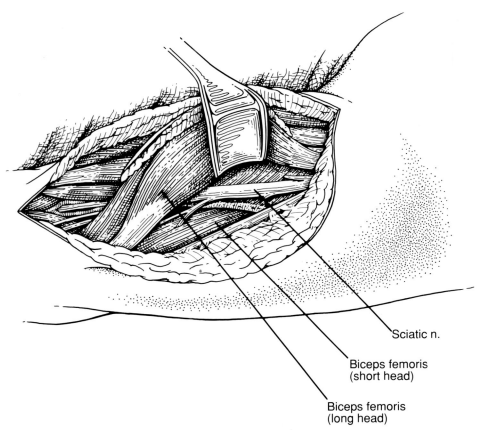

Figure 22–4. **DEFINING THE MUSCLES OF THE POSTERIOR COMPARTMENT.** The extent of the dissection is in part determined by the sarcoma, but resection generally involves the long head of the biceps femoris, semimembranosus, and semitendinosus. It is possible for a portion of the lateral quadriceps mechanism to be included with the specimen. Likewise one or more muscle bundles of the adductor muscle group may be included with the muscle group, if this will afford a more generous margin. The three muscles mentioned are superficial to the sciatic nerve, and their origin is from the ischial tuberosity. A tumor-free margin of resection depends on a plane free of tumor contamination superficial to the posterior limits of this compartment. It is clear that the next adjacent structure is the sciatic nerve itself.

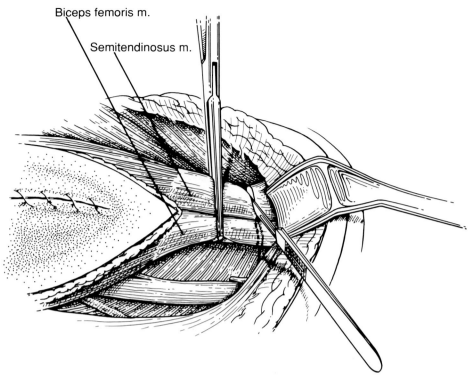

Figure 22–5. TRANSECTION OF MUSCLE ORIGINS. Dissection begins by exposing the ischial tuberosity. This is easily identified on the skin surface. The hamstring muscles are released at their origin from the ischial tuberosity.

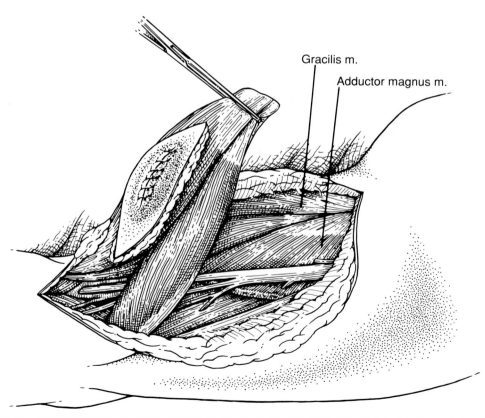

Figure 22–6. DISSECTION OF THE MUSCLE GROUP FROM CEPHALAD TO CAUDAL ASPECTS. The muscle groups are secured with a clamp, and strong traction is placed on the muscle group. Blood vessels and nerves that enter the hamstring muscle are ligated and divided. By a blunt and sharp dissection the entire muscle group is elevated. The sciatic nerve, the short head of the biceps laterally, and the adductor muscles medially form the base of the dissection.

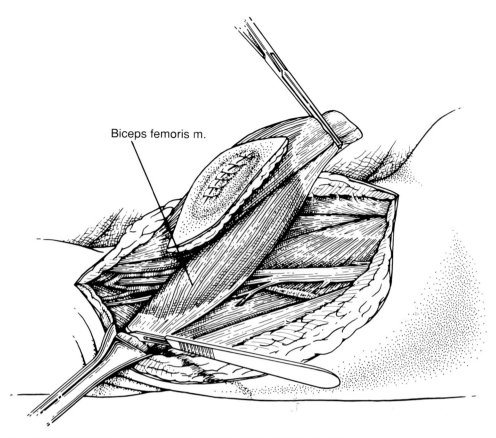

Biceps femoris m.

Figure 22–7. TRANSECTION OF MUSCLE INSERTIONS LATERALLY. The long head of the biceps femoris muscle is transected through its tendinous portion on the lateral aspect of the thigh. One must take care to avoid injury to the common peroneal nerve.

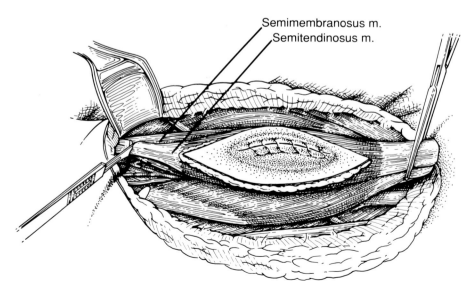

Semimembranosus m.
Semitendinosus m.

Figure 22–8. TRANSECTION OF MUSCLE INSERTIONS MEDIALLY. The insertions of the semimembranosus muscle and semitendinosus are divided through their tendinous portions medially. The medial head of the gastrocnemius muscle is exposed.

304

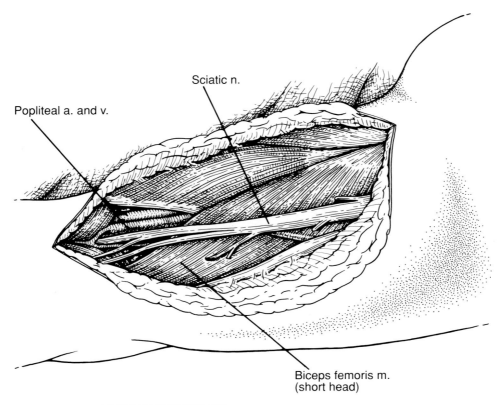

Figure 22–9. THE RESECTION BED.

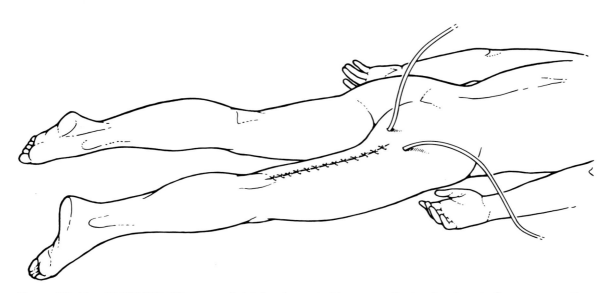

Figure 22–10. CLOSURE. The superficial fascia and skin are meticulously closed. Generous suction drainage is achieved through closed-suction drains. Care should be taken to not make the skin exit sites for the suction drains through the skin flaps. Rather, these should be just above the gluteal crease.

23

Forequarter Amputation

PAUL H. SUGARBAKER, M.D.

OVERVIEW

Forequarter amputation is performed for aggressive tumors of or surrounding the shoulder girdle and proximal humerus. Contraindications to this ablative procedure are distant disease and chest wall involvement. The patient is placed in a lateral position, and all dissection is done from the posterior aspect of the patient. An incision that employs a short anterior and larger posterior flap is fashioned. Skin flaps are constructed to the level of the areola anteriorly and to the edge of the scapula posteriorly. Muscles are detached from the scapula posteriorly, and the shoulder girdle is rolled anteriorly. Just beneath the serratus anterior the neurovascular bundle is dissected free under direct vision, and ligated and divided. After transection of the pectoralis muscles and clavicle, the skin flaps are closed over suction drains.

INTRODUCTION

Forequarter amputation is used to remove bony tumors of the upper half of the humerus and the distal scapula.[1,2] Soft tissue tumors of an advanced stage of the upper arm or shoulder are also ablated with a forequarter amputation (Fig. 23–1). Unless soft tissue tumors occur within the axilla, they can usually be managed by wide local excision and postoperative high-dose wide-field radiation. High-grade tumors that recur in this area after limb salvage treatment may demand a combined forequarter resection with chest wall excision as presented in chapter 24.[3,4]

Osteosarcoma of the proximal humerus frequently requires a forequarter amputation (Fig. 23–2). One should carefully consider a limb-sparing procedure in tumors of the shoulder region. The Tikhoff-Linberg procedure requires adequate margins of excision.[5] Indications for amputation are persistence of tumor after induction chemotherapy in and around the neurovascular bundle at the axilla.

INDICATIONS FOR FOREQUARTER AMPUTATION

Forequarter amputation is used to remove large osteosarcomas of the upper half of the humerus, malignant bony tumors of the scapula, or malignant

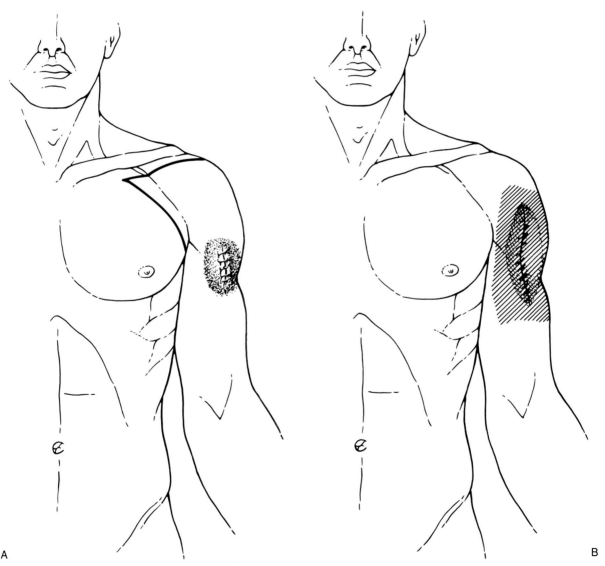

A   B

Figure 23–1. (A) Forequarter amputation for high-grade soft tissue sarcoma involving the proximal upper extremity. (B) In a majority of patients with soft tissue sarcomas of the upper arm or shoulder, wide excision and postoperative radiation therapy are appropriate.

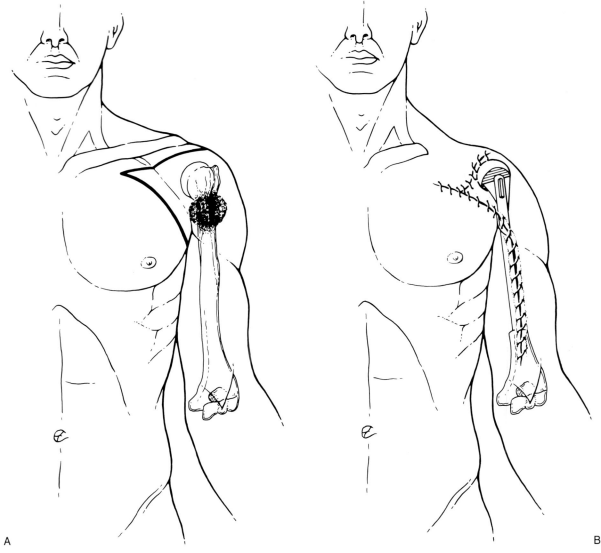

Figure 23–2.   (A) Large malignant tumors of the proximal humerus with soft tissue extension may require forequarter amputation. (B) The Tikhoff-Linberg procedure should always be considered for osteosarcoma of the proximal humerus.

soft tissue tumors in this anatomic area. Amputation is required for these tumors if clinical evaluation following induction chemotherapy shows involvement of the neurovascular bundle or the chest wall. Recurrent high-grade tumors after excision and radiation therapy usually require amputation. This clinical evaluation is necessary before and after induction chemotherapy. Isolated involvement of the axillary vein is not an indication for amputation for there is usually adequate collateral through the cephalic vein and cephalic lymphatics. However, encasement of the axillary artery or the axillary nerves requires forequarter amputation for a curative resection.

Extensive contamination of soft tissue by cancer may occur with tumors in the shoulder or upper arm. This may result from spontaneous rupture of the tumor and bleeding into the soft tissues. Sometimes an open biopsy incision will continue to bleed and extensively contaminate the tissues of the entire shoulder. A pathologic fracture can have the same results.

Skeletal immaturity that may cause length discrepancy with a prosthetic replacement or with radiation therapy to an epiphysis is not generally a consideration in upper-extremity amputations. Length discrepancy is usually tolerated well and does not interfere with upper-extremity function.

Infection may be a major problem, especially if one is considering a Tikhoff-Linberg procedure. This involves the use of prosthetic materials and is not likely to succeed as an approach in a contaminated operative site.

CLINICAL CONSIDERATIONS FOR FOREQUARTER AMPUTATION

The timing for the surgical procedure is important. Both physiological and psychological factors must be optimized. If the patient has received preoperative chemotherapy, it is essential that both leukocytes and platelets be permitted to return toward normal. Significant deficits of red blood cell mass should be corrected by preoperative transfusion. Although vascular insufficiency is rarely a complicating factor of forequarter amputation, suboptimal wound healing may be a problem in patients who have radiation therapy. Also, associated poor nutrition from nausea and vomiting induced by preoperative chemotherapy may further compound wound-healing problems. Hematoma must be avoided by the adequate use of closed-suction drainage. One should defer removal of skin sutures for at least three weeks, especially if the skin closure was under tension.

REHABILITATION AND EMOTIONAL SUPPORT

The cancer patient who requires a forequarter amputation faces unique psychological problems. Not only is there a threat to the loss of the upper extremity and shoulder, but there is also a threat to life itself. Rehabilitation of a patient undergoing a major amputation begins at the same time as the staging studies. The entire health care team must develop an honest relationship with the patient and include him or her in the early stages of decision making. Building upon this, the patient will better be able to accept the amputation and set realistic goals.

All patients undergoing a forequarter amputation will experience some phantom limb sensation. The phantom limb pain and sensations are not as severe as with hemipelvectomy, but they remain the most bothersome postoperative problem. There is no definite solution or remedy for phantom limb pain. The patient's willingness to deny the problem seems to be the best defense against a potentially debilitating situation. Phantom limb pain should always be discussed with the patient prior to surgery. The patient needs to understand that this is an expected sensation that can be treated with analgesics. The patient should be reassured that phantom limb pain will decrease in its severity over time. The patients who report severe pain are often those who find it most difficult to adapt to surgery and to the malignant process.

Although successful rehabilitation depends to a great extent on the patient's attitude, the rehabilitation team can help tremendously in these efforts. A *positive attitude* toward functional recovery augmented by early return to activity helps the patient move rapidly toward personal goals. A prosthesis is rarely used in patients who have forequarter amputation. A soft shoulder pad helps them to wear store-bought clothes.

A positive approach in the forequarter amputation is greatly amplified by contact with other patients who have successfully met some of the rehabilitative challenges. This can provide an immeasurable psychological boost to the patient. The oncologist, rehabilitation therapist, and others involved in the postoperative care must coordinate their efforts carefully, realizing the possibility of conflicting demands on the patient's time. Also, different interpretations of the same clinical information that is presented to the patient by different members of the care team may occur. The entire team must be supportive and positive about complete rehabilitation that can be achieved following forequarter amputation. Even if the dominant upper extremity is removed, function with one upper extremity is excellent and compatible with a normal quality of life in a majority of patients.

Attempts to fashion an upper-extremity prosthesis allowing elbow flexion and a pinched grasp have been moderately successful. Yet it is an unusual patient who can successfully use this apparatus. The prosthesis most patients consistently use is the shoulder mold.[1,3] This light, comfortable prosthesis allows the patient to be fitted with regular-sized clothing without alterations (see chapter 4).

LEVEL OF AMPUTATION

For tumors of the shoulder and axilla, forequarter amputation is usually the procedure of choice. Occasionally a soft tissue sarcoma of the upper arm may be treated with a shoulder disarticulation. However, there is no functional advantage with the shoulder disarticulation compared with the forequarter amputation. However, this is usually not a major consideration because the margins of excision are so much improved with the complete forequarter amputation.

RADIOLOGIC STUDIES

The difficult choice is frequently between forequarter amputation and the shoulder girdle resection with limb sparing. Osteosarcoma of the proximal humerus may have considerable soft tissue extension into the axilla. Computerized tomography, MRI, arteriography, and venography are all of help. However, these studies may show considerable deviation of the neurovascular bundle, but they cannot determine, in most instances, actual invasion of these crucial structures.

PROCEDURE

Unless the patient has a large tumor mass, a mold of the involved shoulder should be made preoperatively. This simplifies construction of a suitable permanent shoulder prosthesis.

According to several other texts, forequarter amputation is generally performed with the surgeon standing anterior to the patient; after the skin incision is made and skin flaps are constructed, the clavicle is divided so that the neurovascular bundle can be secured. However, in the modification described here, the surgeon is positioned posterior to the patient. The procedure moves from posterior to anterior, with the extremity being rolled anteriorly as the muscles are released. Ligation and division of the neurovascular bundle are the last step of the dissection and are performed with a wide exposure.

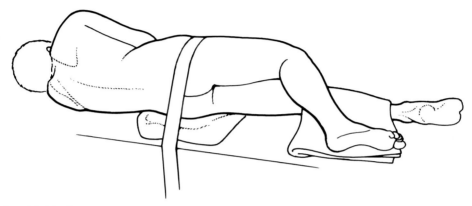

Figure 23–3.   **POSITION.** Intravenous lines are secured, and a Foley catheter is placed in the bladder. The patient is placed in a full lateral position and secured at the hips with tape. Alternatively, a VAC pak can be used to secure the torso. An axillary roll is placed under the axilla to allow full excursion of the chest, and a sponge rubber pad is placed under the hip to prevent ischemic damage to the skin in this area. The skin is prepared, and the tumor-bearing extremity is draped free.

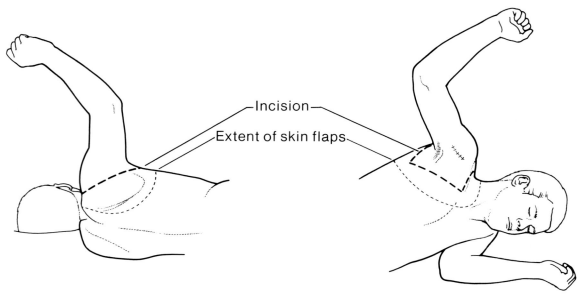

Figure 23–4. **INCISION AND SKIN FLAPS.** The incision starts over the clavicle about 1 in lateral to the sternoclavicular joint. The medial line of incision is in or near the deltopectoral groove; the lateral line crosses the tip of the acromion. These lines meet below the axilla; the surgeon must be sure to excise all of the skin bearing axillary hair. The position of the lines of excision will vary with tumors in different positions. In the patient shown, a hematoma over the deltoid muscle anteriorly required that the anterior skin flap be moved further forward than usual. Because of the excellent blood supply to the skin in this region, long anterior or posterior flaps uniformly survive even though closed under considerable tension. If a tumor mass has extensive skin involvement, the flaps that remain should be secured to the chest wall with absorbable suture material, and the remaining defect covered with a split-thickness skin graft.

The surgeon stands posterior to the patient. The posterior skin flap is usually constructed first. The flaps are constructed as thick as possible so that dissection is usually on muscle fascia. It is usually possible to widely sacrifice skin around a tumor mass or previous biopsy site so that thin skin flaps are unnecessary. Hematoma that results from the biopsy should always be included within the operative specimen. The posterior skin flap is elevated back to the medial border of the scapula. If a long posterior skin flap is required, this dissection may go back to the vertebral spines. The anterior skin flap is elevated back to the anterior axillary line. If a long anterior flap is required, the flap can extend back to the mid-sternum.

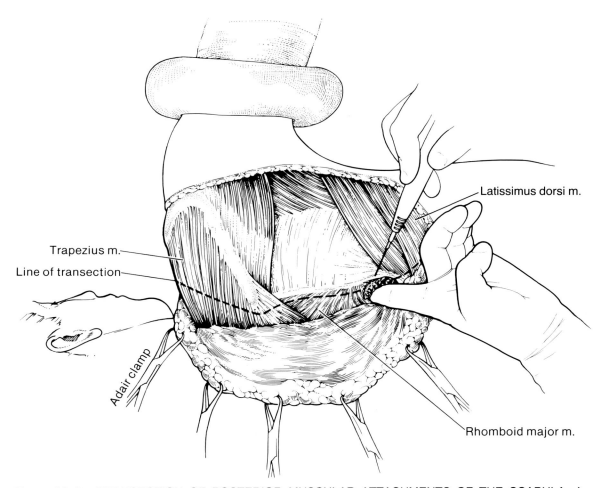

Figure 23–5. **TRANSECTION OF POSTERIOR MUSCULAR ATTACHMENTS OF THE SCAPULA.** An incision in the deep fascia at the mid-portion of the posterior border of the scapula allows the surgeon to pass a finger beneath the scapula. Electrocautery is then used to divide the rhomboid muscles (major and minor), trapezius muscle, and levator scapulae muscle as they insert onto the scapula. Moving caudally, the surgeon transects the latissimus dorsi.

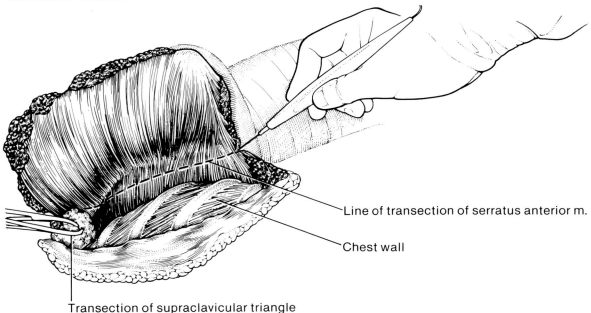

Figure 23–6. **DIVISION OF CONTENTS OF THE SUPRACLAVICULAR TRIANGLE AND SERRATUS ANTERIOR MUSCLE.** Elevation of the scapula allows the structures of the supraclavicular triangle to be divided between hemostats. This includes the transverse cervical and transverse scapular arteries, many lymphatic channels, and the omohyoid muscle. Care is taken to sweep the contents of the axilla into the surgical specimen. The serratus anterior muscle is divided at its origin on the chest wall. This clearly exposes the neurovascular bundle.

313

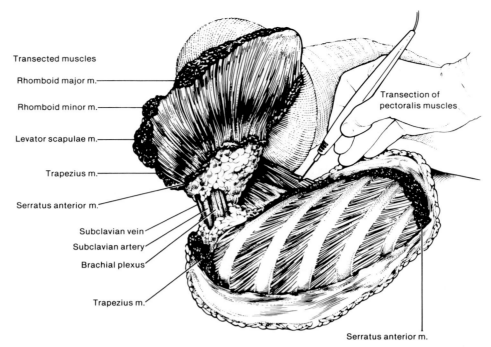

Transected muscles

Rhomboid major m.———

Rhomboid minor m.———

Levator scapulae m.———

Trapezius m.———

Serratus anterior m.———

Subclavian vein———

Subclavian artery———

Brachial plexus———

Trapezius m.———

Transection of
pectoralis muscles

Serratus anterior m.

Figure 23–7. TRANSECTION OF THE PECTORALIS MUSCLES, CLAVICLE, AND NEUROVASCULAR BUNDLE. Anteriorly the pectoralis major and pectoralis minor muscles are divided. Elevation of the inferior angle of the scapula allows these muscles to be divided under tension by using electrocautery with minimal blood loss. The clavicular head of the sternocleidomastoid muscle is severed from this bone. The clavicle is disarticulated from its sternoclavicular joint. Subclavian vein and artery are ligated, divided, and then suture-ligated. The three large nerve bundles are ligated and then transected.

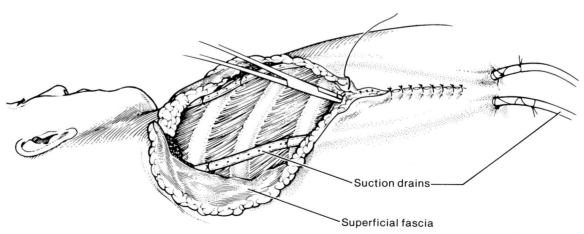

Suction drains———

Superficial fascia

Figure 23–8. CLOSURE. The area is copiously irrigated. Generous suction drainage under the anterior and posterior skin flaps is secured. A marked inequality of the anterior and posterior skin flaps exists. Marked redundancy of the skin may present an unacceptable cosmetic appearance unless the skin flaps are carefully approximated. The mid-portion of the long posterior skin flap is closed to the mid-portion of the anterior flap. Halving the closure in this way pleats the longer posterior skin flap and prevents unsightly folds of skin. A two-layered closure of superficial fascia and then skin is used. Suction drains are removed when serous drainage is minimal.

DISCUSSION

Forequarter amputation is technically much simpler than hemipelvectomy or hip disarticulation. Certainly it does not present the surgical challenge represented by the Tikhoff-Linberg procedure. In performing the dissection, one delays transection of the neurovascular bundle until the posterior dissection has been completed, as described by Littlewood. Exposure of the large vascular trunks is complete, and the vascular cuffs are adequate for in-continuity ligation and then division. No uncontrolled hemorrhage should occur with this approach.[6] The alternative is an anterior approach. It is preferred only if the tumor is on the posterior aspect of the shoulder girdle.[7] One should try to avoid dissection of the neurovascular bundle with poor exposure caused by a large tumor mass.

Because the vascular supply of the skin in this region is excellent, despite tension on the skin flaps with closure, healing is nearly always primary. Suction drains can be removed on the third or fourth day postoperatively rather than after several weeks, as in lower-extremity amputations. Lymphatic drainage from dissections in the upper extremity ceases more quickly than from the lower extremity. Presumably this is because of lower pressure within the lymphatic channels.

A careful neurologic examination may give as much information as the radiologic studies when an optimal surgical approach to shoulder girdle tumors is selected. If there is neurologic impairment, it is very likely that the neurovascular bundle has been invaded. Not infrequently, an exploration of the proximal axilla is required before the extent of tumor and encroachment on the neurovascular bundle can be determined accurately. One must be prepared to go on to a definitive excision at the time of this exploration.

A similar dilemma may exist for advanced tumor of the scapula. Choosing between scapulectomy, Tikhoff-Linberg procedure, and forequarter amputation may be difficult. In some patients the only approach is to explore the limits of a limb salvage procedure prior to deciding on the indicated procedure. If the dissection proceeds without encountering tumor, the limb-sparing procedure can proceed. If tumor is encountered within the crucial anatomic planes, then this incision is closed and one moves the incisions more proximally and proceeds at the same setting with a forequarter amputation (see chapter 28).

Phantom limb pains and sensations are not as severe with forequarter amputation as with hemipelvectomy, but they remain the most bothersome postoperative problem. No solution or remedy for phantom limb pain is available, and the patient's willingness to deny the problem seems to be the best defense against a potentially debilitating situation. Even if the dominant upper extremity is removed, function with one upper extremity is excellent and compatible with good quality of life in a majority of patients. Attempts to fashion an upper-extremity prosthesis allowing elbow flexion and a pinch grasp have been moderately successful. It is an unusual patient who can successfully use this apparatus. The prosthesis most patients consistently use is the shoulder mold.[8] This light, comfortable prosthesis allows patients to be fitted with regular-sized clothing without alterations (chapter 3).

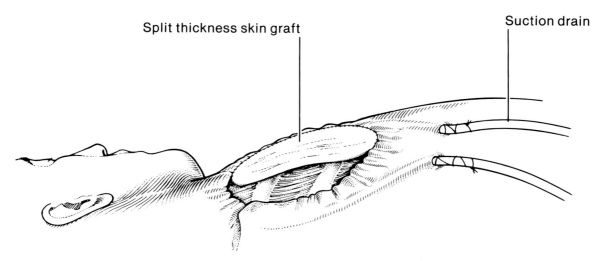

Split thickness skin graft

Suction drain

Figure 23–9. Split-thickness skin graft used to cover the chest wall in tumors with skin infiltration over a wide area.

Occasionally, a large tumor will involve skin to such an extent that skin closure is impossible. If this occurs, the abbreviated skin flaps should be secured to the chest wall and a split-thickness skin graft used to cover the remaining defect. The neurovascular bundle should be covered by skin flaps to avoid late hemorrhagic complications (Fig. 23–9).

REFERENCES

1. Fanous N, Didolkar MS, Holyoke ED, et al: Evaluation of forequarter amputation in malignant diseases. *Surg Gynecol Obst* 1976;142:381–384.
2. Sim FH, Pritchard DJ, Ivins JC: Forequarter amputation. *Orthop Clin N Am* 1977;8:921–931.
3. Mansour KA, Powell RW: Modified technique for radical transmediastinal forequarter amputation and chest wall resection. *J Thorac Cardiovasc Surg* 1978;76:358–363.
4. Wurlitzer FP: Improved technic for radical transthoracic forequarter amputation. *Ann Surg* 1973;177:467–471.
5. Marcove RC, Lewis MM, Huvos AG: En bloc upper humeral interscapulothoracic resection. The Tikhoff-Linberg procedure. *Clin Orthop* 1977;124:219–228.
6. Littlewood H: Amputation at the shoulder and at the hip. *Br Med J* 1922;1:381–383.
7. Sugarbaker PH: *An Atlas of Surgical Oncology: Fundamental Procedures.* Boca Raton, Fla, CRC Press, 1983, vol 2.
8. Blumenfeld I, Schortz RH, Levy M, et al: Fabricating a shoulder somatoprosthesis. *J Prosthet Dent* 1981;45:542–544.

24

Radical Forequarter Amputation with Chest Wall Resection

JACK A. ROTH, M.D.
PAUL H. SUGARBAKER, M.D.
ALAN R. BAKER, M.D.

OVERVIEW

Forequarter amputation with resection of the chest wall is indicated for primary bony and soft tissue tumors involving the shoulder girdle, axilla, and chest wall, and radiation recurrent breast cancer in the axilla. We describe a modification of this procedure that includes an initial thoractomy for intraoperative staging and a median sternotomy incision that avoids individual division of the anterior ribs and clavicle. The skin incision is fashioned to widely encompass the tumor and biopsy site. The incision must allow for an exploratory thoracotomy and an assessment of tumor spread along the thoracic inlet. Skin flaps are initially fashioned to provide coverage for the resultant defect. After the chest is entered through the fifth or sixth intercostal space, the pulmonary parenchyma, pleural surface of the chest wall, and the hilum of the lung are evaluated for metastatic tumor spread. If the tumor seems operable, the back muscles are divided, the intercostal bundles are secured posteriorly, and the ribs are divided. The anterior portion of the specimen may be detached by performing a median sternotomy and resecting one half of the sternum along with the attached ribs. Following division of the strap muscles, the innominate vein, subclavian artery, and brachial plexus nerve roots are dissected free and divided. Division of the anterior, medial, and posterior scalene muscles allows removal of the specimen. Reconstruction of the chest wall defect with prosthetic material is optional.

When malignant bony or soft tissue tumors of the upper arm, shoulder, scapula, or axilla involve the chest wall, forequarter amputation alone is contraindicated. Stafford and Williams first described a modification of the forequarter amputation technique that included chest wall resection, thus rendering such tumors amenable to complete excision.[1] Several modifications of this technique have been described, differing primarily in the addition of a median sternotomy incision to resect the anterior portion of the ribs and the method of reconstruction used.[2–4] The following technique has been particularly useful in resecting bulky tumors involving the scapula with extension into the axilla and chest wall. The following surgical principles will be emphasized:

1. A thoracotomy should be performed early in the procedure to assess resectability at the thoracic inlet and the presence or absence of pulmonary metastases.
2. Division of the posterior ribs and sternum facilitates ligation of the vessels and nerve roots by enhancing mobility of the specimen and thus improving exposure.

INDICATIONS

Tumors that are locally recurrent in the axilla following radiation therapy may require chest wall resection and forequarter amputation for total extirpation. Recurrent breast cancer or locally persistent cystosarcoma phyllodes are tumors that commonly present with this problem. Bony tumors of the scapula or clavicle that involve portions of the chest wall also may require this procedure for local control. Soft tissue sarcomas arising in the axilla, beneath the pectoralis muscle, or beneath the scapula are frequently adherent to the chest wall. If these tumors extend into the axilla and involve the nerve roots and vessels, forequarter amputation and chest wall resection will be indicated. Primary tumors arising in the chest wall and involving structures of the thoracic inlet or axilla may also require this procedure.

It is imperative to obtain a preoperative biopsy for appropriate diagnosis. Depending on the histology of the tumor, preoperative chemotherapy or radiation therapy may be indicated. Low-grade malignancies may not require such a radical approach. Noninvasive imaging studies should be obtained to detect distant metastases. Preoperative arteriograms visualizing the subclavian and vertebral arteries and venograms visualizing the innominate vein and subclavian vein are extremely useful to determine the involvement of these vessels by tumor. Pulmonary function tests are useful in determining the value of reconstructive procedures to stabilize the chest wall.

PROCEDURE

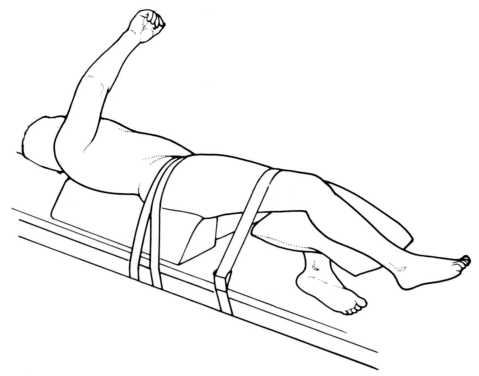

Figure 24–1. POSITION. The patient is placed in the lateral position (torso at 60° to the operating table) and the arm is draped free. Moving the arm so as to keep tissues being transected under tension expedites the dissection. Rolling the table toward or away from the surgeon will often improve exposure. The surgeon should be positioned on the anterior aspect of the patient.

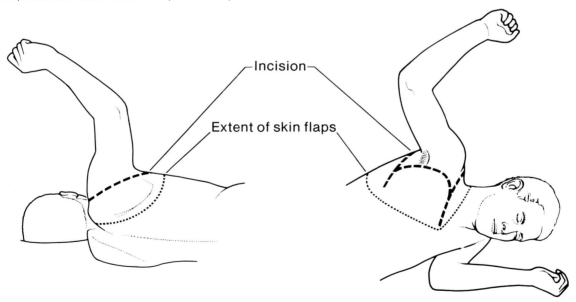

Incision

Extent of skin flaps

Figure 24–2. INCISION AND SKIN FLAPS. The incision must be fashioned to encompass tumor and biopsy site, and to allow for an exploratory thoracotomy. The incision begins over the clavicle medially and extends in the deltopectoral groove, then bisects the shelving edge of the pectoralis major muscle to encompass all axillary hair. The posterior incision courses over the surgical neck of the scapula to join the anterior incision below the axilla. The lateral margins of the incision may be extended anteriorly to form an anterior subcutaneous flap. Alternatively, a posterior flap can be fashioned extending up the arm if the anterior chest wall skin is involved with tumor.

The skin flaps are dissected to the sternoclavicular junction anteriorly and to the medial border of the scapula posteriorly. Superiorly they must expose the supraclavicular fossa to the base of the neck (anterior cervical triangle). Inferiorly the lymphatic contents of the axilla must be exposed so that they can be included within the specimen.

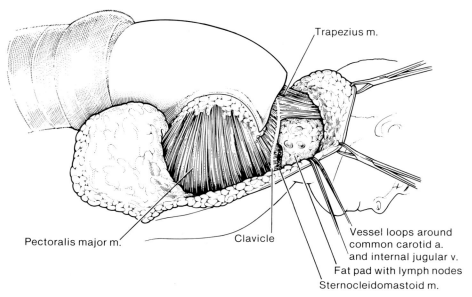

Figure 24–3. EXPLORATION OF THE ANTERIOR CERVICAL TRIANGLE. The sternocleidomastoid muscle is divided at its insertion into the clavicle to expose the junction of the internal jugular vein and subclavian vein. The brachial plexus is exposed to determine if the anterior margin of resection on the neurovascular bundle is clear. Inspection of the cervical lymph nodes is performed so that nodal metastases can be detected. The internal jugular vein and common carotid artery are identified, and vessel loops are passed around them.

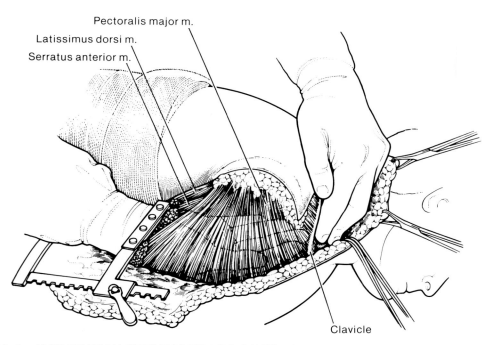

Figure 24–4. EXPLORATION OF THE THORACIC CAVITY. A sufficiently caudad interspace is chosen to enter the chest so that tumor is not violated. Blunt dissection in the free tissue planes beneath the pectoralis major muscle should be avoided. The extracostal muscles are divided over this interspace. The electrocautery is used to elevate the periosteum and intercostal muscle bundle from the superior edge of the sixth rib. Higher interspaces may be chosen for smaller tumors. The sixth rib should be traced to its posterior extent to make sure that this structure does not pass beneath the tumor. The chest is entered, and a chest retractor is inserted. The lung parenchyma is carefully inspected and palpated for pulmonary metastases. If the lung is the only site of metastases, these can be resected provided that adequate functioning lung remains. The pleural surface beneath the tumor mass is inspected for full thickness invasion. The thoracic inlet should be visualized from within the chest. With one hand in the chest and one hand palpating the anterior cervical triangle, palpation of the structures of the thoracic inlet is possible. This allows accurate assessment of the proximal tumor margin relative to the brachial plexus and subclavian vessels.

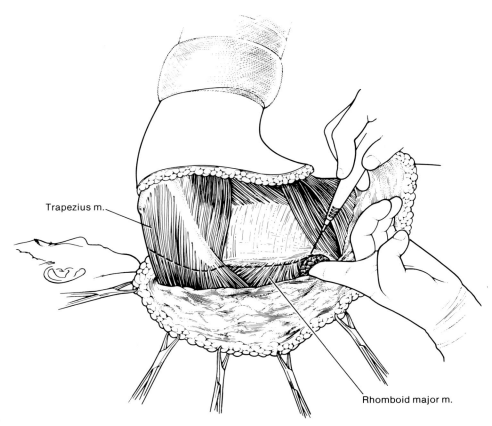

Figure 24–5.   DIVISION OF MUSCULAR ATTACHMENTS OF THE SCAPULA. If the tumor is determined to be operable, the remainder of the muscular attachments of the scapula are divided from below upward. This includes the latissimus dorsi, rhomboids, trapezius, and levator scapulae. Care is taken not to elevate the scapula off the chest wall because this may expose the tumor and result in tumor contamination of the operative field.

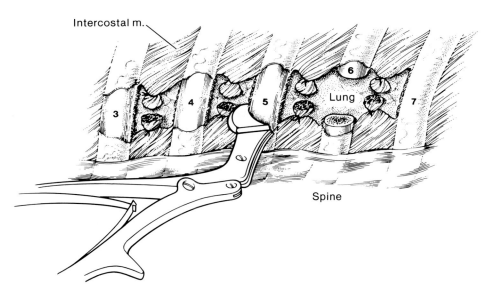

Figure 24–6.   SECURING THE INTERCOSTAL BUNDLES AND TRANSECTING THE RIBS POSTERIORLY. The ribs are scored crosswise with the electrocautery at the point of transection. The periosteum is lifted from the superior and inferior margins of the ribs at the point of transection with the periosteal elevator. Intercostal muscle, nerves, and vessels are dissected free of the ribs with a right-angle clamp. The intercostal bundle is ligated in continuity and then divided. Intercostal vessels are secured from below, working upward. As the ribs become thicker, wider, and closer together toward the apex of the chest, this maneuver becomes more difficult.

The ribs are transected from inferior to superior. Ribs 1 to 5 are divided easily by using the guillotine rib cutter. A 1-cm section of each rib is removed to facilitate mobility of the specimen.

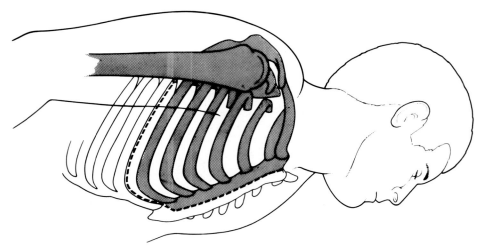

Figure 24–7.   MEDIAN STERNOTOMY INCISION. The portion of the specimen made up of the anterior chest wall is mobilized by median sternotomy incision. The internal mammary vessels are ligated at the lowest interspace to be transected. The sternum is then split with a saw to the same level, and this half of the sternum with attached ribs is detached.

Alternatively, the individual intercostal bundles can be severed at the anterior aspect of the dissection and the ribs individually transected. It is also necessary to divide the clavicle and remove its proximal portion to expose the underlying subclavian and innominate vein if this approach is used.

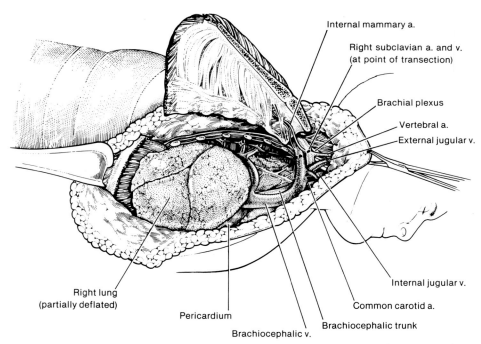

Internal mammary a.

Right subclavian a. and v.
(at point of transection)

Brachial plexus

Vertebral a.

External jugular v.

Internal jugular v.

Common carotid a.

Brachiocephalic trunk

Brachiocephalic v.

Pericardium

Right lung
(partially deflated)

Figure 24–8.   DIVISION OF MUSCLE INSERTIONS ON FIRST RIB AND DIVISION OF VESSELS AND NERVES. Electrocautery and the periosteal elevator are used to skeletonize the first rib as it attaches to the manubrium. The strap, sternohyoid, and sternothyroid muscles are divided in their lower third to expose the innominate vein. The subclavian artery is mobilized, ligated, and divided in continuity distal to the takeoff of the vertebral artery. This is best done by dissecting the artery from within the thorax. The enhanced mobility of the specimen at this point readily permits dissection of the artery along its entire length. The subclavian vein is similarly divided. The cords of the brachial plexus are individually ligated and divided as the dissection proceeds. The medial and posterior scalene muscles are transected to deliver the specimen. Care must be taken to preserve the vagus and phrenic nerves and to ligate the thoracic duct in specimens resected from the left side. It may be necessary to transect the innominate vein at its junction with the subclavian vein to adequately expose the subclavian artery. Excessive blood loss will not occur into the specimen if the subclavian artery is then immediately clamped.

322

Drainage catheter

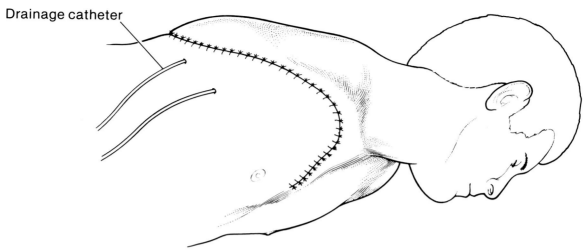

Figure 24–9. CLOSURE. The defect may be closed simply by approximating the skin and subcutaneous tissues. Alternatively the defect may be covered with prosthetic mesh to provide some additional stabilization. A chest tube is inserted along with closed-suction subcutaneous drainage catheters. The subcutaneous catheters must be removed before the chest tube to avoid a pneumothorax. Prolonged ventilatory support (one to five days) was required for all patients undergoing this procedure at our institution.

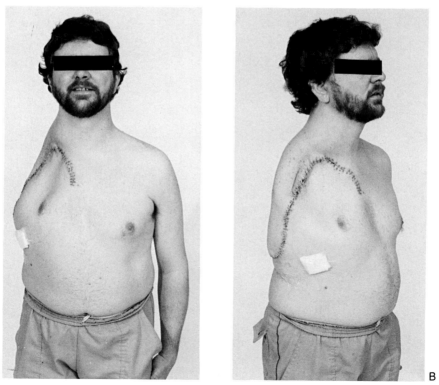

A   B

Figure 24–10. (A) Anterior and (B) oblique views of a patient following forequarter amputation and chest wall resection. Ventilatory support is required postoperatively for most patients. Despite the extensive resection of tissue, recovery is uniformly rapid and complications are few.

DISCUSSION

The postoperative appearance of a patient who underwent this procedure is shown in Figure 24–10. The patient can wear a molded plastic shell under his clothing to improve postoperative cosmesis (chapter 4).

The forequarter amputation with chest wall resection described here is one of the most radical resections that is performed. The arm, shoulder girdle, and chest wall are removed from the angle of the ribs posteriorly to the mid-sternum. Often the attachment of a tumor mass to the chest wall is more limited; then only a small segment of adherent chest wall must be removed en bloc with the specimen. If the first rib is not involved, the procedure is greatly simplified. The great vessels and brachial plexus are intimately related to the first rib. If the first rib must be removed, release of the specimen anteriorly by a median sternotomy greatly simplifies the procedure and does not, in our experience, increase the morbidity of the procedure or the patient's disability.

Considerable controversy concerns the use of prosthetic mesh to close the chest wall defect; we recognize some potential disadvantages of this technique. The paradoxical motion of the covering skin flap is not appreciably reduced by mesh. If infection of the mesh occurs, the entire skin flap may need to be revised to remove the infected prosthetic material. Furthermore, if subsequent thoracotomy is required for pulmonary metastases, the adhesions between pulmonary parenchyma and mesh make exploration of the thoracic cavity difficult. However, some additional chest wall stability may be gained for patients, thus improving postoperative pulmonary function. For patients with marginal pulmonary reserve, this could be significant. Carefully controlled prospective studies determining preoperative and postoperative ventilatory mechanics will be necessary to resolve this point.

REFERENCES

1. Stafford ES, Williams GR, Jr: Radical transthoracic forequarter amputation. *Ann Surg* 1958;148:699–703.
2. Nadler SH, Phelan JT: A technique of interscapulothoracic amputation. *Surg Gynecol Obstet* 1966;122:359–364.
3. Mansour KA, Powell RW: Modified technique for radical transmediastinal forequarter amputation and chest wall resection. *J Thorac Cardiovasc Surg* 1978;76:358–363.
4. Wurlitzer FP: Improved technique for radical transthoracic forequarter amputation. *Ann Surg* 1973;177:467–471.

25

Above-Elbow Amputation

PAUL H. SUGARBAKER, M.D.
MARTIN M. MALAWER, M.D.
ALAN R. BAKER, M.D.

OVERVIEW

Above-elbow amputation is indicated for advanced primary or recurrent soft tissue sarcomas of the forearm. The level of amputation will vary with the location of the tumor in the forearm, at the elbow joint, or even in the lower portion of the arm. The location of the tumor mass medially (surrounding the neurovascular bundle) v lateral (in soft tissue) may, in large part, determine if amputation or limb-salvage surgery should be recommended. During the procedure, muscle flaps are tapered and then closed tautly in two layers over the end of the humerus. If an unusual muscle resection or skin flaps were required, cosmetic-appearing pleats, as opposed to unsightly skin folds along the wound closure, can be ensured by individually placing sutures that divide the open incision. A rigid dressing applied immediately postoperatively decreases pain and edema and begins to mold the stump.

INTRODUCTION

Soft tissue sarcomas of the upper extremity are common. Approximately one fourth of all soft tissue sarcomas occur in the upper extremity, and about half of these occur in the forearm and arm. Primary bone sarcomas are less common at this site.

Limb-sparing surgery in conjunction with radiation therapy and chemotherapy have proven to be a safe and effective alternative to above-elbow amputation for many patients with soft tissue sarcoma of the forearm. More problematic are those soft tissue sarcomas that are intimately related to the elbow joint or involve the neurovascular bundle in the lower aspect of the arm. The success of limb-sparing surgery has further been augmented by the development of new endoprosthetic devices that allow replacement of the distal humerus. Both of these surgical alternatives to amputation offer the patient the possibility of satisfactory limb function after surgery.

Nonetheless, above-elbow amputation retains a clear-cut and definitive role in the management of bone and soft tissue sarcomas of the upper extremity. Above-elbow amputation is required for sarcomas of the forearm and distal arm that cannot be removed with a negative margin of resection. Unresectable forearm sarcomas are treated by a standard (diaphyseal) above-elbow amputation (Fig. 25–1). Tumors occurring around the elbow or within the distal arm require a high above-elbow amputation.

A major responsibility for the orthopedic and surgical oncologist is to determine which patients with

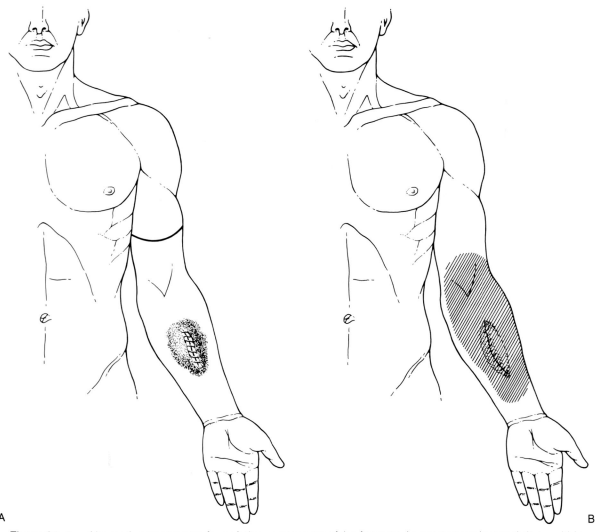

A   B

Figure 25–1.   Alternative treatments for soft tissue sarcoma of the forearm. Large tumors located deep within the muscle bundles and infiltrating structures in the forearm usually require amputation (**A**). Smaller tumors, especially those of lower grade malignancy, are treated by wide local excision plus radiation therapy (**B**).

upper-extremity sarcoma will benefit by amputation and which would benefit most from limb-sparing surgery. Such decisions need to be made on a case-by-case basis. All patients today should be considered and evaluated for limb-salvage surgery, and the decision to proceed with amputation should be made only after this option has been ruled out. Guidelines are based on the surgical stage, tumor grade, and anatomic location of the primary tumor.

INDICATIONS FOR AMPUTATION

Amputations are usually performed for high-grade sarcomas in which wide local excision results in a positive *margin of resection*. *Recurrent high-grade* sarcomas in the absence of systemic disease should be treated by amputation. Rarely should a grade I sarcoma that is not expected to metastasize be initially treated by amputation. Rather, a trial of limb- salvage surgery alone or combined with local radiation therapy should be attempted as long as a functional extremity remains behind.

Major *vascular involvement* may require amputation. In the arm the neurovascular bundle is tightly integrated in a closed anatomic space. Major vessel involvement may require sacrifice of the entire extremity. The incidence of morbidity and failure associated with the resection and reconstruction is significantly higher if a vascular graft is required. The cephalic vein usually provides sufficient collateral if resection of the axillary or brachial vein is required. However, tumor encasement of the brachial artery usually mandates an amputation. Occasionally the tumor mass can be delicately dissected off of the brachial artery and the limb spared.

Major *nerve involvement* may occur. In general, one nerve may be removed, and a two-nerve deficit is tolerated. Sacrifice of the entire brachial plexus leaves the patient with a functionless extremity that is better amputated. Again, the higher on the extremity the tumor is located, the more likely is the need for sacrifice of major nerve trunks. Nerve grafting for replacement of a section of median, ulnar, or radial nerve has not been associated with reasonable return of function.

Extensive local *soft tissue contamination* occurs all too frequently. Large tumor size with sarcomas of the forearm or arm is usually associated with extensive contamination of the muscle compartments. The muscle compartments of the arm and forearm are not as well defined by dense fascial planes as are those of the lower extremity. Tumor spread as a result of the biopsy or attempts at resection of tumor through its pseudocapsule may be associated with extensive soft tissue contamination by tumor.

Pathologic fracture through the humerus or ulna usually results in extensive hematoma formation. This may cause tumor contamination throughout the muscle compartments of the arm or forearm. If this occurs, reliable local control may be impossible to achieve without amputation.

Infection of the tumor itself or of the biopsy site may negate any attempt at local resection. Infection will, of course, prohibit the use of a prosthetic device. It may also interfere with preoperative and/or postoperative chemotherapy.

High doses of radiation therapy in young patients with skeletal immaturity may result in limb-length discrepancy in the upper extremity, as in the lower. However, this rarely results in a significant interference with function. A greater problem may be contractures secondary to radiation therapy around the elbow. Early intensive physical therapy should prevent this complication.

CLINICAL CONSIDERATIONS

Utilization of induction chemotherapy may result in profound tumor shrinkage. Many of these tumors will have a well-defined vascular supply that can be cannulated through a transfemoral route. This means that regional chemotherapy can be used to shrink the tumor prior to definitive surgery. In other patients systemic chemotherapy plus local radiation can be utilized to convert a malignancy thought to require an obvious amputation to a limb-salvage procedure.

TIMING OF THE SURGICAL PROCEDURE

If the patient has received a recent course of chemotherapy, it is essential that both leukocyte and platelet counts be permitted to return toward normal. Significant deficits in red blood cell mass should be corrected by preoperative transfusion. Vascular insufficiency is rarely a complicating factor in these patients, but suboptimal wound healing may be a problem, particularly if patients have received preoperative radiation therapy or chemotherapy. Associated nausea and vomiting may contribute to nutrition and weight loss, which will further compound wound-healing problems. Because of potential healing difficulties, stump wound closure must be meticulously performed. Hematoma must be avoided by the generous use of closed-suction drainage. If possible, one should defer removal of skin sutures for as long as three weeks. If unusual muscle excision or skin flaps were utilized for the resection, extra time for the stump to mold and mature may be required.

REHABILITATION

The cancer patient faces a unique psychological problem. Not only is there a threat to his or her life, but in this situation there may be the loss of a dominant extremity. Although this is well tolerated in the long run, it represents a tremendous loss for the patient, and a grief process must be expected. Because of this, rehabilitation of a patient undergoing above-elbow amputation needs to begin at the time of the staging studies. The entire health care team must develop a relationship with the patient and include him or her in the early stages of all decision making. Building upon this, the patient will be better able to accept the need for an amputation and its consequences. It is important that realistic rehabilitation goals be set even prior to the amputative procedure.

It is the responsibility of all persons who interact with the amputation patient to recognize emotional problems as they arise and to provide as much assistance as possible. Professional psychological intervention and the use of psychotropic agents may be required before or after surgery. All patients undergoing an amputation, especially a high amputation such as an above-elbow amputation, experience phantom limb pain. This must be discussed with the patient prior to surgery. The patient should understand that this is to be expected, and that it can be treated with analgesics and pain-management therapy. It will subside with this level of amputation over time. The care team should realize that the patient who reports severe pain (10% to 15% of all cases) prior to surgery is often the one who finds it most difficult to adapt to amputation and to being a cancer patient. It is important to distinguish stump pain that is well localized and confined to a specific location from phantom pain. Problems with the amputation are usually signaled by stump pain. Recurrence may be signaled by an increasing severity of phantom limb pain late in the patient's course.

The rehabilitation therapist can be of tremendous help preoperatively in preparing the patient. A *positive attitude* toward functional recovery and the use of a prosthesis are necessary. The prosthesis must often be readjusted several times before stump stability is achieved. This requires patience and persistence on the part of the rehabilitation team. Seeing other patients who have successfully met some of the rehabilitation challenges similar to the ones experienced by the patient can result in an immeasurable psychological boost to the patient. The surgical or orthopedic oncologist, rehabilitation therapist, and others involved in the postoperative care must coordinate their efforts carefully, realizing the possibilities of conflicting demands on the patient's time and conflicting messages being delivered by different caregivers.

LEVEL OF AMPUTATION

The highest-priority consideration for any amputative procedure is the avoidance of local recurrence. For soft tissue sarcoma a full 5 cm of normal tissue above the macroscopic proximal extent of the cancer must be sacrificed. The same margin of normal marrow is required above the radiologic deficit seen with an osteosarcoma.

PREOPERATIVE RADIOLOGIC EVALUATION

The major contraindications for limb-sparing resection in the arm or forearm are tumor size, major nerve or blood vessel involvement (especially in the antecubital location), and extensive tumor contamination in the muscle compartments from biopsy or local removal of a high-grade sarcoma. One must be aware that tumors that arise adjacent to a major nerve or blood vessel may extend quite far in the proximal direction. The muscle compartments of the arm and forearm are not as well defined as those of the lower extremity, and the extent of tumor spread may be more difficult to determine by radiologic studies. The computerized tomogram and MRI of the arm may be of considerable value in determining the extent of soft tissue involvement. A bone scan can often indicate bone involvement by cancer. An arteriogram is often of great importance to determine vascular involvement and vascular displacement by the tumor mass.

A CT scan of the chest should be used to rule out lung metastases, and a bone scan should be performed to rule out skeletal metastases.

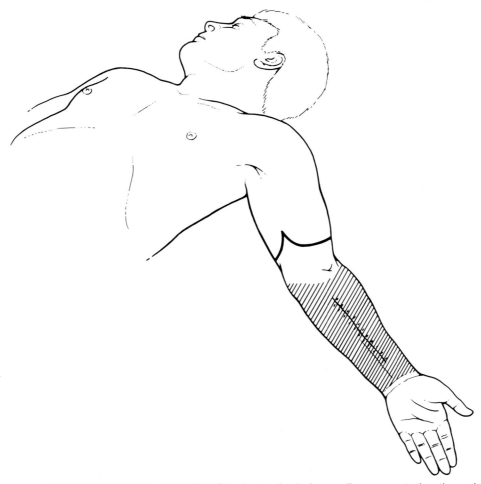

Figure 25–2.   **PATIENT POSITION AND INCISION.** A standard above-elbow amputation through the bony diaphysis is performed for a tumor recurring at the proximal end of the scar following wide excision and radiation therapy of a forearm sarcoma.

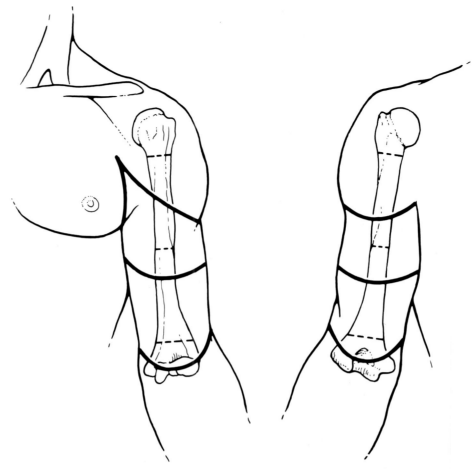

Figure 25–3.   SKIN INCISION AND OSTEOTOMY FOR PROXIMAL HUMERUS (METAPHYSEAL), DIAPHY-
SEAL, AND SUPRACONDYLAR AMPUTATION. High above-elbow amputations are those proximal to the
deltoid tuberosity. Patients who undergo amputations proximal to the deltoid tuberosity and pectoralis major
insertion have far greater problems adjusting to their prosthesis than to those who have undergone more distal
above-elbow amputations. The longest stump possible that is considered oncologically safe should be
utilized. In a young child a high-level amputation should be performed in lieu of a disarticulation, since 80% of
humeral growth occurs proximally.

    Standard anterior/posterior flaps are utilized; occasionally, medial/lateral flaps are needed. Wound healing
is almost never a problem with upper-extremity amputation.

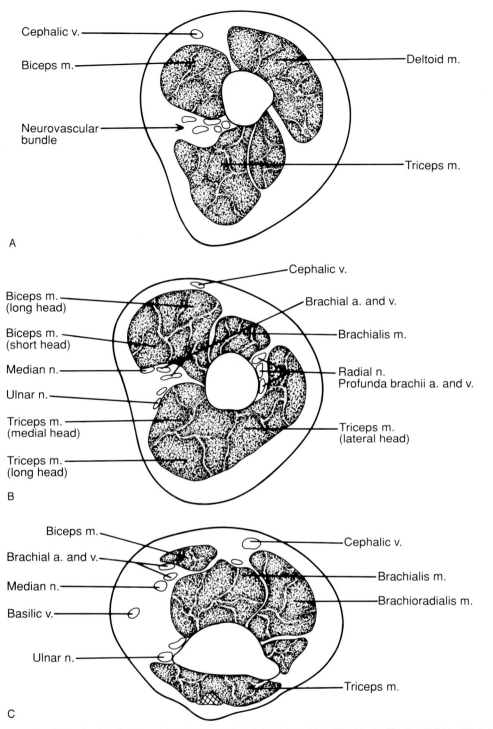

Figure 25–4.   CROSS-SECTIONAL ANATOMY. (**A**) PROXIMAL HUMERAL AMPUTATION, (**B**) DIAPHY-SEAL AMPUTATION, (**C**) SUPRACONDYLAR AMPUTATION.

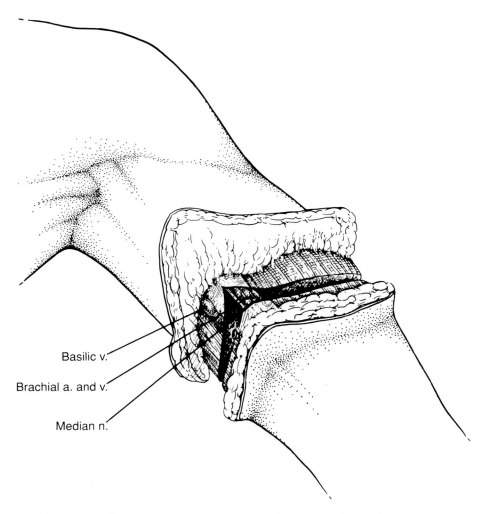

Basilic v.

Brachial a. and v.

Median n.

Figure 25–5. TAPERING OF THE MUSCLE INCISION. The skin, superficial fascia, and subcutaneous tissue are divided perpendicular to the skin surface. The muscles are tapered. Large blood vessels are ligated in continuity and then suture-ligated.

The nerves are handled delicately. They are pulled approximately 2 cm from their muscular bed, doubly ligated with nonabsorbable monofilament suture, and cut with a knife. The area around the nerve is infiltrated with a long-acting local anesthetic agent.

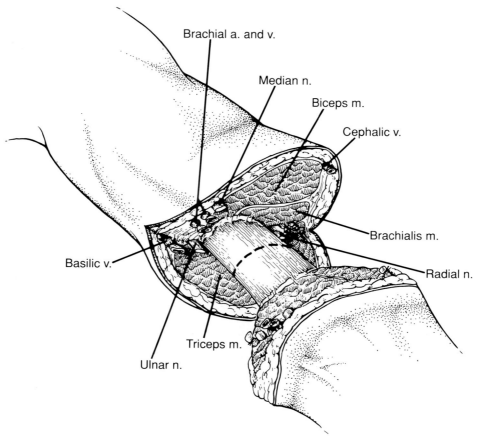

Figure 25–6.   TRANSECTION OF MUSCLE AND BONE.

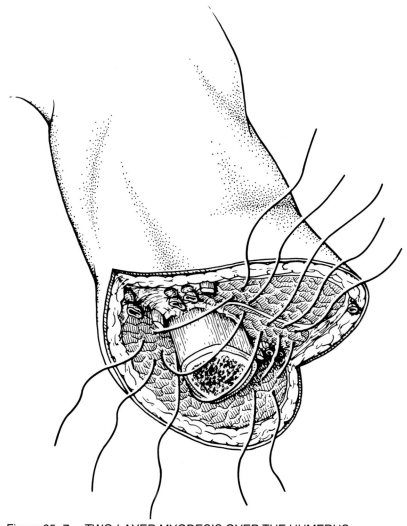

Figure 25–7.   TWO-LAYER MYODESIS OVER THE HUMERUS.

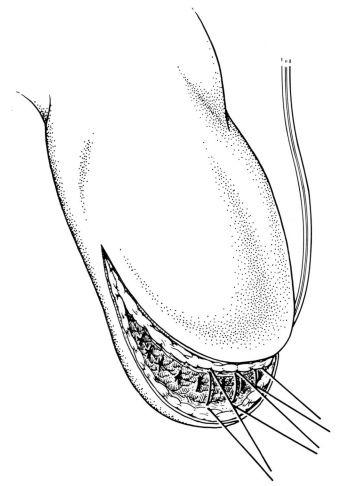

Figure 25–8. CLOSURE OF SUPERFICIAL FASCIA AND SKIN OVER CLOSED-SUCTION DRAINS.

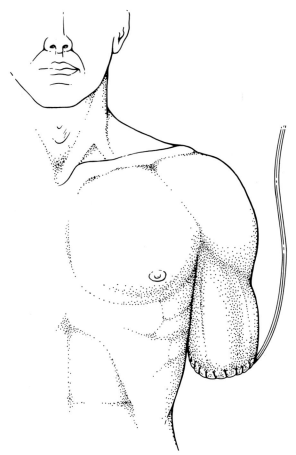

Figure 25–9.   SKIN CLOSURE.

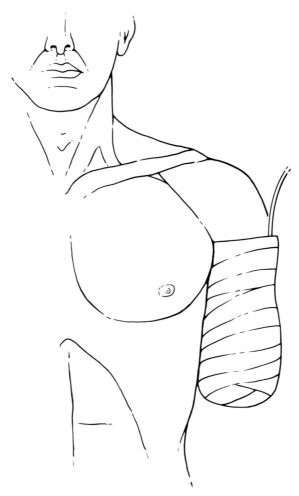

Figure 25–10.   APPLICATION OF THE RIGID DRESSING. A rigid dressing helps decrease pain and edema. Attention should be paid to padding the anterior portion of the humerus, which is essential for adequate force transmission within a prosthesis. Prosthesis training should begin as soon as possible after surgery. Stump edema is rarely a problem in the upper extremity.

SHOULDER DISARTICULATION

Shoulder disarticulation is rarely used in patients undergoing an amputation for cancer. There is a cosmetic benefit to sparing the shoulder over performing a forequarter amputation. However, there is almost always a decided oncologic advantage to performing the forequarter amputation. With a light prosthesis to fill out the shoulder, patients with this amputation can wear regular clothes and have the same functional capabilities as patients with a shoulder disarticulation.

26

Scapulectomy: Type III Shoulder Girdle Resection

TAPAS K. DAS GUPTA, M.D., Ph.D.

OVERVIEW

Scapulectomy is indicated for soft tissue tumors located superficial to the scapula and for primary malignant tumors of this bone. A generous oblique incision is made, and skin flaps are constructed to visualize the limits of the scapula. After reflecting trapezius and deltoid muscles from the spine, muscular attachments on the vertebral border are released; then superior and lateral muscle groups are severed from the scapula. Traction on the tip of the scapula will keep muscles to be transected under tension and will facilitate their division. By elevation of the scapula, the subscapularis muscle is divided. An osteotome is used to divide the acromion, and a Gigli saw is used to divide the neck of the scapula. Muscles are reapproximated, and the skin is closed over suction drainage. Complications are few, and rehabilitation usually is complete.

Scapulectomy for removal of tumors in the scapular region was described originally by Syme in 1864.[1] In his monograph he described three patients on whom he had performed this operation. Although he did not clearly define the indications for scapulectomy, he showed the procedure to be feasible and practical. In his presidential address to the American Surgical Association Meeting in 1909, de Nancrede categorically stated that scapulectomy was an inferior operation.[2] It thus fell into disrepute in this country, and the results of this operation were reported only occasionally thereafter.[3] In 1958, Pack and Ariel mentioned this procedure but did not elaborate either in favor of or against it.[4] Thus, it is apparent that the indications for scapulectomy have never been defined clearly; consequently, the end results have been unsatisfactory. It should be emphasized that scapulectomy has a limited role in surgery for neoplastic disease. Strict criteria must be established for its performance, or a perfectly suitable operative procedure will not be utilized. However, it may be considered as an alternative to interscapulothoracic amputation or the Tikhoff–Linberg operation in carefully selected patients (chapters 23 and 27).

INDICATIONS

A scapulectomy is indicated in the following types of tumor:

A. Soft tissue tumors
   1. Low-grade fibrosarcoma invading the scapular muscles
   2. Desmoid-type tumor infiltrating the scapular muscles
   3. Liposarcoma arising from the adipose tissue in the scapular region where an adequate soft tissue excision necessitates excision of part or all of the scapula
   4. Deeply invasive carcinoma of the skin for which there must be wide excision including the scapula
B. Bone tumors
   1. Primary malignant bone tumor arising in the scapula is rare. However, scapulectomy may be useful in unusual cases of low-grade chondrosarcoma or of giant cell tumor of the scapula.
   2. Solitary metastatic lesion is a very rare tumor. Although scapulectomy for this lesion was reported by Ryerson, it is rarely, if ever, indicated for metastatic scapular lesions.[3]

Scapulectomies in carefully selected patients have been performed with long-term cure and excellent functional results. The majority of these patients were able to resume normal activity with reasonable use of the arm shortly after the operation.

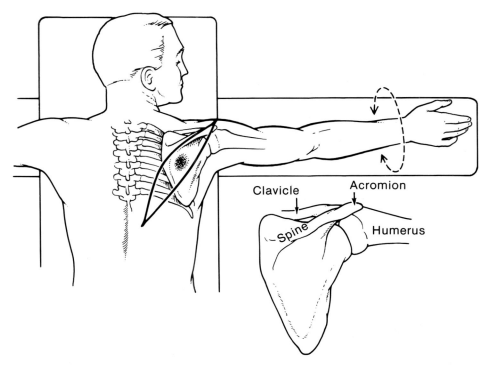

Figure 26–1.   POSITION AND INCISION. The patient is placed in the prone position with the arm resting in 90° abduction on an arm board. The arm should be draped so that an assistant can move it as required during the operation.

An elliptical skin incision is then made, encompassing the tumor and extending from the tip of the acromion superolaterally to the paravertebral region inferomedially. The lower end of the incision can be extended to cross the midline if the tumor is so large as to make this necessary.

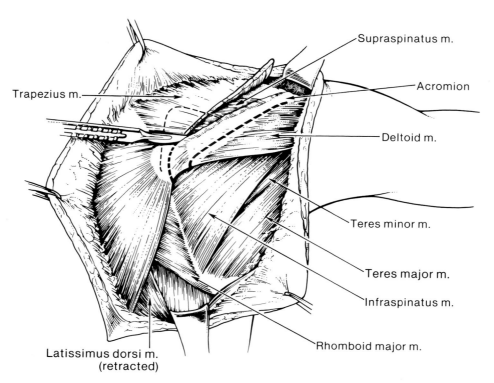

Figure 26–2. CONSTRUCTION OF SKIN FLAPS AND RELEASE OF TRAPEZIUS AND DELTOID MUSCLES. The medial and lateral skin flaps are raised as in a standard radical mastectomy. The superficial dorsal muscular attachments to the scapula are identified. The attachment of the trapezius muscle to the scapular spine is completely resected and retracted superomedially, exposing the supraspinatus muscle. The attachment of the deltoid muscle to the lateral tip of the scapular spine is similarly resected and reflected laterally. At this stage the rhomboid major muscle at the vertebral border, the latissimus dorsi inferiorly, the teres major and minor muscles laterally, and the infraspinatus muscle can be identified easily.

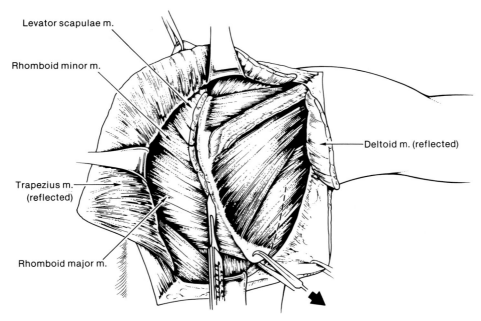

Figure 26–3. RELEASE OF MUSCLES ATTACHED TO VERTEBRAL BORDER OF SCAPULA. The insertion of the latissimus dorsi muscle at the tip of the scapula is then excised, and the muscle is retracted downward, exposing the tip. The scapular tip is then held by an assistant with a straight towel clip and pulled inferolaterally. This provides traction to the muscles at the vertebral border, and excision of their scapular attachment is simplified.

The muscular attachments in the superior angle of the scapula are then resected along the vertebral border of the scapula. The levator scapulae and the rhomboids, easily delineated, are then cut. This maneuver can be quite simple if the assistant maintains constant traction at the tip of the scapula.

341

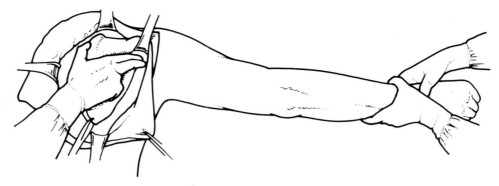

Figure 26–4. INSPECTION OF THE AXILLARY CONTENTS. The inferior tip of the scapula is then rotated, and a medial pull is applied while the arm is abducted. This permits easy access to and identification of the axillary contents. The contents are then retracted out of the operating field.

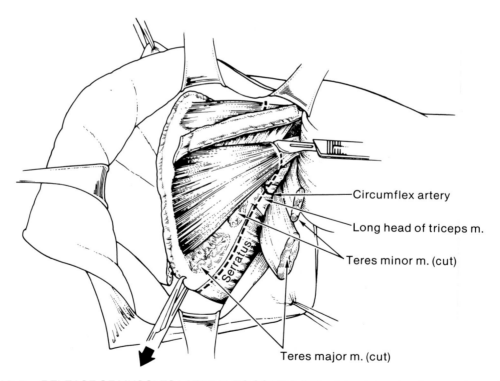

—Circumflex artery

—Long head of triceps m.

—Teres minor m. (cut)

serratus

Teres major m. (cut)

Figure 26–5. RELEASE OF MUSCLES LATERAL TO SCAPULA. The lateral muscles, teres major and minor, and the long head of the triceps are cut. Next, the supraspinatus and infraspinatus tendons and the attachment of serratus anterior muscles are released from the scapula.

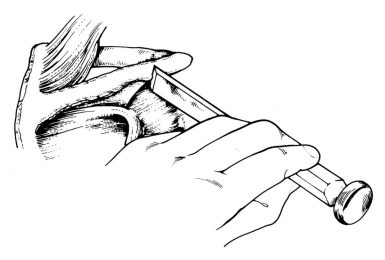

Figure 26–6. OSTEOTOMY OF ACROMION. The shoulder joint is then exposed and identified, and the spine is cut near the acromion process with an osteotome.

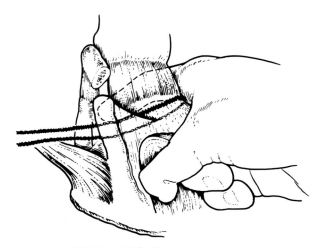

Figure 26–7. RELEASE OF SUBSCAPULARIS. The only muscle remaining attached to the scapula, humerus, and shoulder joint is the subscapularis, which is resected under the guidance of the operator's finger.

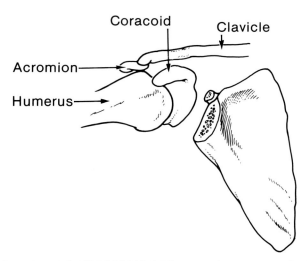

Coracoid   Clavicle

Acromion

Humerus

Figure 26–8. OSTEOTOMY OF NECK OF SCAPULA. The scapular osteotomy is viewed here from its anterior aspect. A Gigli saw is then passed around the neck of the scapula, avoiding the glenohumeral joint. The scapula is resected and the specimen removed, care being taken to avoid injury to the glenohumeral joint.

343

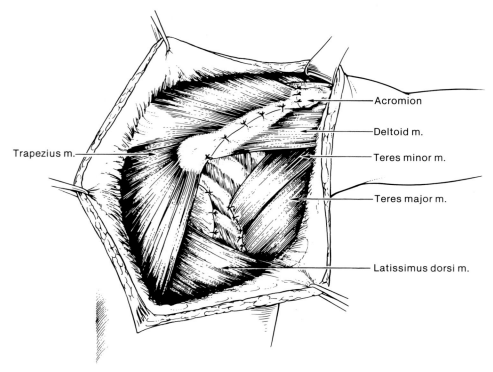

Figure 26–9. MUSCLE RECONSTRUCTION. After proper hemostasis is achieved, the cut edge of the trapezius muscle is sutured to the deltoid muscle at the line of the previous position of the spine of the scapula. The lateral margins of these muscular stitches incorporate the remnant of the acromion process. The teres major and minor muscles are sutured to the chest wall.

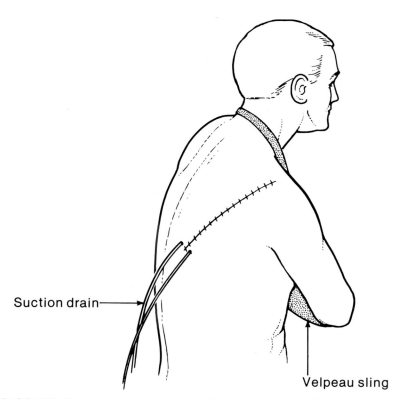

Figure 26–10. CLOSURE. The suction catheter beneath each skin flap is then brought out through normal skin, the wound is closed by interrupted subcutaneous 3–0 chromic catgut sutures, and the skin margins are apposed by interrupted 3–0 Dermalon stitches. The suction catheters are then attached to a continuous suction device. A dressing is applied and the arm is placed in a Velpeau sling.

DISCUSSION

The patient should be allowed to ambulate early. The dressing is removed after 48 hours and replaced by an ordinary collar and cuff sling. The patient is instructed to keep the arm in this sling during the day and support the arm on a pillow at night. By the end of the seventh day or when suction catheters have been removed, active exercise, such as attempts at abduction, should be encouraged.

The patient should be seen by a physical therapist at this time for instruction in active and passive exercises. The suction catheters are removed by the eighth or ninth day, and the skin stitches are removed by the tenth to twelfth days.

A carefully organized physiotherapy program begun early after the operation ensures maximum use of the extremity. In most instances the patient can return to normal work within 8 to 12 weeks after the operation.

REFERENCES

1. Syme J: *Excision of the Scapula.* Edinburgh, Edmonston and Douglas, 1864.
2. de Nancrede CBG: The end results after total excision of the scapula for sarcoma. *Ann Surg* 1909;50:1.
3. Ryerson EW: Excision of scapula. *JAMA* 1939;113:1958.
4. Pack GT, Ariel IR: *Tumors of the Soft Somatic Tissues.* New York, Paul B. Hoeber, 1958.

27

Shoulder Girdle Resections: The Tikhoff-Linberg Procedure and Its Modifications

MARTIN M. MALAWER, M.D.
PAUL H. SUGARBAKER, M.D.

OVERVIEW

The Tikhoff-Linberg resection and its modifications are limb-sparing surgical options to be considered for bony and soft tissue tumors in and around the proximal humerus and shoulder girdle. Careful selection of patients whose tumor does not involve the neurovascular bundle or chest wall is required. Portions of the scapula, clavicle, and/or proximal humerus are resected in conjunction with all muscles inserting and originating from the involved bones. Optimal function is achieved by muscle transfer and skeletal reconstruction. A custom prosthesis is used to maintain length and stabilize the distal humerus following resection of sarcomas of the proximal humerus. Function of the hand and forearm following most shoulder girdle resections should be nearly normal; elbow flexion plus stability of the shoulder may be achieved without the need of an orthosis. Approximately 80% of patients with high-grade sarcomas of the shoulder girdle can be treated by a limb-sparing resection. A recently proposed classification system of the various shoulder girdle resections is described. The Tikhoff-Linberg procedure and its modifications should continue to be used for limb salvage in selected patients with tumors in or around the shoulder girdle.

In 1928, Linberg described a procedure for resection of the shoulder girdle in selected patients with primary bone or soft tissue sarcomas. The resection consisted of en bloc removal of the scapula, clavicle, and proximal humerus with preservation of the hand and forearm. Suspension of the remaining extremity was accomplished by attaching the biceps tendon to the periosteum of the rib or the remaining pectoralis major muscle. Linberg credited Professor Tikhoff with the development of this technique, which was proposed in lieu of forequarter (interscapulothoracic) amputation. The procedure has been designated the Tikhoff-Linberg resection.

Approximately 25 Tikhoff-Linberg resections have been reported in the English literature up to 1983. Seventeen of these were reviewed by Marcove, Lewis, and Huvos.[1-7] Within the past decade, limb-sparing surgery for primary bone and soft tissue sarcomas of the extremities has become increasingly popular. Tumors of the proximal humerus may be removed by en bloc resection; however, local control requires a long segmental resection of the humerus with the surrounding musculature. Brief technical descriptions of this procedure have been included with previous reports. However, a systematic approach to the surgical problems encountered with tumors of the upper humerus and shoulder girdle has not previously been available. Resection of tumors of the proximal humerus has created surgical problems not encountered with the classical Tikhoff-Linberg resection. A large intercalary defect is created, which requires the use of a prosthesis. Also, means to suspend the arm, to ensure soft tissue coverage, and to allow optimal motor reconstruction are needed.

We describe a modified technique of the Tikhoff-Linberg resection and comment on the modification that tumors in different locations require.[8] An "extended" procedure in which a major portion of the humerus is resected is described for sarcomas of the proximal portion of this bone. A new method of reconstruction using a custom prosthesis and muscle transfers gives improved function after resection. A proposed classification of the various shoulder girdle resections is described.[2,9]

INDICATIONS

Indications for limb-sparing procedures include high-grade and some low-grade bone and soft tissue sarcomas of the shoulder girdle. Selection of patients for this procedure is based on the anatomic location of the cancer and on a thorough understanding of the natural history of osteosarcomas and soft tissue sarcomas. Absolute contraindications include extension of tumor to *involve the neurovascular bundle* or to the *chest wall*. Relative contraindications may include *pathologic fracture*, extensive involvement of the shaft of the humerus, or *tumor contamination* of the operative area from hematoma following biopsy or unwise placement of the biopsy incision. Pathologic fracture through the tumor may result in extensive tumor-contaminated hematoma disseminating into the operative field.

PREOPERATIVE STUDIES

Useful preoperative evaluations include the physical examination, computerized tomogram of the shoulder girdle, arteriogram and venogram, and bone scan; more recently, the MRI has been utilized. Neurovascular involvement may be suggested by the position of the tumor at the shoulder, by an abnormal neurological examination, or by absent pulses. However, these symptoms may be produced by tumor compression as well as by invasion by tumor. The computerized tomogram and MRI are especially useful for assessing chest wall involvement. They will also show the position of the tumor mass and suggest the amount of soft tissue extension.

The arteriogram and venogram are used to assess the interval between tumor and neurovascular structures. The bone scan is used to determine the extent of intramedullary involvement of the humerus site through which the humerus is to be transected and to determine the prosthesis length. The humerus is resected to 6 cm beyond the area of technetium uptake. MRI is useful to determine intraosseous extent and skip metastases.

CLASSIFICATION OF SHOULDER GIRDLE RESECTIONS

Recently a classification system for resections of both bony and soft tissue neoplasms involving the shoulder girdle has been developed (Fig. 27–1).[10] Types I–VI are classified according to the bony structures removed during surgery and their relationship to the glenohumeral joint. Types I–III and IV–VI are performed intra-articularly and extra-articularly, respectively. The major variable is the presence or absence of the major motor group, the abductor mechanism. In the classification system, A denotes that the shoulder abductors have been spared, and B denotes that abductor muscles are partially or completely resected. In general, the loss of any component of the abductor mechanism (rotator cuff and or/deltoid muscle) creates a similar functional dis-

SURGICAL CLASSIFICATION OF SHOULDER GIRDLE RESECTIONS

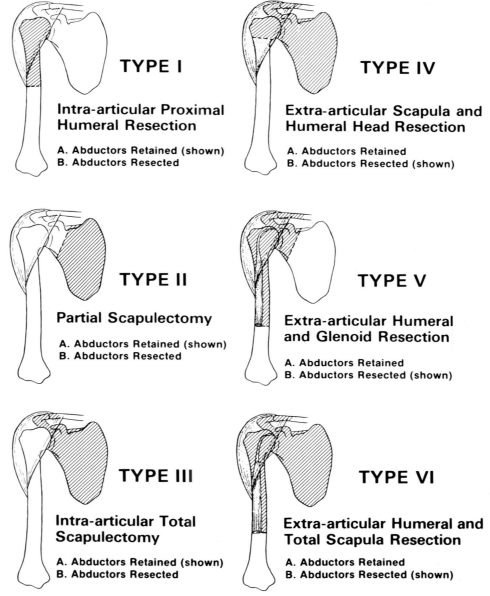

TYPE I

Intra-articular Proximal Humeral Resection

A. Abductors Retained (shown)
B. Abductors Resected

TYPE II

Partial Scapulectomy

A. Abductors Retained (shown)
B. Abductors Resected

TYPE III

Intra-articular Total Scapulectomy

A. Abductors Retained (shown)
B. Abductors Resected

TYPE IV

Extra-articular Scapula and Humeral Head Resection

A. Abductors Retained
B. Abductors Resected (shown)

TYPE V

Extra-articular Humeral and Glenoid Resection

A. Abductors Retained
B. Abductors Resected (shown)

TYPE VI

Extra-articular Humeral and Total Scapula Resection

A. Abductors Retained
B. Abductors Resected (shown)

Figure 27–1. Surgical classification of shoulder girdle resections (see text) (from Malawer et al[8]).

ability. The abductor mechanism is almost always resected when there is extraosseous extension of a bone tumor in this area. Procedures that are type A (abductors preserved) accomplish an intracompartmental resection, type B procedures (abductors resected) an extracompartmental resection.

In general, Types I, II, and III resections are performed for benign or low-grade lesions of the proximal humerus or scapula. Types IV, V, and VI are most often used for the treatment of high-grade sarcomas of the scapula and humerus. In this system, the original Tikhoff-Linberg resection is classified as Type IV-B. The most common procedure for high-grade sarcomas (especially osteosarcoma of the proximal humerus) is Type V-B and is illustrated in this chapter. In summary, this proposed system considers the status of the structures removed (bone/abductor mechanism), the type of resection (intracompartmental *v* extracompartmental) performed, reflects the status of the glenohumeral joint (intra-articular *v* extra-articular), denotes the type of surgical margin achievable (marginal, wide, or radical), and indicates the increasing surgical magnitude of the resection and, thus, the type of reconstruction required.

PROCEDURE

Biopsy

The biopsy site should be carefully selected. If possible, it should be through the deltoid muscle and away from the major vessels and nerves. The biopsy site should be placed so it can be widely excised by the definitive excision.

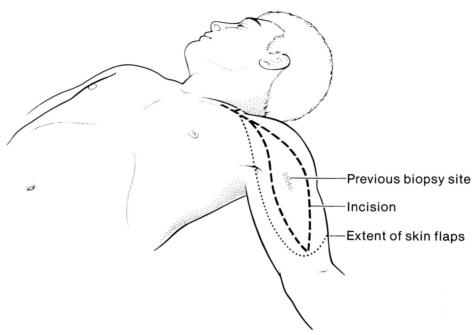

Figure 27–2. **POSITION AND INCISION.** Antibiotics are begun preoperatively and continued until suction drains are removed. The patient is placed in an anterolateral position, which allows some mobility of the upper torso. A Foley catheter is placed in the bladder, and an intravenous line is secured in the opposite extremity. The skin is prepared down to the level of the operating table, to the umbilicus, and cranially past the hairline. The incision starts over the junction of the inner and middle thirds of the clavicle. It continues along the deltopectoral groove and then down the arm over the medial border of the biceps muscle. The biopsy site is excised, leaving a 3-cm margin of normal skin. The posterior incision is not opened until the anterior dissection is complete.

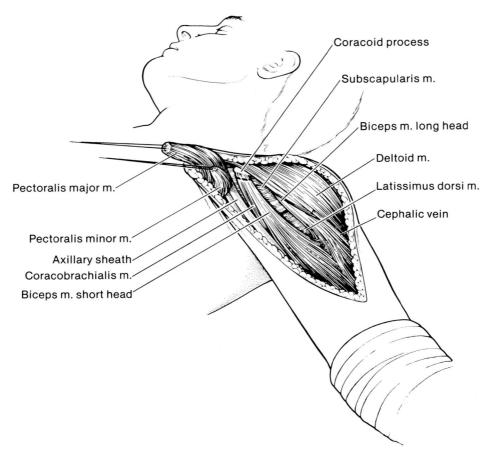

Coracoid process

Subscapularis m.

Biceps m. long head

Deltoid m.

Latissimus dorsi m.

Cephalic vein

Pectoralis major m.

Pectoralis minor m.

Axillary sheath

Coracobrachialis m.

Biceps m. short head

Figure 27–3. EXPLORATION OF THE AXILLA TO DETERMINE RESECTABILITY. The skin is opened through the superficial fascia, but care is taken to preserve the deep fascia on muscles. Anteriorly the skin flap is dissected off the pectoralis major muscle to expose its distal third, and the short head of the biceps muscle is uncovered. The pectoralis major muscle overlying the axilla is dissected free of axillary fat so that its insertion on the humerus can be visualized; this muscle is divided just proximal to its tendinous insertion on the humerus, and the portion of the muscle remaining with the patient is tagged with a suture. The axillary sheath is now identified and the coracoid process visualized. In order to expose the axillary sheath along its full extent, the pectoralis minor, short head of the biceps, and coracobrachialis muscles are divided at their insertion on the coracoid process. Again, all proximal muscles are tagged with a suture for their later identification and use in the reconstruction.

Prior to exploration of the neurovascular bundle, the skin flaps are minimally developed. The patient's tumor may be found unsuitable for limb-salvage surgery, and more extensive flap dissection at this point would lead to tumor contamination of the anatomic site that would not constitute flaps of a forequarter amputation.

351

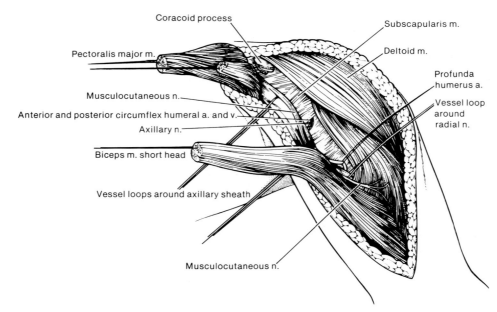

Coracoid process

Subscapularis m.

Pectoralis major m.

Deltoid m.

Profunda humerus a.

Musculocutaneous n.

Anterior and posterior circumflex humeral a. and v.

Vessel loop around radial n.

Axillary n.

Biceps m. short head

Vessel loops around axillary sheath

Musculocutaneous n.

Figure 27–4.   DISSECTION OF THE NEUROVASCULAR BUNDLE. Vessel loops are passed around the neurovascular bundle near the proximal and distal ends of the dissection. Medial traction on the neurovascular bundle allows visualization of the axillary nerve, posterior circumflex humeral artery, and anterior circumflex humeral artery. These three structures are ligated and then divided. If the neurovascular bundle is found to be free of any extension of the tumor, dissection for the limb-salvage procedure proceeds. The musculocutaneous nerve is isolated and carefully preserved. Although sacrifice of this nerve is occasionally required to preserve tumor-free margins of resection, its loss means lack of elbow flexion following surgery. The deep fascia between the short and long heads of the biceps muscle is divided below the tumor mass to maximally separate the short and long heads of the biceps. This permits easy visualization of the musculocutaneous nerve. The radial nerve is identified at the lower border of the latissimus dorsi muscle passing around and behind the humerus into the triceps muscle group. The profunda humerus artery that accompanies this nerve is ligated and divided. The radial nerve passes posterior to the humerus in its midportion (spiral groove). To dissect it free of the bone, a finger is passed around the humerus to bluntly move the nerve away from the bone. Likewise the ulnar nerve is traced down the arm; divide the intermuscular septum between biceps and triceps over the nerve to clearly visualize it.

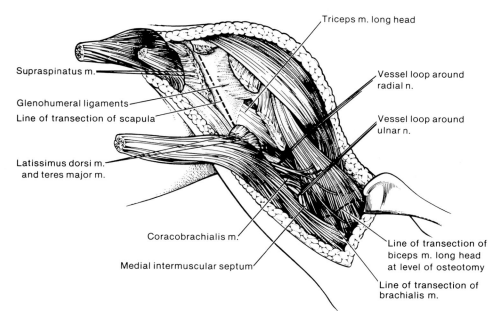

Triceps m. long head

Supraspinatus m.

Glenohumeral ligaments

Line of transection of scapula

Latissimus dorsi m. and teres major m.

Coracobrachialis m.

Medial intermuscular septum

Vessel loop around radial n.

Vessel loop around ulnar n.

Line of transection of biceps m. long head at level of osteotomy

Line of transection of brachialis m.

Figure 27–5. DIVISION OF MUSCLE GROUPS ANTERIORLY TO EXPOSE THE NECK OF THE SCAPULA. The short and long heads of the biceps are widely separated to expose the humerus. Determine the site for the humeral osteotomy, then transect the long head of the biceps and brachialis muscles at this level. The inferior border of the latissimus dorsi muscle is identified, and a fascial incision is made that allows one to pass a finger behind the latissimus dorsi and teres major muscles several centimeters from their insertion into the humerus or scapula. The latissimus dorsi and teres major muscles are transected using electrocautery. External rotation of the humerus exposes the subscapularis muscle, which is transected at the level of the coracoid process. Care must be taken not to enter the joint space. The portions of these muscles that are to remain with the patient are tagged for future reconstruction. By transecting these muscles the anterior portion of the neck of the scapula has been exposed.

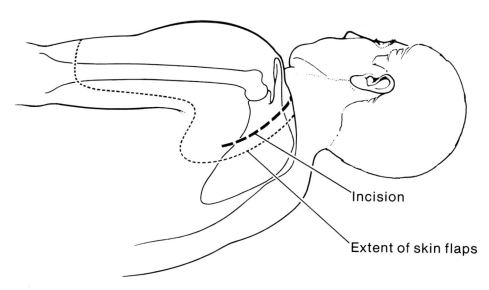

Incision

Extent of skin flaps

Figure 27–6. POSTERIOR INCISION AND LATERAL SKIN FLAP. The surgeon now changes his orientation from the anterior to the posterior aspect of the patient. Rotation of the table away from the surgeon may allow for better visualization. The posterior incision begins anteriorly over the junction of the middle and lateral thirds of the clavicle. It continues down over the lateral third of the scapula until it passes the lower edge of this bone. A skin flap is developed by dissecting the skin and subcutaneous tissue between the anterior and posterior incisions from the underlying deltoid muscle down to the level of the mid-humerus. If the entire scapula is to be removed, this posterior incision is made longer to allow the skin flap to expose muscle over the entire scapula.

353

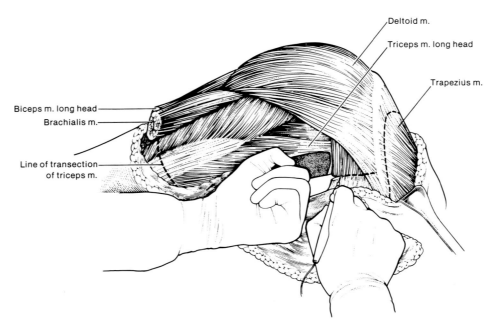

Deltoid m.

Triceps m. long head

Trapezius m.

Biceps m. long head

Brachialis m.

Line of transection
of triceps m.

Figure 27–7. DIVISION OF MUSCLE GROUPS POSTERIORLY. The thick fascia joining the posterior border of the deltoid muscle to the infraspinatus muscle and scapular spine is divided. The deltoid muscle is left intact as a covering over the tumor mass. The trapezius muscle is transected from its insertions on the scapular spine and acromion. The surgeon's index finger is passed beneath the teres minor up to the area of the planned scapular osteotomy. The supraspinatus, infraspinatus, and teres minor muscles are transected over the neck of the scapula; this allows the plane of transection through the neck of the scapula to be exposed. All transected muscles are tagged proximally.

While shielding the radial and ulnar nerves, the triceps muscles are transected at the level selected for the humeral osteotomy.

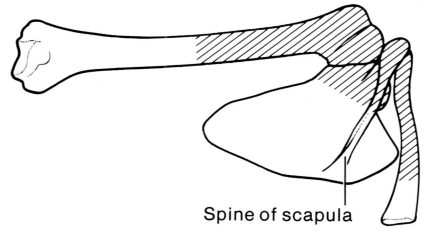

Spine of scapula

Figure 27–8. CLAVICULAR, SCAPULAR, AND HUMERAL OSTEOTOMIES. The clavicle is divided at the junction of its middle and inner one-third. This is usually accomplished with a Gigli saw. The scapula is divided through its surgical neck medial to the coracoid process, also using a Gigli saw. Usually the clavicular and scapular osteotomy are performed prior to the humeral osteotomy.

If the entire scapula is to be resected, the skin flap is taken back to the medial edge of the scapula. After this is accomplished, the rhomboid, levator scapuli, and trapezius muscles are divided from their insertions on the scapula. The teres major, teres minor, supraspinatus, infraspinatus, and subscapularis muscles need not be divided if a full scapula resection is to be performed.

If the procedure is being performed for a sarcoma of the proximal humerus, the humerus is transected 6 cm distal to the tumor as determined by preoperative bone scan. Cryostat sections of tumor margins and touch preparations for cytological examination of the marrow at the site of the osteotomy are obtained. The section of humerus removed is measured and a prosthesis 4 to 6 cm shorter is selected. Some shortening of the extremity allows better soft tissue coverage.

Upon removing the specimen, one should note that a generous amount of soft tissue still covers the tumor. The long and lateral heads of the triceps muscle remain on the humerus. The upper portion of the long head of the biceps and the upper portion of the brachialis muscle remain with the specimen. The entire deltoid muscle covers the tumor. The insertions of the supraspinatus, infraspinatus, pectoralis major, latissimus dorsi, teres major, teres minor, and subscapularis muscles remain covering the tumor and constitute the free margins.

354

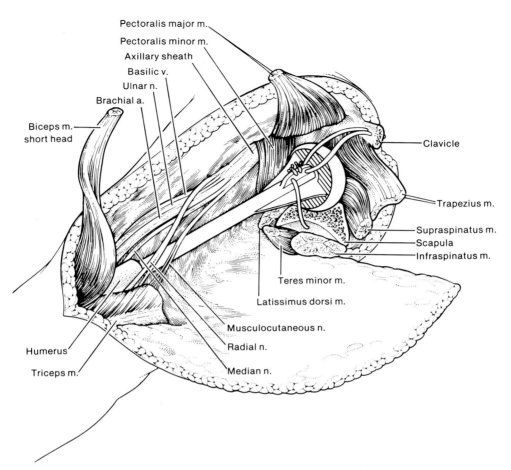

Pectoralis major m.
Pectoralis minor m.
Axillary sheath
Basilic v.
Ulnar n.
Brachial a.
Biceps m.
short head
Clavicle
Trapezius m.
Supraspinatus m.
Scapula
Infraspinatus m.
Teres minor m.
Latissimus dorsi m.
Musculocutaneous n.
Radial n.
Median n.
Humerus
Triceps m.

Figure 27–9.   SECURING THE PROSTHESIS. If a prosthesis is to be used, 5 to 7 cm of distal humerus must be preserved. A power reamer is used to widen the medullary canal of the remaining humerus; it is reamed until it is 1 mm larger than the stem of the prosthesis. The length of the bony specimen is measured so that a prosthesis of appropriate length is used. Methyl methacrylate cement is injected into the medullary canal and the prosthesis is positioned. The head of the prosthesis should be oriented so that it lies anterior to the transected portion of scapula while the arm is in neutral position. The radial nerve should be positioned anterior to the prosthesis so it does not become entrapped between muscle and prosthesis during the reconstruction. Drill holes are made through the scapula at the level of its spine. Drill holes also are made through the distal portion of the transected clavicle. The head of the prosthesis is secured by Dacron tape to the remaining portion of the scapula so that the prosthesis is suspended mediolaterally (horizontal stability). It is suspended in a cranio–caudal direction by a second tape from the end of the clavicle (vertical stability). A 3-mm Dacron tape is used.

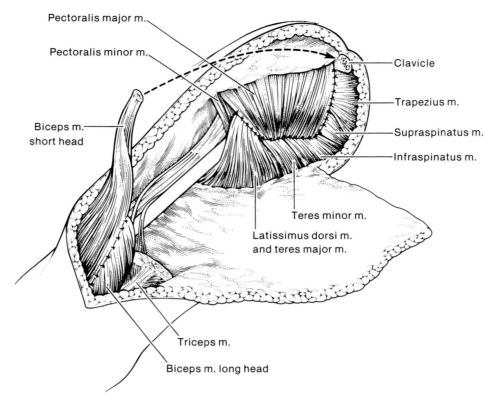

Figure 27–10.   RECONSTRUCTION. The pectoralis minor muscle is sutured to the subscapularis muscle over the neurovascular bundle to protect it from the prosthesis. The pectoralis major muscle is closed over the prosthesis to the cut edge of the scapula and secured by nonabsorbable sutures through drill holes. Following this the trapezius, supraspinatus, infraspinatus, and teres minor are secured to the superior and lateral borders of the transected pectoralis major. The teres major and latissimus dorsi muscles are secured to the inferior border of the pectoralis major muscle. The tendinous portion of the short head of the biceps is secured anteriorly under appropriate tension to the remaining clavicle. The long head of the biceps and brachialis muscles are sutured to the short head of the biceps muscle under appropriate tension so that these two muscles can work through the short biceps tendon. The remaining triceps muscle is secured anteriorly along the lateral border of the biceps to cover the lower and lateral portion of the shaft of the prosthesis. Ideally, when the proximal and distal muscular reconstruction is complete the prosthesis is covered in its entirety by muscle.

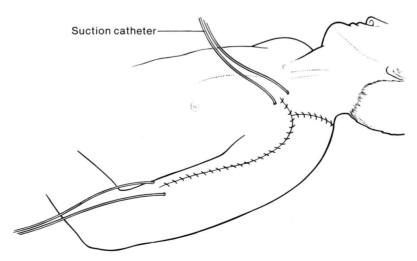

Figure 27–11.   CLOSURE. Large-bore suction catheter drainage is secured. The superficial fascia is closed with absorbable suture and the skin is closed with clips. Povidone-iodine ointment is applied to the incision along with a dry sterile dressing. A sling and swathe are applied in the operating room.

REHABILITATION

Patients undergoing shoulder girdle resection retain hand function and good elbow function, but lose shoulder function. From a rehabilitation perspective it clearly offers an outcome superior to a forequarter amputation or shoulder disarticulation procedure. Further, shoulder girdle resection is less disfiguring and is associated with only minimal pain and edema. Figure 27–12 shows the appearance of a patient after this procedure. In our experience patients' acceptance of the outcome of surgery has been good.

The rehabilitation process begins with a patient orientation program, often showing pictures of patients who have undergone the procedure and demonstrating what one can do postoperatively and what limitations in function are likely to follow surgery. Preoperatively, a shoulder mold is fashioned, using the involved shoulder, provided its contours are not distorted. The cosmetic shoulder helps preserve the symmetry and appearance of the shoulder contour, and can support a bra strap or heavy overcoat.

On postoperative day 1 an arm sling is provided for support and to restrict abduction. The motion restriction should be maintained until the incision is healed; sutures are removed usually after about two weeks. Edema (when present) should be controlled with an elasticized glove or elastic stockinette. At the same time active, maximal head motion is begun to preserve strength and range and to help mobilize edema. Teaching the patient to be aware of proper head and neck positioning and cervical range of motion is initiated when the patient first becomes ambulatory.

If the incision heals per primum and after suction catheters have been removed, active and assistive elbow motion within the confines of the sling is started. At about three weeks the sling is removed for passive shoulder range of motion (ROM) and pronation and supination of the wrist. The sling is used intermittently after the suture line is healed, primarily for upright activities in which arm support increases comfort. Once the arm is out of the sling, full ROM of elbow (flexion, extension, pronation, and supination) should be performed. Passive ROM to the shoulder (flexion, abduction, external and internal rotation) and pendulum exercise should be done with the help of a family member or physical therapist.

Normal daily activities are encouraged, but weights in excess of 20 lb maximum should not be lifted with the arm that has undergone a Tikhoff-Linberg procedure. Pain and shoulder or arm discomfort have not been significant management

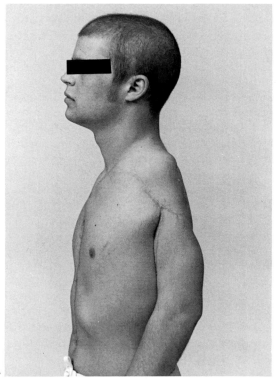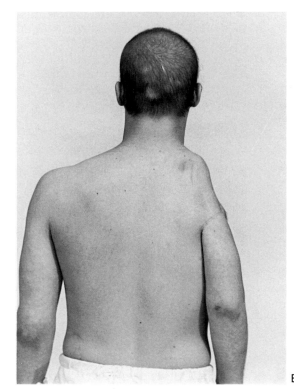

A   B

Figure 27–12.   (A) Lateral and (B) posterior views of cosmetic result after Type V resection.

problems, and control is achieved with minimal analgesia.

DISCUSSION

High-grade sarcomas of the shoulder girdle have been treated traditionally by interscapulothoracic amputation. Nonablative extirpation has been rare. This chapter contains a complete description of the technique for a modified Tikhoff-Linberg procedure in patients with sarcomas of the proximal humerus. Also, modifications of the procedure for tumors at other anatomic sites have been utilized. Proximal humeral lesions require resection of a greater length of humerus and adjacent soft tissues than described in the original Tikhoff-Linberg procedure. Our experience is similar to that of Marcove, who recently reported 17 resections of high-grade malignant tumors, 12 of which involved the proximal humerus.[6]

The technique of resection and reconstruction requires a thorough knowledge of the regional anatomy and technique of musculoskeletal reconstruction. Essential aspects of the treatment plan should be emphasized. The initial biopsy should be performed through the anterior portion of the deltoid muscle for a lesion of the proximal humerus. The deltopectoral interval should not be utilized, because biopsy here would contaminate the deltopectoral fascia, the subscapularis, and pectoralis major muscles and would jeopardize the ability to perform an adequate resection through uninvolved tissue planes. For the definitive resection, the initial incision extends along the medial aspect of the biceps muscle, divides the pectoralis major, and exposes the neurovascular structures, thereby enabling the surgeon to determine resectability early in the dissection. This incision does not jeopardize construction of an anterior skin flap in patients who will require forequarter amputation.

The length of bone resection is determined preoperatively from a bone scan and MRI. To avoid a positive margin at the site of humeral transection, the distal osteotomy is performed 6 cm distal to the area of abnormality on the scan. Segmental reconstruction of the resultant humeral defect is necessary if resection is performed distal to the deltoid tuberosity. Reconstruction is necessary to maintain length of the arm and to create a fulcrum for elbow flexion. Marcove, Lewis, and Huvos reported use of a Kunstcher nail inserted into the medullary canal of the distal humerus for this purpose.[6] Whitehill and colleagues fixed the Kunstcher nail to a U-shaped flange attached to the second rib to maintain proximal stability of the interposition device.[7] In recent procedures we have elected not to use a Kunstcher nail because of the risk of proximal migration, instability, and skin perforation.[6] Rather, a custom prosthesis is fixed distally with methyl methacrylate into the remaining humerus and proximally with Dacron tape to the clavicle and remaining portion of the scapula. Alternatively, good results have been reported with autograft (usually fibulas) or allograft utilized as spacers in obtaining an arthrodesis.

Principles of Shoulder Reconstruction

Proximal soft tissue reconstruction is essential to cover the prosthesis and create shoulder stability. This is accomplished through a technique of "dual suspension" through static and dynamic reconstruction (Fig. 27–13). Dacron tape was utilized to secure the prosthesis horizontally. Vertical suspension is by Dacron tape secured by drill holes in the remaining bony structures (clavicle and scapula or clavicle alone). These two sets of Dacron tapes provide for mediolateral and cranio–caudad stability. This interposition prosthetic device provides a strut between the rib cage and residual humerus for static suspension (Fig. 27–13A). Dynamic suspension provided by transfer of the short head of the biceps muscle to the stump of the clavicle allows elbow flexion (Fig. 27–13B).

Motor reconstruction and soft tissue coverage is as follows. The short head of the biceps brachii is secured to the end of the clavicle. Also, to assist in elbow flexion, the severed long head of the biceps brachii is sutured along the cut edge of its short head. Mobility at the shoulder is provided by preservation and transfer of the pectoralis major, trapezius, supraspinatus, infraspinatus, teres minor, teres major, and latissimus dorsi muscles. Utilization of these muscle groups offers dynamic support, assists in suspension of the prosthesis, and provides soft tissue coverage. Soft tissue coverage is essential in preventing skin problems and secondary infection (Fig. 27–13C).

Preserving the musculocutaneous nerve is important. The short biceps muscle is responsible for elbow flexion postoperatively and is also used for soft tissue coverage of the prosthesis. It is the most important arm muscle remaining after resection. Flexion of the elbow is possible in patients with function of the biceps muscle (Fig. 27–14). Muscle transfer also allows some flexion and extension motion at the shoulder. The pectoralis major muscle allows forward flexion of the shoulder. The trapezius and latissimus dorsi muscles cause posterior motion.

Extra-articular, rather than intra-articular, resec-

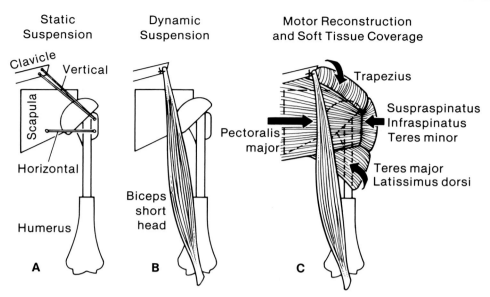

Figure 27–13. **(A)** Static suspension of the prosthesis. The interposition prosthesis is secured horizontally by Dacron tape placed through drill holes in the scapula. Vertical stability is achieved by passing tape through drill holes in the end of the clavicle. **(B)** Dynamic suspension of the prosthesis. Elbow flexion is preserved by transferring the origin of the short head of the biceps muscle to the end of the clavicle. **(C)** Motor reconstruction and soft tissue coverage. The pectoralis major muscle is secured to the scapula to provide forward flexion of the shoulder. Extension of the shoulder occurs through transfer of the trapezius, teres major, and latissimus dorsi muscles.

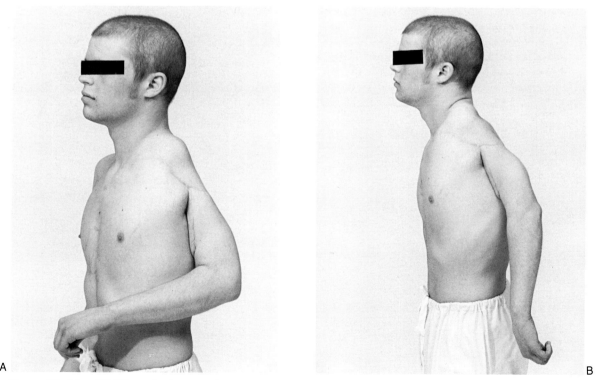

Figure 27–14. **(A)** Elbow flexion may be preserved if the musculocutaneous nerve and its innervation, the short head of the biceps muscle, are spared. **(B)** Backward and forward flexion of the shoulder may be achieved through muscle transfer.

tion of the glenohumeral joint by scapular osteotomy medial to the coracoid is recommended for proximal humeral lesions because it removes en bloc the potentially contaminated extension of the tumor.[6] Scapular osteotomy not only removes the potential for tumor contamination of the operative field but also permits medialization of the prosthesis and a decrease in bulk in the area to be covered.

To minimize the incidence of transient nerve palsies, care should be taken not to place undue traction on nerves during resection. The radial nerve should pass in front of, rather than around, the prosthesis. The scapular osteotomy should be performed before the humeral osteotomy to minimize traction that may occur during manipulation of the extremity.

On follow-up, none of our patients complained of shoulder instability or fatigue. This is attributed to our technique of prosthetic suspension and soft tissue reconstruction. In general, forward and backward shoulder flexion ranges from 30° to 45° with good strength. Shoulder abduction was initially absent, but with scapulothoracic motion (because of the remaining scapula) about 30° was eventually obtained. Elbow strength and motion depended on the status of the remaining biceps. This emphasizes the need for careful preservation, when possible, of musculocutaneous nerve and the short head of the biceps.

The technique of resection and reconstruction as described in this chapter permits a curative, nonablative alternative to forequarter amputation. Despite the magnitude of resection, the surgical morbidity is minimal and functional results are good. We recommend this procedure in carefully selected patients. The proposed classification system allows for accurate description of most limb-sparing surgical procedures of the shoulder region.

REFERENCES

1. Burwell HN: Resection of the shoulder with humeral suspension for sarcoma involving the scapula. *J Bone Joint Surg* 1965;47B:300–303.
2. Francis KC, Worchester JN Jr: Radical resection for tumors of the shoulder with preservation of a functional extremity. *J Bone Joint Surg* 1962;44A:1423–1429.
3. Janecki CJ, Nelson CL: En bloc resection of the shoulder girdle: Technique and indications. *J Bone Joint Surg* 1972;54A:1758.
4. Pack GT, Baldwin JC: The Tikhoff-Linberg resection of shoulder girdle. *Surgery* 1955;38:753–757.
5. Linberg BE: Interscapulo-thoracic resection for malignant tumors of the shoulder joint region. *J Bone Joint Surg* 1928;10:344–349.
6. Marcove RC, Lewis MM, Huvos AG: En bloc upper humeral interscapulo-thoracic resection. *Clin Orthop* 1977;124:219–228.
7. Whitehill R, Wanebo HJ, Mabie KN: Reconstruction after the Tikhoff-Linberg procedure. *Arch Surg* 1982;117:1248–1249.
8. Malawer MM, Link M, Donaldson S: Bone sarcomas, in DeVita VT Jr, Helman S, Rosenberg SA (eds): *Cancer: Principles and Practice of Oncology*, ed 3. JB Lippincott, Philadelphia, chap 41, 1989.
9. Malawer MM, Meller I, Dunham WK: Shoulder girdle resections for bone and soft tissue tumors: Analysis of 38 patients and presentation of a unified classification system, in Yamamura T (ed): *International Symposium on Limb-Salvage in Musculoskeletal Oncology*. New York/Berlin, Springer-Verlag, to be published.
10. Malawer MM, Meller I: Classification of shoulder girdle resections: Analysis of 38 cases. Annual Meeting of the Musculoskeletal Tumor Society (MSTS) Toronto, May 1987.

28

Summary of Alternative Approaches to Forequarter Amputation

PAUL H. SUGARBAKER, M.D.
MARTIN M. MALAWER, M.D.

OVERVIEW

Forequarter amputation is the appropriate treatment for many patients with high-grade malignancy in and around the shoulder girdle. The forequarter amputation is tolerated well as an amputative procedure with few complications. Functionally, patients with a single upper extremity perform surprisingly well. The major problems are those of phantom limb pain, a severe cosmetic deformity, and, occasionally, a devastating psychological defect. Of course, the unnecessary sacrifice of function is always to be avoided unless the probability for long-term survival is jeopardized. The experienced surgical team knows that there are numerous alternatives to this ablative procedure. *Shoulder disarticulation or high above-elbow amputation* can upon occasion replace the forequarter amputation with malignant tumors of the upper or middle humerus. These amputative procedures are seldom indicated because they carry the same functional debit as a forequarter amputation and usually compromise the margins of resection for high-grade malignancies. As experience with *shoulder girdle resections with limb salvage* has become available, this approach has become increasingly popular. Because the functional capacity of the upper extremity is centered in the hand, these shoulder girdle resections leave only a cosmetic deficit in many patients. In patients with more superficial tumors, wide local excision with a negative surgical margin can be combined with shoulder radiation therapy in order to secure an excellent functional and oncologic result. Smaller and more superficial tumors, especially when they are of a lower-grade malignancy, may be treated by surgical excision alone. For shoulder girdle malignancy the treatment alternatives vary with the anatomic location of the malignancy, its biologic grade, and its response to induction chemotherapy.

INTRODUCTION

The alternative approaches to the forequarter amputation are listed below. The limb-salvage procedures are, of course, to be preferred over the amputative procedure. Careful patient selection is required to prevent local treatment failure in this area with complex anatomy. A thorough knowledge of anatomy, technical skill, and experience are required in order to maintain an excellent surgical result in all patients.

1. Forequarter amputation (chapter 23)
2. Radical forequarter amputation with chest wall resection (chapter 24)
3. Shoulder disarticulation
4. High above-elbow amputation (chapter 25)
5. Type I shoulder girdle resection
6. Type II shoulder girdle resection
7. Type III shoulder girdle resection or scapulectomy (chapter 26)
8. Type IV shoulder girdle resection or the Tikhoff-Linberg Procedure
9. Type V shoulder girdle resection
10. Complete resection of the humerus and scapula
11. Combined wide local excision plus high-dose radiation therapy (chapter 6)
12. Wide local excision with negative margins of resection for low-biologic-grade tumors

STANDARD FOREQUARTER AMPUTATION

The indications for a forequarter amputation are high-grade malignancies in or around the shoulder girdle. The major indication for the ablative procedure usually results from a large tumor mass being intimately related to the major nerves or vascular supply to the upper extremity. For osteosarcomas of the humerus, extension of the tumor after induction chemotherapy into the neural vascular bundle in the axilla necessitates an amputative procedure. Not infrequently, evaluation of the workup of the patient prior to induction chemotherapy may suggest that an amputation is required. However, in those patients in whom positive surgical margins are suspected, vigorous chemotherapy prior to exploration of the axilla is a definite requirement before one resorts to the ablative procedure. For soft tissue tumors or other malignancies in this anatomic site, involvement of the brachial plexus requires forequarter amputation. Unless a tumor in and around the brachial plexus is of low biologic grade, infiltration of this structure requires amputation for any hope of curative re-

moval of the disease process. For low-grade tumors, especially aggressive fibromatosis, meticulous piecemeal stripping of the tumor from the brachial plexus, followed by high-dose wide-field irradiation of the entire operative field, may give excellent long-term disease-free results. Other clinical situations that require amputation involve tumors that arise deep in the shoulder girdle so that chest wall involvement is present. Frequently, induction chemotherapy even with radiation therapy does not cause sufficient reduction in primary tumor size for resection with clear margins to occur. In this instance, forequarter amputation is the procedure of choice.

In the standard forequarter amputation, the surgeon may approach the tumor from either the anterior or posterior aspect. If the tumor is located anteriorly, a large posterior skin flap is created, and one dissects around the tumor mass by rolling the scapula off the chest wall by releasing it posteriorly. Using this approach, the surgeon does not have to work over a large tumor mass in the process of securing the subclavian artery and vein. Alternatively, if the tumor mass is located on the posterior aspect of the shoulder girdle, division or resection of the clavicle in order to clearly expose the neurovascular bundle should be the first step of the procedure. After the vessels are secured, dissection along the chest wall and in behind the tumor allows for an orderly approach to tumor resection. Again, one tries to avoid approaching the subclavian artery and vein over the top of a large tumor mass so that accidents incurred through a difficult exposure of these vessels are avoided.

A common indication for forequarter amputation (with or without chest wall resection) is cancer recurrence following wide local excision plus radiation therapy. In order to widely excise the recurrent tumor mass after prior resection, amputation is generally required. Also, in these patients the beneficial effects of systemic or regional chemotherapy to reduce the size of the tumor mass will not occur. These modalities have been exhausted prior to this salvage type of reoperative surgery. Even massive excisions of the chest wall combined with forequarter amputation are well tolerated with the help of postoperative ventilatory support (chapter 24). If a tumor does not disseminate to systemic sites, excellent long-term results of these seemingly heroic procedures have frequently been a reality.

SHOULDER DISARTICULATION

This is an unusual procedure for musculoskeletal cancer. Also, the counterpart of this procedure in the lower extremity—hip disarticulation—has become increasingly unusual. Occasionally, pathologic fracture through the humerus in the mid-portion of this bone with a painful and useless extremity because of pain is an indication. For primary tumors the functional deficit with shoulder disarticulation is equal to that of a forequarter amputation, but usually the margins of surgical incision are compromised. In certain carefully selected patients the cosmetic benefit of shoulder preservation and the lesser severity of phantom limb pain with the more distal transection of the brachial plexus cause this procedure to be selected.

HIGH ABOVE-ELBOW AMPUTATION

The indications for this procedure are usually similar to those for shoulder disarticulation. Occasionally this amputation may be indicated in patients with metastatic disease, even when the procedure is not performed for cure. Indications for the procedure are palliation with a painful extremity in a patient with metastatic disease or an advanced primary bone tumor of the middle half of the humerus.

TYPE I SHOULDER GIRDLE RESECTION

This procedure is an intra-articular proximal humeral resection (Fig. 28–1). It is performed almost exclusively for low-biologic-grade tumors or for primary bone tumors of the upper humerus

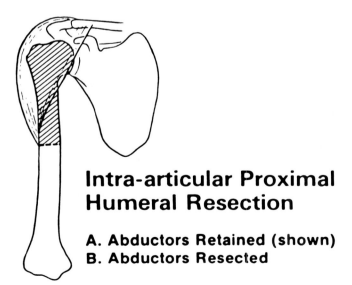

Intra-articular Proximal Humeral Resection

A. Abductors Retained (shown)
B. Abductors Resected

Figure 28–1.   Type I shoulder girdle resection.

(Fig. 28–2). The procedure does not allow for wide margins of resection of muscle tissue on the excised bone specimen. Osteochondromas and low-grade chondrosarcomas are the most frequent lesions. This is usually the least frequently performed of the shoulder girdle resections.

Not infrequently, metastatic disease of the proximal humerus with a pathologic fracture can be treated with resections of the proximal humerus as described for the Type I shoulder girdle resection. The quality-of-life benefit of this procedure in patients with metastatic disease can be most impressive.

TYPE II SHOULDER GIRDLE RESECTION

This procedure involves a partial scapulectomy (Fig. 28–3). Usually the tumors are osseous malignancies

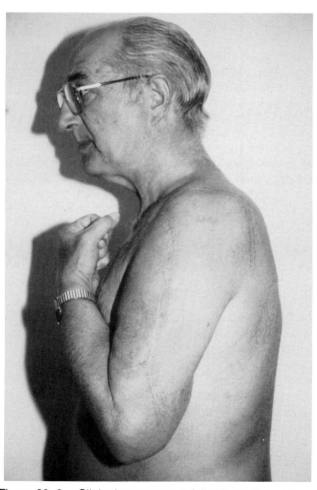

Figure 28–2.   Clinical appearance following a Type I-A resection (intra-articular proximal humeral resection with preservation of the deltoid muscle) for a low-grade chondrosarcoma.

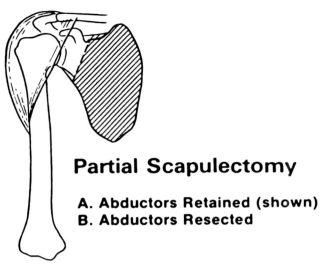

Partial Scapulectomy

A. Abductors Retained (shown)
B. Abductors Resected

Figure 28–3. Type II shoulder girdle resection.

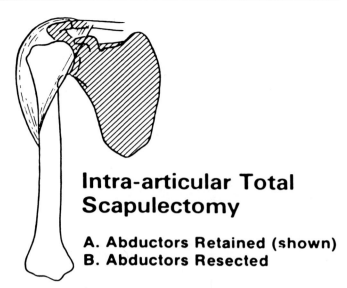

Intra-articular Total Scapulectomy

A. Abductors Retained (shown)
B. Abductors Resected

Figure 28–4. Type III shoulder girdle resection.

of the scapula itself or soft tissue sarcomas superficial or deep to this bone. Occasionally, a limited chest wall resection beneath the partial scapulectomy is required in order to achieve a negative margin of excision. This is usually well tolerated because of the remarkable structural integrity of the skin flaps in and around this anatomic site. Again, most of the lesions removed by partial scapulectomy are a low biologic grade of malignancy. Occasionally, patients with higher-grade lesions with limited margins of excision may merit wide-field postoperative radiation therapy in order to improve local control.

TYPE III SHOULDER GIRDLE RESECTION

The Type II resection is a partial scapulectomy that is extra-articular. In the Type III resection the glenohumeral joint is entered for an intra-articular total scapulectomy (chapter 27). Scapulectomy is indicated for soft tissue tumors located superficial and deep to the scapula and primary malignant tumors of this bone. A low biologic grade of chondrosarcoma or giant cell tumor of the scapula may be effectively treated. Most frequently this procedure is performed for low-grade soft tissue sarcomas invading the scapular muscles or liposarcomas in and around this bone. Occasionally, desmoid tumors may infiltrate the periscapular muscles. If the soft tissue tumor arises deep to the scapula, a localized excision of the chest wall may be indicated.

TYPE IV SHOULDER GIRDLE RESECTION

In this procedure there is an extra-articular en bloc resection of the distal scapula and humeral head (Fig. 28–5). Most malignant tumors of the neck of the scapula require this approach. However, the most common indications are high-grade osteosarcomas of the proximal humerus. For a Type IV resection the tumor must be limited within the head of the humerus (Fig. 28–6). Careful workup with bone scan and MRI in order to rule out involvement of the

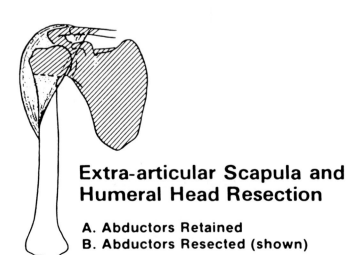

Extra-articular Scapula and Humeral Head Resection

A. Abductors Retained
B. Abductors Resected (shown)

Figure 28–5. Type IV shoulder girdle resection.

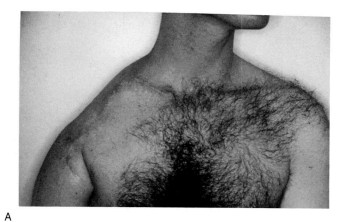

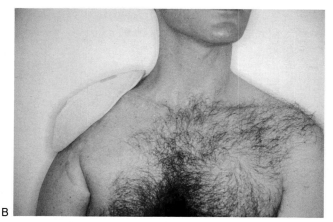

Figure 28–6. (A) Cosmetic appearance following Type IV-B resection (extra-articular glenohumeral total scapulectomy). Classical Tikhoff-Linberg resection for multiple recurrent periscapular soft tissue sarcoma. (B) Custom mold is used to restore symmetry for cosmesis.

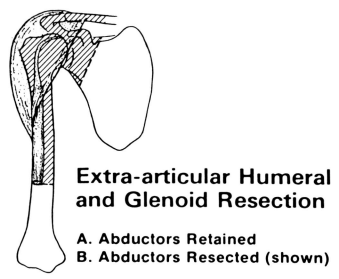

Extra-articular Humeral and Glenoid Resection

A. Abductors Retained
B. Abductors Resected (shown)

Figure 28–7. Type V shoulder girdle resection.

marrow of the remaining humerus are necessary. Pathologic control of the resected specimen is also a necessity.

TYPE V SHOULDER GIRDLE RESECTION

This procedure involves an extra-articular resection of the upper third of the humerus together with the distal scapula (Fig. 28–7). The osteotomy through the scapula is through its surgical neck. This is the original shoulder girdle resection as described by Tikhoff and Linberg. This procedure is indicated for high-grade tumors of the proximal humerus. It is the most common of the limb-salvage procedures in and around the shoulder girdle. If the tumor does not involve the brachial plexus cephalad, the neurovas-

cular bundle medially, and the chest wall medially, this is the procedure of choice for an osteosarcoma of the humerus. Clinical evaluation of the patient by CT scan, magnetic resonance imaging, and arteriography may be required before and after induction chemotherapy in order to gain the maximal amount of clinical information. Not infrequently, exploration of the neurovascular bundle within the axilla is required prior to determining whether an amputation or a limb-salvage procedure is indicated. Not infrequently, the extent of tumor regression induced by induction chemotherapy cannot be adequately accessed through radiologic studies. Only surgical exploration of the margin of resection can provide the necessary information (Fig. 28–8).

TYPE VI SHOULDER GIRDLE RESECTION

This procedure is less frequently performed than Type V resections (Fig. 28–9). Large advanced osteosarcomas of the proximal humerus that have invaded posteriorly in and around the scapula require this resection. Also, high-grade soft tissue tumors located over the glenohumeral joint may require this type of resection.

COMPLETE RESECTION OF THE HUMERUS AND DISTAL SCAPULA

Some osteosarcomas of the proximal humerus will have spread extensively throughout the marrow cav-

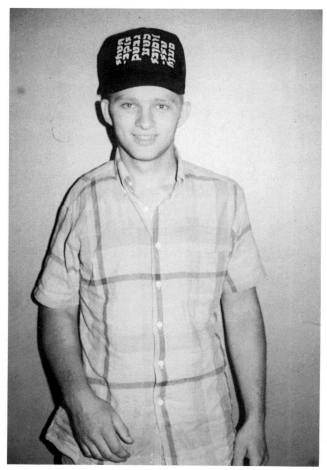

Figure 28–8.   Clinical appearance following Type V resection (extra-articular glenohumeral, proximal humeral resection) for a high-grade osteosarcoma. This patient underwent reconstruction with a custom proximal humeral replacement. Note the good elbow flexion and normal-appearing hand function. Type V resections are generally used for high-grade sarcoma resections.

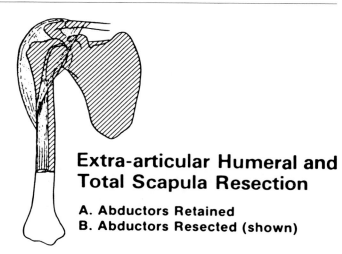

Extra-articular Humeral and Total Scapula Resection

A. Abductors Retained
B. Abductors Resected (shown)

Figure 28–9.   Type VI shoulder girdle resection.

ity of the humerus. In this clinical situation complete excision of the humerus should be undertaken.

COMBINED WIDE LOCAL EXCISION PLUS RADIATION THERAPY FOR SHOULDER GIRDLE SOFT TISSUE SARCOMA

The standard therapy for soft tissue sarcoma of the shoulder girdle is the same as it is in other parts of the body—wide local excision plus radiation therapy. The surgeon should strive to achieve a minimum of 2- to 3-cm margin of normal tissue around the primary soft tissue tumor specimen. If the lesion appears to be well encapsulated and biopsy has shown that it is

of low or moderate malignancy, this margin can be reduced. The procedure involves skin flaps so that one can palpate around the tumor specimen. Then one must repeatedly palpate the tumor mass as the muscles and fascial structures are divided. The surgeon is guided in the dissection by the extent of tumor rather than by anatomic landmarks. Vital structures (both vascular and neural) are dissected away from the tumor mass with as much margin as possible. In some instances there will be only a few cell layers between these vital structures and the tumor mass. Only if there is a gross invasion into the vital structures should they be sacrificed. The margins of dissection are marked with metal clips in order to help plan the field of irradiation. It is of utmost importance to involve the radiation therapist in the treatment planning prior to resection of the malignant process (chapter 6).

WIDE EXCISION FOR LOW-GRADE TUMORS

Occasionally, small malignant tumors or even large biologically low-grade malignancies can be excised by surgery alone as a wide excision. One does not expect low-grade lesions, especially liposarcomas or fibrosarcomas, to recur even if the margins of excision are minimal. An exception to this is aggressive fibromatosis. One needs to achieve a negative margin with this procedure. Nerve and vascular structures should be skeletonized meticulously but should not be sacrificed. A wide field of radiation should be applied to encompass the tumor mass as clinically defined with a 2- to 3-cm margin of irradiated normal tissue.

29

Below-Elbow Amputation

PAUL H. SUGARBAKER, M.D.
MARTIN M. MALAWER, M.D.
ALAN R. BAKER, M.D.

OVERVIEW

Below-elbow amputation is performed for unresectable tumors of the hand and distal forearm. The hand and forearm are relatively common sites for synovial, epithelioid, and clear cell sarcomas. The amputation should be performed to maximize the margin of resection while preserving as much length as possible of both radius and ulna. Muscles are secured over the cut ends of the bone to facilitate stump mobility. Postoperatively a rigid dressing is utilized to minimize swelling and to begin to mold the stump.

INTRODUCTION

Below-elbow amputation is performed for unresectable tumors of the hand and distal forearm. The hand and forearm are relatively common sites for soft tissue sarcomas. Synovial, epithelioid, and clear cell sarcomas frequently occur at these sites. These lesions, fortunately, tend to be small and are resectable under ideal conditions, especially if there has been no prior surgical intervention. Combinations of preoperative and postoperative radiation therapy or infusional chemotherapy have proved to be safe and effective alternatives to amputations for many patients with hand or wrist sarcomas (Fig. 29–1).

Nonetheless, amputation retains a clear-cut and definitive role in the management of hand and wrist sarcomas. Amputation is often required due to the restricted anatomic compartments of the hand. Amputations are needed because the sarcomas may infiltrate, in a clinically occult fashion, surrounding normal tissues at some distance from the primary tumor mass. In these circumstances, procedures that entail anything less than a wide resection will be associated with an unacceptably high rate of local recurrence.

A major responsibility of the orthopedic and surgical oncologist is to determine which patients are candidates for amputation and which may benefit from a limb-sparing surgical procedure. Such decisions must be made by an interdisciplinary group on a case-by-case basis. All patients should be considered and evaluated for limb-sparing surgery, and the decision to proceed with amputation should be made only after this option has been ruled out. Guidelines

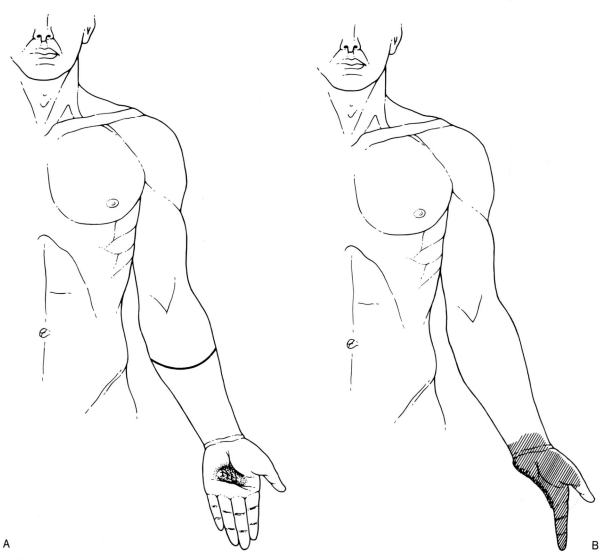

Figure 29–1.   Below-elbow amputation is required as treatment for sarcomas that extensively involve the hand (**A**). In some patients wide local excision plus radiation therapy can provide an excellent functional result (**B**).

for these decisions are based upon (1) surgical stage and tumor grade, and (2) the anatomic location of the tumor.

GENERAL INDICATIONS FOR AMPUTATION

Amputations are most commonly performed for high-grade sarcomas that infiltrate the tissues making up the complex anatomy of the hand. Often the indication for ablative surgery is the recurrence of a high-grade sarcoma despite radiation and chemotherapy in conjunction with surgical removal of the tumor mass. Low-grade tumors are removed by amputation only if there is a recurrence that cannot be removed with preservation of hand function.

Major *vascular or nerve involvement* may necessitate an amputation. The compact nature of the vascular and nerve supply to the hand through the wrist makes involvement of radial and ulnar arteries possible. In this instance, the incidence of morbidity and failure associated with resection and reconstruction using a vascular graft of one of these vessels is prohibitively high. In general, one or even two nerves to the hand can be sacrificed. Often a two-nerve deficit results in poor function of the hand, and a prosthesis may give a better functional result.

Extensive *soft tissue contamination* is a frequent indication for below-elbow amputation. Local contamination often occurs due to prior surgery, or it may result from a poorly planned biopsy. Hand anatomy make both lateral and longitudinal extensions of the tumor commonplace. Often patients who originally had a local resection option require amputation because of prior injudicious biopsy or tumor removal through its pseudocapsule.

Pathological fracture can occur with osteosarcomas at the wrist and results in hematoma formation that causes tumor contamination far beyond the local area. Pathologic fracture is usually an indication for amputation rather than limb-salvage surgery. Fortunately, primary bone sarcomas do not often occur in this region. Reports of limb salvage for distal radial or ulnar bony sarcomas are rare.

Infection, usually of the tumor itself or of a biopsy site, will often negate any attempt at local resection.

OTHER CLINICAL CONSIDERATIONS

Timing of the surgical procedure is important. Both physiological and psychological factors must be op-

timized. If the patient has received a course of preoperative chemotherapy, it is essential that both leukocyte and platelet counts be permitted to return to normal. Significant deficits in red blood cell mass should be corrected by preoperative transfusion. Vascular insufficiency is rarely a complicating factor of upper-extremity amputation. Suboptimal wound healing may be associated with preoperative chemotherapy, poor nutritional intake associated with nausea and vomiting, or chemotherapy or pain from an indolent and protracted treatment course prior to the definitive amputation. Because of potential healing difficulties, stump wound closure must be meticulously performed. Hematoma and seroma must be avoided by the use of adequate closed-suction drainage. If possible, one should defer removing skin sutures for approximately three weeks after the operation. If unusual muscle excision or unconventional skin flaps were required, it may take months to properly mold and mature the stump.

REHABILITATION AND EMOTIONAL SUPPORT

Cancer patients face a unique psychological problem in that they not only face a threat to their lives, but they also may lose a hand. Loss of the dominant hand is even more frightening. Therefore the rehabilitation of a patient undergoing a major amputation, especially a cancer patient, begins at the time of the staging studies. The entire health care team must develop a trusting and honest relationship with the patient and include him or her in the early stages of all decision making. Building upon this interaction, the patient will be better able to accept the amputation and set realistic goals for return to a normal existence. The patient's family, significant peers, and each member of the care team are crucial to this adjustment. It is a responsibility of all persons who interact with the cancer/amputation patient to recognize problems as they arise and to provide as much assistance through the care team as is possible. Professional psychological intervention may sometimes be required before or after surgery. The use of psychotropic drugs may be of immense help in the depressed patient.

All patients undergoing an amputation may experience phantom limb pain. This is not nearly so severe with distal amputations as it is with proximal amputations. Nonetheless, it should be discussed with the patient prior to surgery. The patient should understand that it is normal and that, if uncomfortable, it can be treated with analgesics and other therapy. It will usually subside completely in patients who have below-elbow amputations. It is important to distinguish between stump pain and phantom limb pain. Stump pain is well localized and confined to a specific area; it may indicate complications from the amputation.

Successful rehabilitation depends to a great extent on a patient's attitude. The rehabilitation therapist can aid tremendously in developing a *positive attitude* toward functional recovery. This may be greatly helped in the early postoperative period with a below-elbow amputation by immediate postoperative cast application and early training with a prosthetic device. The prosthesis must often be readjusted several times before stump stability is achieved. This requires patience on both the part of the patient, rehabilitation personnel, and prosthetist. Seeing other patients who have successfully met some of the rehabilitative challenges can provide an immeasurable psychological boost to the patient. Surgical and orthopedic oncologists, rehabilitation therapists, and others involved in the postoperative care must coordinate their efforts carefully, realizing the possibility of conflicting demands on the patient's time and of mixed messages given by different care providers.

LEVEL OF AMPUTATION

The overriding consideration in planning the level of amputation is local recurrence. A generous margin of normal soft tissue must be achieved. We suggest a full 5 cm of normal tissue beyond the tumor mass. Tumors that tend to spread longitudinally along the extremity may require a greater margin. For example, neurosarcomas may track many centimeters along the nerve bundle from which the primary tumor arose. Large tumors may force their way along tendon sheaths.

RADIOLOGIC EVALUATION

Staging studies in the forearm and hand are less accurate than those in more proximal locations. MRI tends to be more accurate for the hand than does computerized tomography. A careful physical examination is often the most accurate of all examinations. Bone scans can be used to determine the likelihood of involvement of bone by a soft tissue sarcoma mass. If a primary bone sarcoma is present, a bone scan is required to determine the level of marrow involvement. The MRI is also of great value in this respect.

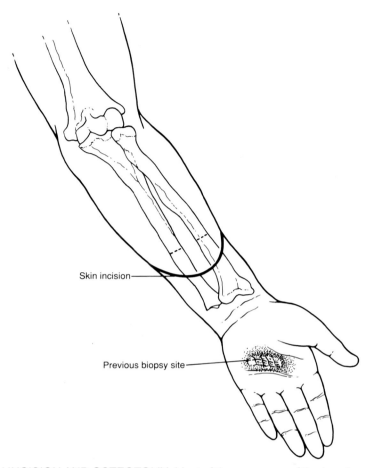

Skin incision

Previous biopsy site

Figure 29–2.   SKIN INCISION AND OSTEOTOMY. Most of the sarcomas of the hand and forearm should be explored with a tourniquet to determine resectability. One should not proceed immediately to an ablative procedure despite a radiologic workup that suggests the need for below-elbow amputation. This anatomic location with its complex structure demands a surgical exploration by an experienced hand surgeon. Biopsy should be performed and a frozen-section diagnosis established at a single operative setting. Resection should proceed if at all possible at the same time to avoid contamination of the operative field by an exploratory procedure.

The osteotomy should be performed to preserve maximal length of both the radius and ulna. Tumors of the hand are treated by a standard below-elbow amputation. Tumors of the distal forearm may require a high below-elbow amputation, and warrant special consideration. A minimum of 2.5 to 3 cm of bony stump, measured from the radial tuberosity, is required to preserve function. Additional length in the very short stump can be obtained by releasing the biceps tendon; the brachialis muscle will flex the stump.

A sterile tourniquet is placed proximal to the tumor to prevent the adjacent tumor from contaminating the operative site.

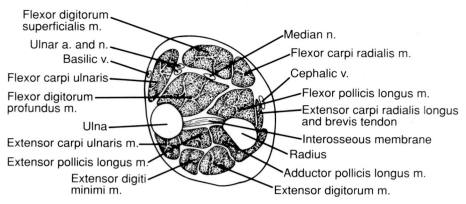

Figure 29–3. CROSS-SECTIONAL ANATOMY.

Labels (clockwise from upper left):
- Flexor digitorum superficialis m.
- Ulnar a. and n.
- Basilic v.
- Flexor carpi ulnaris
- Flexor digitorum profundus m.
- Ulna
- Extensor carpi ulnaris m.
- Extensor pollicis longus m.
- Extensor digiti minimi m.
- Median n.
- Flexor carpi radialis m.
- Cephalic v.
- Flexor pollicis longus m.
- Extensor carpi radialis longus and brevis tendon
- Interosseous membrane
- Radius
- Adductor pollicis longus m.
- Extensor digitorum m.

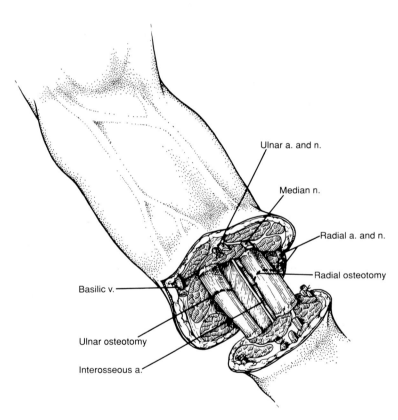

Labels:
- Ulnar a. and n.
- Median n.
- Radial a. and n.
- Radial osteotomy
- Basilic v.
- Ulnar osteotomy
- Interosseous a.

Figure 29–4. SOFT TISSUE AND BONE TRANSECTION. The skin, superficial fascia, and subcutaneous tissue are divided perpendicular to the skin surface. Then the muscle flaps are beveled to allow closure of soft tissue over the bone. The flaps are modified as required to give the maximal margin on tumor combined with optimal preservation of tissue and, likewise, function. The bones are transected at equal lengths.

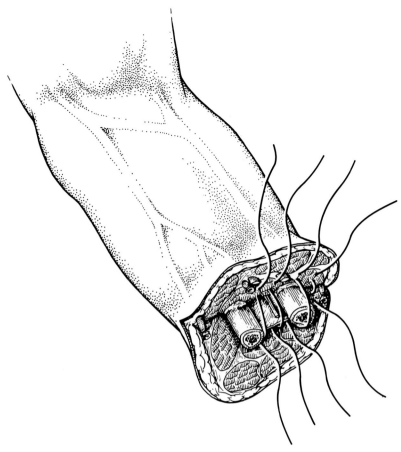

Figure 29–5.   TWO-LAYER MYODESIS OVER TRANSECTED RADIUS AND ULNA. It is important for the optimal function of the prosthesis that muscle be positioned tightly and securely cover the transected bone ends.

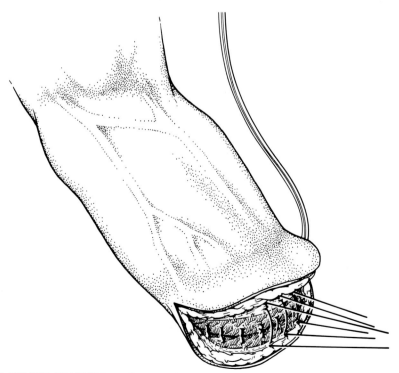

Figure 29–6.   CLOSURE OF SUPERFICIAL FASCIA OVER CLOSED-SUCTION DRAINS. The muscle as well as the skin should always be closed by dividing the incision in half with each suture. Therefore when unusual skin flaps are created, there will be no unsightly folds of tissue. Rather neat and manageable pleats will occur when a long skin flap is opposed to a shorter flap.

373

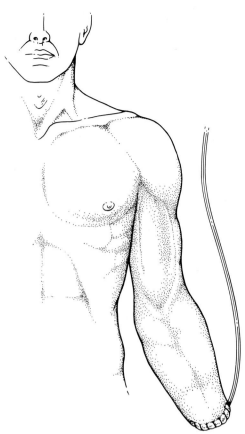

Figure 29–7.   SKIN CLOSURE. The skin is meticulously closed with interrupted sutures. The closed-suction drains should not be entered to the skin so that they can be removed without removal of the rigid dressing.

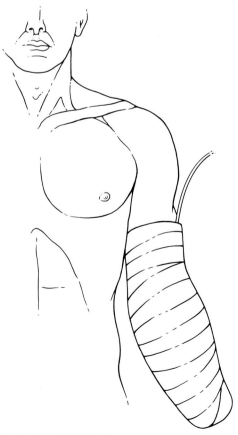

374   Figure 29–8.   POSTOPERATIVE RIGID DRESSING. A cast is used in the immediate postoperative period extending above the elbow. Serial munsterlike casts are often utilized. Care must be taken to adequately protect the skin that directly overlies the bone.

30

The Surgical Treatment of Metastatic Bone Disease

RENÉ P. H. VETH, M.D.
HARALD J. HOEKSTRA, M.D.
HEIMEN SCHRAFFORDT KOOPS, M.D.
DINESH M. MEHTA, M.D.
PAX H. B. WILLEMSE, M.D.

OVERVIEW

Improvements in the oncologic management of patients suffering from cancer and metastatic disease have resulted in an increased survival rate. Metastatic cancer of the skeletal system is the most common neoplasm.[1] It is encouraging that these bone lesions can be managed rather adequately in a multidisciplinary way. Consequently, the patient can look forward not only to a longer survival than before but an acceptable quality of life can be guaranteed. Improvements in imaging, such as bone scintigraphy, computed tomography, and magnetic resonance imaging permit early detection of bone lesions. Moreover, these tools are aids in the therapeutic planning and follow-up observations. Ever since the development of polymethyl methacrylate (PMMA) and joint prostheses, large tumor defects and pathologic fractures have been a challenge to the orthopedic surgeon,[2-4] who is in charge of the treatment of these patients. Much experience has been gathered from the field of limb-saving procedures in primary tumors of the musculoskeletal system.[5] Cemented osteosynthesis,[2] ordinary joint prostheses, custom-made[5] or modular megaprostheses,[6] and spinal instrumentation[7,8] are orthopedic tools in the treatment of metastatic defects. They offer rewarding techniques, but the results of these procedures depend largely on interdisciplinary communication—on the treatment of the patient by an entire team.

INCIDENCE AND LOCALIZATION OF SKELETAL METASTASES

The upper extremity is the least commonly involved part of the skeleton in metastatic bone disease. Figures gathered from the literature vary from 10% to 15%.[9,10] The axial skeleton and the lower extremities, in particular the hip region, are most frequently affected.[11] According to Abrams,[12] the sites of the primary tumors associated with bony metastases are breast (73.1%), lung (32.5%), kidney (24%), rectum (13%), pancreas (13%), stomach (10.9%), colon (9.3%), and ovary (9%). Other tumors frequently associated with skeletal metastasis are carcinoma of the prostate and multiple myeloma. The vertebral column is involved in 69% of the cases, the pelvis in 41%, and the hip region in 25%.[9] Pathologic fractures that require surgical instrumentation occur in 9% of the patients who suffer from metastatic bone disease. Most frequently, the femur, hip, and humerus are affected in this way.

MECHANISMS AND PATHWAYS OF METASTASIS

The manifestations of blood borne metastasis in bone represent the outcome of a series of interactions between the tumor and the host. The way in which this process occurs is poorly understood. However, several steps can be recognized:

1. Invasion of the surrounding tissues by the primary tumor cells in order to gain access to blood and lymph vessels[13]
2. Release of tumor cells into the circulation
3. Arrest of these cells in vessels in bone marrow
4. Extravasation of tumor cells and subsequent multiplication
5. Growth of vascularized stroma into the new metastatic bone tumor[14,15]

It has been suggested that the high incidence of skeletal metastasis of the lumbar spine is due to the vertebral venous system,[16] which communicates freely with the pelvic and intracostal veins. This paravertebral venous system may also be the source of the frequent involvement of the pelvis.

Tumor cells may destroy bone directly by osteolysis or by producing bone ischemia.

Bone resorption can also be osteoclast-dependent. A number of different substances stimulate osteoclast proliferation, such as osteoclast activating factor (OAF), prostaglandins (PGE₂), and tumor growth factor (TGF). It has been shown that these substances can be produced and released by tumor cells.[17]

RADIOLOGY OF SKELETAL METASTASES

The imaging techniques presently available for the detection and monitoring of skeletal metastases include conventional radiography, scintigraphy, computer tomography (CT), and magnetic resonance imaging (MRI). A radiographic skeletal survey is now largely obsolete as a screening method of metastases in patients with malignant disease. Bone scintigraphy is the method of choice in most cases, with the exception of multiple myeloma patients, in whom bone scintigraphy is often falsely negative. Conventional radiographs are highly accurate in differentiating metastatic bone lesions from primary bone tumors. The most frequently affected parts of the skeleton are the vertebral column, the hip, the femur, and the humerus. The patterns of bone destruction are recognized[18] and have been referred to as geographic, moth-eaten, and permeative. Geographic destruction consists of large, well-defined lytic areas, which are greater than 1 cm in diameter; there is a distinct and sclerotic rim. Moth-eaten destruction contains smaller (2–5 mm) lytic areas with ill-defined margins. Permeative lesions of destruction are characterized by multiple, small (1-mm) areas, principally in cortical bone. Geographic destruction is associated with slow-growing tumors, moth-eaten with moderately aggressive lesions and permeative with highly aggressive tumors. Apart from these lytic lesions, osteoblastic and mixed-type metastases should be recognized radiographically. The osteoblastic component is not neoplastic, but should be interpreted as a reaction of normal bone to the metastatic cancer. Primary tumors of the prostate and GI tract may account for a blastic response. Lytic lesions are frequently observed in metastases of kidneys, melanoma, breast, and lung tumors. Mixed-type lesions are found in metastases secondary to primary tumors of the breast, GI tract, and reproductive system.

Bone scintigraphy is an excellent method for the early detection of skeletal metastases, especially in cases where bone lesions remain radiologically occult. Today Tc 99m-labeled polyphosphonates are preferred in bone scans. According to Galasko[13] bone scans can detect metastatic lesions 2–18 months earlier than can conventional radiographs. The least accurate for diagnosis are multiple myeloma, leukemia, and lymphoma. Pitfalls in the interpretation of bone scans are trauma, infection, and miscellaneous factors, such as preexistent disease (eg, osteosclerosis, rheumatoid arthritis). The finding of a lesion at scintigraphy should induce an additional evaluation, such as CT and probably the performance of a biopsy. The density discrimination of CT is superior to conventional radiography.[18] Soft tissue changes are thus well demonstrated. This has clinical implications in defining the extent and operability of these tumors. It may also be helpful in the determination of the appropriate fields in radiation therapy of metastatic lesions. In the past, angiography was performed to assess both the vascularity and the soft tissue extension of the tumor. Enhanced CT has largely replaced angiography in this respect. However, angiography and embolization are still important in the preoperative assessment and treatment of vascular tumors.[19]

Magnetic resonance imaging provides[20] soft tissue contrast superior to that of computed tomography. Images can be obtained in the axial, coronal, and sagittal planes, which allow for a clear demonstration of the extent of the lesion, especially the bone marrow involvement. There is evidence that MRI is more sensitive and can detect the extent of the disease more rapidly than isotope studies can. It should, however, be emphasized that MRI studies have to be correlated with other studies.

PREOPERATIVE STAGING AND BIOPSY

The clinical history includes a thorough review of symptoms and a profound examination of the patient.[10] Bone metastasis is often associated with pain. The discomfort is often worst at night. In extensive bone disease, multiple and migratory areas of pain are recorded. Examples of diagnostic pitfalls are pain in metastatic disease of the spinal column, which is treated as a lumbar disk syndrome, and discomfort around the knee, which is due to a metastasis in the region of the hip. Important laboratory studies include those of blood, enzymes, proteins, and minerals.[10] Serum protein immune electrophoresis should be performed routinely to exclude multiple myeloma. Hypercalcemia may be found in patients with bony metastases. Other markers are serum alkaline and acid phosphatase, which is elevated in patients who exhibit large lytic lesions and serum prostate specific acid phosphatase, which is associated with cancer of the prostate. Carcinoembryonic antigen (CEA) is another indicative test, especially in GI tumors.

Preoperative staging studies also include conventional radiographs, bone scintigraphy, computer tomography, and magnetic resonance imaging. A biopsy should be considered in the following situations: to confirm metastatic disease in a patient with a known primary tumor, to evaluate a lesion as shown on conventional radiographs or on bone scintigraphy, and to obtain tissue for special studies.

Prior to the performance of the biopsy, the surgeon should be well aware of the clinical, immunologic, and hematologic condition of the patient. This group of patients is highly susceptible to infection and hemorrhage. One should therefore perform a biopsy with great care. Adequate blood replacement should be available, for instance, in metastases of carcinoma of the kidney.

Needle aspiration and cytologic evaluation may confirm the diagnosis of cancer. However, in skeletal lesions, biopsy is preferred.[21] Fluoroscopic guidance is often useful; a radiograph should be made to document that the correct area has been sampled. Bacteriologic cultures and frozen sections should be made to rule out infection and to evaluate the reliability of the sample. If special techniques are required by the pathologist, the appropriate measures should be taken. In excessive bleeding the lesion can be packed with Gel-foam or PMMA. The site of the biopsy should always be in line with the definitive incision.

PRINCIPLES OF SURGICAL TREATMENT IN METASTATIC DISEASE OF THE SKELETON

Major progress has been made in the surgical management of metastatic skeletal disease over the past 20 years. Many techniques have been developed to treat bone defects. The surgical procedures carried out most frequently in our hospital are

1. Tumor curettage and cemented osteosynthesis: intracapsular resection of the tumor combined with internal fixation (bone plates, screws, and intramedullary rods) and polymethyl methacrylate (PMMA).[22]
2. Tumor curettage and spinal instrumentation: intracapsular resection of the tumor, followed by interposition of PMMA or some kind of biomaterial (hydroxylapatite), bone grafting, and spinal anterior and/or posterior stabilization.[7,8,23]
3. Tumor resection and joint replacement[5,6]: intracapsular or marginal resection of the tumor and the involved joint, followed by implantation of an endoprosthesis.[4,24,25] This technique is used most frequently in the hip region. PMMA is often used for fixation.
4. Segmental resection and reconstruction[5,6,26,27]: marginal or intracapsular resection of the tumor together with a large segment of bone, followed by implantation of a custom-made or modular mega endoprosthesis. PMMA is often used for fixation purposes. Nowadays this technique is used more often than in the past, especially when reconstruc-

tion with an ordinary endoprosthesis is impossible due to the absence of functional bone remnants.

5. Cryosurgery[4,25,28,29]: This technique can be used to obtain better margins without resection of great amounts of bone. It can also be useful in the treatment of tumor hemorrhage.

6. Amputation: This procedure is seldom required. In our view it is not in agreement with the goals of the palliative type of treatment, which should be used in these patients.

In addition to this synopsis of different types of treatment that are available for patients with skeletal defects due to metastases, we would like to focus on several points of interest. The primary goals of treatment are relief of pain, restoration of function, and facilitation of nursing care. As much tumor-destroyed bone as possible should be removed, and the risk for a second procedure should thus be eliminated. Guidelines to the treatment of these lesions are the risk for failure of fractures to unite, the shortened life expectancy of the patients, and the weakened bone in the vicinity of the tumor.[30] Further criteria for treatment are inadequate reaction of the lesion to adjuvant therapy, a lytic lesion more than 2.5 cm in diameter, and destruction of the cortex exceeding 50% of the circumference.[30]

In lesions of the lower extremity, which require partial weight bearing, the treating physician should be well informed about the upper extremities of the patients, since lesions in these areas may preclude the use of walking aids. The nutritional condition of the patient should be optimal. Perioperative antibiotics are obligatory, for instance a combination of gentamycin and cefamandol. For vascular lesions, preoperative embolization is advisable. Generally, all patients receive chemotherapy and/or radiotherapy preoperatively and postoperatively in order to diminish the risk for soft tissue seeding and the occurrence of a local recurrence. In major bone defects, especially in the hip region, a marginal resection is always performed.[26] The plane of resection is chosen 3 cm distally or proximally (knee region) of the radiographically recorded boundaries of the tumor. The resection is followed by the implantation of a mega endoprosthesis, with the aid of cement. By this technique the risk for further bone destruction in the area of the bone prosthesis interface is diminished to a large extent. Figure 30–1A shows a lytic lesion of the

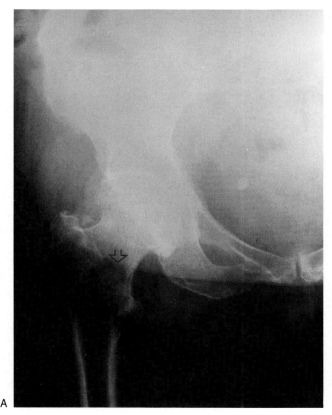

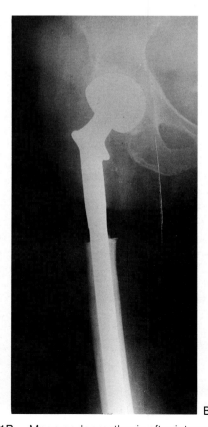

Figure 30–1A. Metastatic lytic lesion of the proximal femur, due to carcinoma of the kidney.

Figure 30–1B. Mega endoprosthesis after intracapsular resection of the tumor.

proximal femur that has been treated by resection–reconstruction with an endoprosthesis (Fig. 30–1B).

In the diaphyseal area of long bones, a cemented osteosynthesis with an IM rod and PMMA is preferred to an internal fixation with a plate, screws, and PMMA.[13] Figure 30–2A shows a lytic lesion in multiple myeloma that has been treated by radiotherapy, intracapsular resection, IM osteosynthesis, and PMMA implantation (Fig. 30–2B).

In the metaphyseal area a cemented osteosynthesis is often performed after intracapsular resection. An example of this procedure is shown in Figure 30–3. The patient was suffering from carcinoma of the kidney and secondary skeletal metastasis. The bony lesion (Fig. 30–3A) had been treated by radiotherapy, embolization, intracapsular resection, and cemented osteosynthesis (Fig. 30–3B). During the operation bacteriologic cultures of the wound are always taken and are used in the postoperative treatment of the patient. An extensive vacuum drainage is always provided for.

Postoperatively, bed rest is prescribed for 48 hours. Afterwards a rehabilitation program is started, initially with the aid of a continuous passive-motion apparatus. The aim of this program is to make the patient walk with the aid of crutches at least two weeks postoperatively. Radiotherapy and chemotherapy are resumed three weeks postoperatively.

NONOPERATIVE TREATMENT OF SKELETAL METASTASIS

Radiotherapy is an effective method of treatment for cancer and skeletal metastasis.[25,30] The primary aim is relief of pain, restoration of function, and arrest of tumor growth. In patients who exhibit multiple lesions, it is reasonable to use radiotherapy for the most symptomatic areas. We recommend a total of 30 Gy in 10 fractions, 3 Gy daily, for palliative purposes. Sometimes a single 8-Gy treatment is given to patients with a very short life expectancy. If effective chemotherapy and/or hormonal therapy is available, it should be employed.[25]

As the majority of patients with bone metastases suffer from breast cancer, empirical treatment with tamoxifen or combination chemotherapy is usually given. Additional treatment with a diphosphonate such as APD or EHDP has been proven to prevent a number of events, defined as fractures or the necessity of additional radiotherapy,[31] and may induce sclerosis of lytic bone lesions. Diphosphonate will be effective in the treatment of hypercalcemia, and can inhibit osteoclast activity by mechanisms still unknown. Inhibition of bone mineralization may be a problem in the long run, but not in cancer patients. Most diphosphonates are resorbed poorly, and should be given on an empty stomach to prevent binding to calcium salts present in food. Ample water should be taken to prevent local ulceration. Acute hypercalcemia can be treated by a single infusion of APD 1 mg/kg over 2 hours IV.[32,33]

Bone lesions not amenable to surgery should be monitored and treated with great care. For lesions in the spinal region the prescription of a brace is often justified. Due to tumor progression and the effects of radiotherapy, the vertebral body may collapse, and a brace will mostly prevent excessive axial deviation. In other cases, such as diaphyseal lesions of the upper extremity, a brace may prevent the occurrence

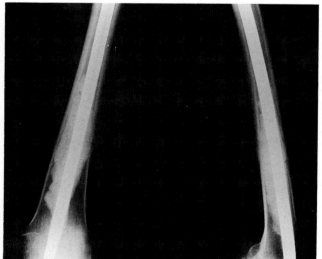

A

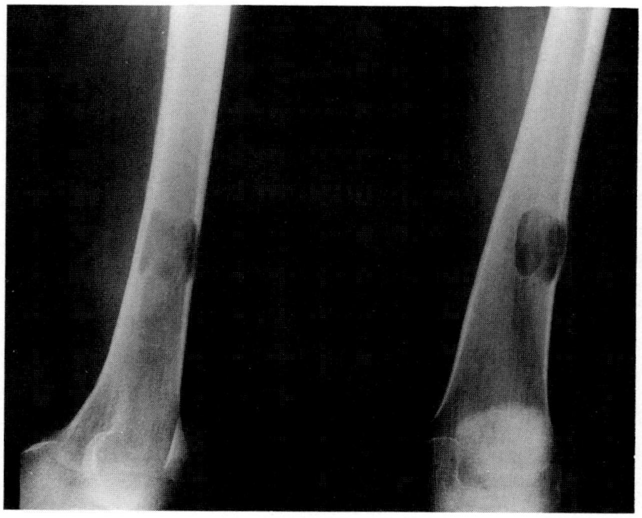

Figure 30–2A. Lytic bone lesion in the distal part of the femur, due to multiple myeloma.

B

Figure 30–2B. Cemented osteosynthesis with the aid of an intramedullary rod after intracapsular resection.

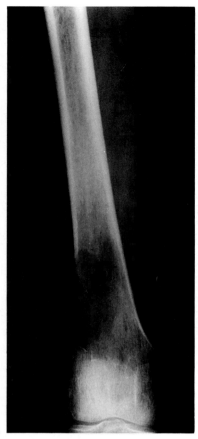

A

Figure 30–3A. Metastatic lytic lesion in the distal part of the femur, due to carcinoma of the kidney.

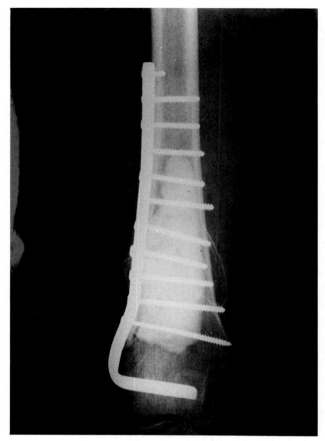

B

Figure 30–3B. Cemented osteosynthesis with the aid of a plate and screws.

of a pathologic fracture; in lesions of the lower extremity, partial weight bearing is often obligatory. Radiotherapy and chemotherapy not only affect the tumor, but they also may have adverse effects on the adjacent normal bone. Finally the healing potency of bone is diminished.

In some cases of metastatic disease of the skeleton, radioactive isotopes are used to palliate pain. Iodine-131 can provide for pain relief in patients with osseous metastases due to thyroid carcinoma, and it may halt tumor progression.

PROGNOSTIC FACTORS IN SKELETAL METASTASES

The prognosis of the patient who suffers from skeletal metastasis plays a major role in the therapy concept. In case of a short life expectancy, major surgery should be avoided. Factors contributing to an unfavorable prognosis are aggressive primary tumor, short recurrence-free interval after primary

treatment, radiographic absence of bone sclerosis in metastases initially and after systemic therapy, multiple bone lesions, involvement of more than one organ by metastases (especially the liver), high overall tumor burden, and poor general condition.

Factors contributing to a more favorable prognosis are moderately progressive primary tumor (prostate cancer), long recurrence-free interval after primary treatment, radiographic presence of sclerosis in bone metastases initially and after systemic treatment, a solitary bone lesion, preferably of a geographic type, low overall tumor burden (preferably bone only), and good general condition of the patient. The optimal way to treat a patient with skeletal metastasis should be assessed by multidisciplinary consultation.

CONCLUSIONS

The multidisciplinary treatment of patients who suffer from metastatic disease of the skeleton is rewarding. To restore defects of the bone due to metastatic tumor involvement, the presence of an orthopedic surgeon as a member of the team is of great importance. Improvements in the oncologic management of the disease have resulted in an increased survival rate for a number of patients. New developments in the orthopedic field have often given access to a better quality of life.

REFERENCES

1. Behr JT, Dobozi WR, Badrinath K: The treatment of pathologic and impending pathologic fractures of the proximal femur in the elderly. *Clin Orthop* 1985; 198:173.
2. Harrington UD: New trends in the management of lower extremity metastasis. *Clin Orthop* 1982;169:53–61.
3. Harrington UD, Sim FD, Eris JE, et al: Methylmethacrylate as an adjunct in internal fixation of pathological fractures. *J Bone Joint Surg* 1985;38:1047.
4. Malawer MM, Marks A, McChacney D: The effect of cryosurgery and PMMA in dogs with experimental bone defects, comparable to tumor defects. *Clin Orthop* 1988;226:299–310.
5. Scales JT, Wright KWJ: Major bone and joint replacement using custom implants, in Chao EYS, Irin IC (eds): *Tumor Prosthesis for Bone and Joint Reconstruction, the Design and Application.* Stuttgart, Thieme Verlag, 1983, pp 149–168.
6. Sim FH: Lesions of the pelvis and hip, in Sim FH: *Diagnosis and Management of Metastatic Bone Disease.* New York, Raven Press, 1988, pp 183–199.
7. Fidler MW: Anterior decompression and stabilisation of metastatic spinal fractures. *J Bone Joint Surg* 1986;68B:83–90.
8. Fidler MW: Posterior instrumentation of the spina: an experimental comparison of various possible techniques. *Spine* 1986;11:367–372.
9. Clain A: Secondary malignant disease of bone. *Br J Cancer* 1965;19:15–29.
10. Enneking WF: Metastatic carcinoma, in Enneking WF (ed): *Musculoskeletal Tumor Surgery.* New York, Churchill Livingstone, vol 2, p 1541.
11. Willis RA: The spread of tumors in the human body, ed 3. London, Butterworth, 1973, pp 177–178.
12. Abrams ML, Spiro R, Goldstein N: Metastases in carcinoma. Analysis of 1000 autopsied cases. *Cancer* 1950;23:74–85.
13. Galasko CSB: Skeletal metastases. *Clin Orthop* 1986;210:18–30.
14. Springfield DS: Mechanisms of metastasis. *Clin Orthop* 1982;169:15.
15. Stoll BA: Natural history prognosis and staging of bone metastases, in Stoll BA, Pahbao S (eds): *Bone Metastasis.* New York, Raven Press, 1983; pp 1–21.
16. Batson OV: Role of vertebral veins in metastatic processes. *Ann Int Med* 1942;16:38–45.
17. Trump DL: Mechanisms of bone destruction by cancer, in Stoll BA, Pahbao S (eds): *Bone Metastasis.* New York, Raven Press 1983; pp 39–47.
18. Adams JE, Isherwood I: Conventional and new techniques in radiological diagnosis, in Stoll BA, Pahbao S (eds): *Bone Metastasis.* New York, Raven Press, 1983; pp 107–149.
19. Johnsson U, Ichnell O: Preoperative angiography in patients with bone metastases. *Acta Radiol Diag* 1982;23:485–489.
20. Berquist Th H: Bone and soft tissue tumors, in Berquist Th H (ed): *Magnetic Resonance of the Musculoskeletal System.* New York, Raven Press, 1987, pp 85–109.
21. Heeten GJ den, Oldhoff J, Oosterhuis JW, et al: Biopsy of bone tumours. *J Surg Oncol* 1985;28:247–251.
22. Wilkins RM, Sim FH: Lesions of the femur, in Sim FH (ed): *Diagnosis and Management of Metastatic Bone Disease.* New York, Raven Press, 1988, pp 199–205.
23. Harrington UD: Anterior cord decompression and spinal stabilisation for patients with metastatic lesions of the spine. *J Neurosurg* 1984;61:107–117.
24. Lane JM, Sculca TP, Zdan S: Treatment of pathological fractures of the hip by endoprosthetic replacement. *J Bone Joint Surg* 1980;62A:954–959.
25. Malawer MM, Delaney TF: Treatment of Metastatic Cancer to Bone, in DeVita VT, Hellman S, Rosenberg SA (eds): *Cancer Principles and practice of oncology,* ed. 3. Philadelphia, JB Lippincott, 1989, pp. 2298–2316.
26. Veth RPH, Nielsen HKL, Oldhoff J, et al: Megaprostheses in the treatment of primary malignant and metastatic tumors in the hip region. *J Surg Oncol* 1989;40:1214–1218.
27. Veth RPH, Nielsen HKL, Oldhoff J, et al: Resection of tumors of the pelvis and proximal femur, in Yamamuro T (ed): *New Developments for Limb Salvage in Musculoskeletal Tumors.* Tokyo, Springer Verlag, 1989, pp 419–425.
28. Marcove RC, Miller TR: Treatment of primary and metastatic bone tumors by cryosurgery. *JAMA* 1969;207:1890.
29. Oeseburg HW, Oldhoff J: Cyrosurgery in the treatment of tumors (Chirurgische mogelijkheden bij de behandeling van tumoren). *NTvG* 1973;117:1296–1297.
30. Oda MAS, Schurmany DJ: Monitoring of pathological fractures, in Stoll BA, Pahbao S (eds): *Bone Metastasis.* New York, Raven Press, 1983, p. 271.
31. Holten-Verzantvoort ATH van, Bijvoet OLM, Hermans J, et al: Reduced morbidity from skeletal metastases in breast cancer patients during long-term biphosphonate (APD) treatment. *Lancet* 1987;2:983–985.
32. Body JJ, Pot M, Borkowski A, et al: Dose/response study of aminohydroxypropylidene bisphosphonate in tumor-associated hypercalcemia. *Am J Med* 1987; 82:957–963.
33. Thiébaud D, Jaeger Ph, Jacquest AF, et al: Dose-response in the treatment of hypercalcemia of malignancy by a single infusion of biphosphonate AHPrBP. *J Clin Oncol* 1988;6:762–768.

Index